Medical LLMs and AI in Healthcare:

Ethics, Trust, and Clinical Applications

Fernando Ortiz-Rodriguez
https://orcid.org/0000-0003-2084-3462
Tamaulipas Autonomous University, Mexico

Mrignainy Kansal
https://orcid.org/0009-0005-2610-040X
Netaji Subhas University of Technology (NSUT), Delhi, India

Rajesh Kumar Dhanaraj
https://orcid.org/0000-0002-2038-7359
Symbiosis International (Deemed to be) University, India

Firoz Khan
Ball State University, USA

IGI Global
Scientific Publishing
Publishing Tomorrow's Research Today

Vice President of Editorial	Melissa Wagner
Director of Acquisitions	Mikaela Felty
Director of Book Development	Jocelynn Hessler
Production Manager	Mike Brehm
Cover Design	Jose Rosado

Published in the United States of America by
IGI Global Scientific Publishing
701 East Chocolate Avenue
Hershey, PA, 17033, USA
Tel: 717-533-8845 | Fax: 717-533-7115
Website: https://www.igi-global.com E-mail: cust@igi-global.com

Library of Congress Cataloging-in-Publication Data

LCCN: 2026026706 (CIP Data Pending)
ISBN13: 9798260021736
Isbn13Softcover: 9798260021743
EISBN13: 9798260021750

British Cataloguing in Publication Data
A Cataloguing in Publication record for this book is available from the British Library.

Table of Contents

Detailed Table of Contents

The Large Language Models (LLMs) are at the core of a transformation in artificial intelligence (AI) and medical applications. The large amount of clinical information can be processed and analyzed for medical decision making. The healthcare professionals get diagnostic and administrative help enhancing their capacity. They enhance the outcome of medicine, data science and linguistic intelligence. This chapter first introduces the basics of LLMs, how they are designed and how to use them safely in the treatment of patients and in medical research. Moreover, it addresses the ethical and legal issues that LLMs are used for enhancing patient safety. LLMs begins by demonstrating the evolution of natural language processing (NLP) in medicine. At the start, rule-based systems supported by fixed knowledge bases were used but these were not able to identify the nuances of the context in clinical data. The statistical methods improved pattern recognition but a fixed vocabulary was a major concern.

Artificial Intelligence (AI) has become a groundbreaking technology in the field of medicine during the last decade, and the opportunities this specific area of application remain substantial as ANI may be used to automate the process of diagnosis, treatment, and disease prognosis. This paper explores the ethical issues surrounding

The sudden spike in Artificial Intelligence (AI) attention has prompted investigations of its uses in healthcare domain, specifically in medical imaging and diagnostics. In this chapter, a qualitative case study explores the level of trust healthcare providers have in diagnostic artificial intelligence systems and the factor behind this case is described. The study provides essential preconditions of achieving clinical confidence in the form of the interviews with the participants working in various clinical positions and experience levels. The results demonstrate that the degree of trust depends on personal experience, but the high level of trust is usually provided under the condition of the meeting of some certain conditions. The main assumptions of such findings lie in the fact that AI is not a substitute tool to human judgment, but a decision stressor.

The use of Large Language Models (LLMs) in the medical field, especially in clinical safety evaluation, has substantial prospective advantages to enhance the diagnostic performance, clinical decision-making process, and patient outcomes. Although these advantages exist, there are complicated ethical, legal, and governance issues with the introduction of AI in healthcare. This chapter critically reviews ethical implication of the use of LLM with special reference being given to clinical autonomy, algorithmic bias, informed consent, and accountability. It draws on real-life case studies to emphasize the role of biased training data and lack of transparency in decision-making in promoting health disparities and undermining trust between clinicians and patients. The analysis also outlines some of the crucial failure points in current legal and regulatory frameworks particularly on the aspect of the distribution

literature, and both researchers and practitioners of medical LLMs benefit from the presented findings.

The generation of diagnostic reports from chest X-ray images is a complex task that requires both accurate medical image interpretation and clear clinical language. Manual reporting is time-consuming, expertise-intensive, and susceptible to fatigue. Although deep learning–based systems have been developed to support this process, most traditional approaches treat image analysis and report generation as separate tasks, leading to inconsistencies and loss of critical details. Recent vision–language models offer a more unified solution by linking visual understanding with natural language generation. This chapter proposes an end-to-end framework that integrates a Swin Transformer image encoder with a Q-Former and a fine-tuned BioMedLM for producing accurate and clinically meaningful reports. Experiments on a curated chest X-ray dataset demonstrate improved pathology coverage, reduced errors, and enhanced report clarity, supporting reliable and efficient clinical decision-making.

This changed with transformers, which promised a sea change in medical imaging particularly image segmentation and automatic decision-making tasks. Later, their expertise in natural language processing thus, instead of known transformers has successfully transferred to computer vision tasks (including medical imaging) where they can take in global context and dependencies at long range, a significant step up from traditional convolutional neural networks. In medical image segmentation, transformers have good results even by bringing local and global features together, frequently supplementing this with CNNs to improve accuracy in distinguishing lesions or body parts such as organs-there is nothing like the precision possible on land that will benefit from a blended signal in this way.

The adoption of Large Language Models (LLMs) and artificial intelligence-driven clinical decision-support systems into the field of health care has led to hype about the efficiency, scalability, and personalised care. However, their use in the context of physiotherapy and rehabilitation is characterised by peculiar challenges because of the nature of clinical reasoning and the need to conduct physical examination and responsiveness of patients to therapeutic measures. The current chapter describes two areas that are prerequisites of the safe implementation of LLMs in rehabilitation environments: model interpretability and the existence of human-in-the-loop (HITL) validation.It is suggested to use a physiotherapy-specific conceptual framework of integrating HITL validation into clinical practise that would focus on clinician supervision, ongoing monitoring, and context-based decision making. This chapter lays down the future trends of the explainable AI in rehabilitation, along with policy-relevant and are in line with the international perspectives of regulation.

The present report describes a multimodal approach to the management of gestational diabetes mellitus (GDM) using LLM-enabled technology. This approach will combine the use of Internet of Things (IoT) sensor data, electronic health record data, and patient-reported outcome data in a single integrated platform. The major goals of this integrated solution are to improve clinical outcomes through continuous monitoring and real-time predictive analytics of GDM, to predict patient subtypes of GDM with increased accuracy, to provide personalized recommendations and

Preface

INTRODUCTION

The rapid advancement of artificial intelligence (AI) and large language models (LLMs) has ushered in a transformative era for healthcare systems worldwide. From clinical diagnostics and medical imaging to patient engagement and personalized treatment planning, AI-driven technologies are increasingly reshaping the foundations of modern medicine. As healthcare institutions seek to improve efficiency, accessibility, and clinical accuracy, LLMs have emerged as powerful tools capable of processing vast amounts of medical information, synthesizing clinical knowledge, and supporting evidence-based decision-making. However, alongside these remarkable opportunities come significant ethical, legal, and societal challenges that demand careful examination and responsible governance.

The edited volume *Medical LLMs and AI in Healthcare: Ethics, Trust, and Clinical Applications* was conceived to address this critical intersection between technological innovation and human-centered healthcare. While much of the global discourse surrounding AI emphasizes technical performance and computational capabilities, there remains an urgent need to evaluate how these systems influence trust, transparency, accountability, patient safety, and healthcare equity. Medical AI systems do not operate in isolation; rather, they interact directly with clinicians, patients, institutions, and regulatory environments. Consequently, their successful implementation depends not only on technological sophistication but also on ethical alignment, interdisciplinary collaboration, and public confidence.

This volume brings together contributions from researchers, clinicians, engineers, legal scholars, and healthcare practitioners across multiple countries and academic disciplines. The chapters collectively explore the foundations, methodologies, ethical frameworks, clinical applications, and emerging research directions associated with medical LLMs and AI-enabled healthcare systems. By combining theoretical insights with practical case studies and application-driven research, the book offers readers a comprehensive understanding of how AI technologies are evolving within healthcare environments and the responsibilities that accompany their deployment.

A central theme running throughout this book is the concept of trust. Healthcare has always relied upon trust between patients and providers, institutions and communities, and science and society. As AI systems increasingly participate in clinical workflows, questions surrounding explainability, transparency, bias, accountability, and human oversight become fundamental concerns. Several chapters in this collection therefore focus specifically on ethical governance, human-in-the-loop validation, multilingual accessibility, legal implications, and the responsible integration of AI into sensitive medical domains. These discussions highlight that technological advancement alone cannot guarantee better healthcare outcomes unless it is supported by robust ethical and regulatory frameworks.

At the same time, this volume demonstrates the extraordinary potential of AI to improve clinical efficiency and patient care. From radiology report generation and medical image segmentation to gestational diabetes management and rehabilitation decision support, the contributors illustrate how AI-driven models can augment healthcare delivery, accelerate medical research, and provide personalized insights that support both clinicians and patients. These applications reveal the growing convergence of language intelligence, computer vision, predictive analytics, and multimodal healthcare systems in shaping the future of medicine.

The editors hope that this book will serve as a valuable scholarly resource for researchers, healthcare professionals, policymakers, graduate students, and industry practitioners interested in the future of AI-enabled healthcare. Beyond offering technical and conceptual perspectives, the volume encourages critical reflection on the broader implications of integrating intelligent systems into healthcare ecosystems. Ultimately, the responsible adoption of medical AI requires a balanced approach—one that embraces innovation while preserving the ethical principles, professional standards, and human values at the core of healthcare practice.

CHAPTER OVERVIEW

Chapter 1, *Foundations of LLMs in Medicine and Healthcare: LLMs in Healthcare*, introduces the foundational concepts behind large language models and their integration into healthcare systems. The chapter explores the evolution of natural language processing in medicine, examines the architecture and capabilities of

LLMs, and discusses their role in clinical decision-making, medical research, and patient safety while emphasizing ethical and legal considerations.

Chapter 2, *Integrating Artificial Intelligence into Healthcare: Ethical Imperatives, Data Bias, and the Challenges of Clinical Implementation*, investigates the ethical dilemmas associated with AI-assisted healthcare systems. Drawing from qualitative research and stakeholder interviews, the authors analyze institutional acceptance, data bias, transparency concerns, and the practical barriers to integrating AI into clinical settings.

Chapter 3, *Principles and Applications of LLMs in Healthcare - Methods, Models, Data Privacy, New Medical Treatments, and Challenges*, provides a detailed examination of LLM methodologies and healthcare applications. The chapter highlights how LLMs support patient care, clinical research, and treatment discovery while also addressing issues related to data privacy, safety, and healthcare analytics.

Chapter 4, *Navigating Trust and Acceptance: Exploring Healthcare Professionals' Perspectives on AI-Assisted Diagnostic Tools*, focuses on healthcare professionals' perceptions of AI-driven diagnostic systems. Through qualitative case studies, the chapter examines the factors that influence clinical trust, acceptance, and confidence in AI-assisted decision-making tools.

Chapter 5, *Ethical and Legal Implications in Medical AI*, critically evaluates the ethical, legal, and governance-related challenges of deploying AI systems in medicine. Topics such as clinical autonomy, informed consent, algorithmic bias, liability distribution, and data privacy are explored through contemporary examples and regulatory perspectives.

Chapter 6, *Ethical Implications of LLMs Use in Sensitive Clinical Domains*, examines the deployment of LLMs in high-stakes healthcare environments, including oncology, mental health, pediatrics, emergency medicine, and end-of-life care. The chapter emphasizes the ethical risks associated with bias, transparency, accountability, and professional responsibility while discussing governance strategies for responsible implementation.

Chapter 7, *On Multilingual Medical LLMs*, presents a comprehensive survey of multilingual medical language models and their growing importance in global healthcare systems. The authors discuss existing multilingual medical LLMs, identify research gaps, and propose future directions for inclusive and linguistically adaptable healthcare AI systems.

Chapter 8, *End-to-End Radiology Report Generation from Chest X-rays Using Vision–Language Models*, explores the integration of vision-language architectures for automated radiology report generation. By combining advanced transformer-based image encoding with biomedical language modeling, the chapter demonstrates improvements in pathology coverage, report clarity, and diagnostic efficiency.

Chapter 9, *Transformer Models in Medical Image Processing: A Review of Image Segmentation and Automatic Decision Making for Medical Images*, reviews the role of transformer architectures in medical image segmentation and automated clinical decision-making. The chapter discusses how transformers enhance contextual understanding and improve precision in medical imaging tasks.

Chapter 10, *Model Interpretability and Human-in-the-Loop Validation in Physiotherapy and Rehabilitation Practice: Bridging Artificial Intelligence with Evidence-Based Rehabilitation Decision-Making*, addresses the integration of explainable AI and human oversight within physiotherapy and rehabilitation settings. The authors propose frameworks for clinician supervision, model interpretability, and evidence-based rehabilitation support.

Chapter 11, *Transforming Gestational Diabetes Management Through LLM-Enabled Multimodal Healthcare*, examines how LLM-enabled multimodal systems can improve gestational diabetes management through the integration of IoT data, electronic health records, predictive analytics, and personalized clinical recommendations.

Chapter 12, *Hybrid Soft Set and Manifold Learning Frameworks for Diabetes Risk Classification and Visualization*, concludes the volume by presenting hybrid machine learning models for diabetes risk prediction and visualization. The chapter combines soft set–based feature engineering with manifold learning techniques to improve interpretability, predictive performance, and intelligent clinical decision support.

CONCLUSION

The chapters presented in this volume collectively demonstrate that medical LLMs and AI technologies are no longer experimental concepts confined to research laboratories; they are becoming integral components of contemporary healthcare systems. Their applications span diagnostics, clinical documentation, rehabilitation, medical imaging, disease prediction, multilingual healthcare communication, and personalized medicine. These developments signify a profound transformation in the ways healthcare knowledge is generated, interpreted, and delivered.

At the same time, the contributions within this book underscore that the adoption of AI in healthcare cannot be viewed solely through a technological lens. Ethical responsibility, transparency, fairness, explainability, and human oversight remain indispensable to ensuring that AI systems support rather than compromise patient care. The discussions surrounding algorithmic bias, data privacy, legal accountability, and clinician trust highlight the necessity of multidisciplinary collaboration among engineers, healthcare professionals, policymakers, and ethicists.

Another important insight emerging from this volume is the growing importance of human-centered AI design. Across multiple chapters, the contributors emphasize that AI systems should augment clinical expertise rather than replace human judgment. Human-in-the-loop validation, explainable decision-making, and clinician supervision are essential for maintaining patient safety and fostering trust in AI-assisted healthcare environments. As AI capabilities continue to evolve, the preservation of empathy, ethical integrity, and patient-centered care must remain at the forefront of healthcare innovation.

The editors believe that this book contributes meaningfully to the ongoing global dialogue surrounding responsible AI integration in medicine. By combining foundational theories, ethical analysis, technical advancements, and real-world clinical applications, the volume provides readers with both a broad conceptual understanding and practical insights into the opportunities and challenges associated with medical AI systems.

We extend our sincere appreciation to all contributing authors, reviewers, and academic collaborators whose expertise and dedication made this volume possible. Their scholarly contributions reflect the interdisciplinary spirit required to address the complexities of AI-driven healthcare transformation. We also thank the research communities and institutions worldwide that continue to advance knowledge in this rapidly evolving field.

Finally, we hope that *Medical LLMs and AI in Healthcare: Ethics, Trust, and Clinical Applications* inspires future research, innovation, and thoughtful dialogue on the responsible use of AI in medicine. As healthcare systems continue to evolve in response to technological progress, the collective challenge before us is not merely to build more intelligent systems, but to ensure that these systems remain ethical, trustworthy, inclusive, and fundamentally aligned with the well-being of humanity.

Chapter 1
Foundations of LLMs in Medicine and Healthcare

Karthic Sundaram
http://orcid.org/0000-0002-0968-8468
SRM Institute of Science and Technology, India

N. Maheswaran
SRM Institute of Science and Technology, India

T. Sumathi
http://orcid.org/0000-0002-7833-0152
Dr. Mahalingam College of Engineering and Technology, India

Kamaraj Kanagaraj
Manipal Institute of Technology, India

ABSTRACT

The Large Language Models (LLMs) are at the core of a transformation in artificial intelligence (AI) and medical applications. The large amount of clinical information can be processed and analyzed for medical decision making. The healthcare professionals get diagnostic and administrative help enhancing their capacity. They enhance the outcome of medicine, data science and linguistic intelligence. This chapter first introduces the basics of LLMs, how they are designed and how to use them safely in the treatment of patients and in medical research. Moreover, it addresses the ethical and legal issues that LLMs are used for enhancing patient safety. LLMs begins by demonstrating the evolution of natural language processing (NLP) in medicine. At the start, rule-based systems supported by fixed knowledge bases

DOI: 10.4018/979-8-2600-2173-6.ch001

were used but these were not able to identify the nuances of the context in clinical data. The statistical methods improved pattern recognition but a fixed vocabulary was a major concern.

1. INTRODUCTION

The integration of AI in healthcare has revolutionized the working of health care domain. Apart from the medical breakthroughs, AI has also enhanced the patient care, optimized clinical workflows and speeded up biomedical research (Shool et al., 2025). NLP is the AI subfield that allows machines to grasp, analyze and produce human language. It is essentially the core engine of AI application in medical research. LLMs and NLP techniques are drastically changing the ways medical data is handled and analyzed for decision making (Qiu et al., 2024).

With the advantage of transformer-based architectures, LLMs are able to go deep into large unstructured data like clinical annotations, health records, scientific publications and diagnostic images and extract key information seamlessly. To perform context-aware reasoning LLMs can assist a clinician in making a diagnostic decision and can also perform administrative tasks. Such models make a significant difference from traditional rule-based systems which lacked the capacity to interpret clinical language. The DL models can comprehend complex and Another challenge to medical LLMs is that a lot of medical data is often scattered across different sources and in various formats such as electronic health records (EHRs), scientific literature and patient letters (Zhou et al., 2024). The LLMs can assist healthcare professionals in effectively utilizing the data and enables them to extract valuable insights that can guide diagnosis, and efficient treatment plan. Extracting the essentials of clinical notes, medical coding, report preparation and conducting patient communication in real time via conversational AI interfaces are some of the functions (Luo et al., 2025) (Panagoulias et al., 2024). In addition to enhancing the efficiency of healthcare services, embedding LLMs in clinical decision support systems also improves the evidence-based medicine practice by handling a diverse range of medical information.

The important application of LLMs in medicine goes beyond their technical capabilities. It can empower healthcare practitioners with safe and effective tools. Medical LLMs must actually solve some fundamental issues. For example, the success of medical LLMs heavily relies on the nature of the data they get trained on. If there is a lack of sufficient and unbiased data, these AI systems will make errors and suggest wrong treatments for particular patients. Furthermore, data privacy plays a vital part and the need to comply with laws such as HIPAA and GDPR

. Complying these laws are essential for ensuring patients' trust and for following ethical standards (Alissa, 2025).

The biggest ethical issue with LLMs in healthcare is the ethical concern. Patients can be directly threatened by prejudice, misinformation, and hallucinations (Ahmad et al., 2025). Thus, models need to go through intensive testing and explainability, hence a decision becomes transparent and can be checked by the user. They must involve constant monitoring, routine audit and human-in-loop control to guarantee clinical safety (Uddin, 2025). The chapter provides the background of LLMs in healthcare by analyzing its key design characteristics, applications, and weaknesses. It follows the connection between primitive rule-based systems and the recent deep-learning models and underlines the changes of data that facilitated this development. The training and retraining methods adhered to by the medical use and the ethical, privacy, and regulatory issues that should be taken care of are also described in the chapter. Lastly, it examines the future possibilities including multimodal, federated, as well as edge AI methodologies that would provide additional improvements to the system. On the whole, the chapter provides a thorough overview of medical LLMs, which helps researchers understand the background of such technologies and predict the problems that policymakers and clinicians will encounter upon the implementation of the latter.

2. EVOLUTION OF LANGUAGE MODELS IN MEDICINE

Theprogress of Language Models (LMs) in the medical field has been mostly driven by breakthroughs in computational methods. This requires a better understanding of the complexities of medical language. Initially, the rule-based approaches were devised and DL models took the lead. LMs evolution has been guided by the growing need for methods that are able to process large amounts of unstructured medical data and provide healthcare professionals with valuable insights. The section highlights the achievement of medical language models with an emphasis on the transition from rule-based systems to transformer based architectures and the launch of domain-specific . Figure 1 illustrates the timeline of LLMs in the healthcare sector.

Figure 1. Evolution of LLMs in Medicine

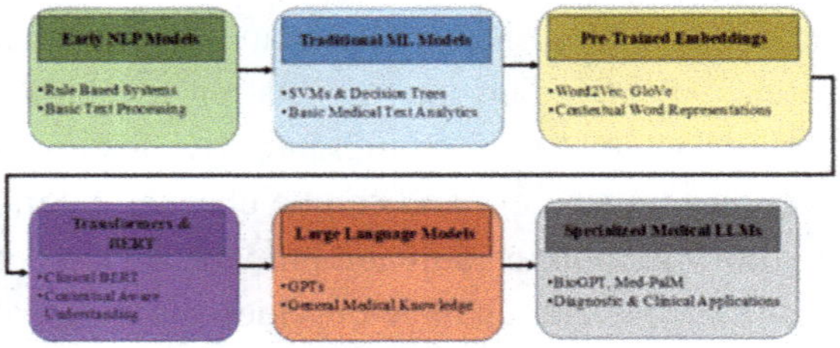

2.1 Early Rule-Based Systems and Statistical NLP

The language models in medicine focused mostly on rule-based systems that were heavily reliant on manual input from human experts. These models acted as the human-defined rules and expert-curated bodies of knowledge to detect particular patterns in medical texts, e.g., clinical notes or patient history, and correspond them to a list of possible diagnoses (Harshavardhan et al., 2025). The rule based systems also possessed some issues; they were extremely strict and unable to understand the peculiarities of the medical language such as abbreviations, homonyms, and complicated structures of the sentences. Without human intervention they were not able to adjust to new situations and were unrealistic in real-world settings where medical language is constantly changing. Rule-based systems revealed the need for more versatile and sophisticated methods of text analysis and thus can be regarded as the first step leading to the development of more advanced models.

The statistical NLP methods like Hidden Markov Models (HMMs) and Conditional Random Fields (CRFs) introduced a probabilistic aspect to text analysis during 1990s. These models were able to locate the patterns in clinical text with a better accuracy rate as they learned from the data and predicted the most likely meaning of a medical term or phrase based on the context in which it was used. However, statistical models still lagged in understanding the meaning of the text and stayed limited by fixed vocabularies and feature sets.

2.2 Neural Networks and Word Embeddings: The Shift Toward Deep Learning

The evolution of language models witnessed a significant milestone after the evolution of neural networks and word embeddings. During 2010s, the researchers began incorporating DL techniques to derive representations of words, phrases and sentences in a continuous vector space referred as word embeddings. The models were previously based on manually constructed features. It was replaced by word embeddings that enabled models to extract rich, context-dependent representations from massive text information. Such development has opened the prospect of operating with complicated medical terminology, abbreviations, and synonyms, in effect (Akbar et al., 2022).

Word2Vec and GloVe (Global Vectors of word representation) are the two models that have altered how text can be processed by AI models in the healthcare sector. Such models produce linguistically correct as well as semantically meaningful word representations. They expose how words relate to one another depending on their context of use as opposed to human regulations. This development was a basis of coming up with advanced NLP applications in health care industry that enhances the execution of results. It has been used in activities like classification of clinical texts, medical entity identification and relation mining. Table 1 presents the stages of evolution

Table 1. Stages of language models in medicine

Stage	Model Used	Key Features	Contributions to Healthcare
Early Rule-Based Systems	Expert Systems, RNNs	Handcrafted rules, limited learning ability	Early systems for decision support; could process predefined rules but lacked flexibility and contextual understanding.
Statistical NLP	HMMs, CRFs, TF-IDF	Probabilistic models, pattern detection, fixed vocabularies	Improved pattern recognition in medical text (e.g., clinical notes); still constrained by static vocabularies and inability to learn context.
Word Embeddings	Word2Vec, GloVe	Distributed word representations, context-based learning	Enabled semantic understanding of medical terms; better handling of synonyms, abbreviations and context.
Neural Networks and Deep Learning	Deep Learning Models	Multi-layer networks for feature extraction	Advanced medical text classification, sentiment analysis and entity recognition (e.g., diagnosis extraction from clinical records).
Transformer Architecture	BERT, GPT, BioBERT, ClinicalBERT	Attention mechanisms, parallel processing, large-scale pretraining	Breakthrough in understanding contextual relationships in medical language; fine-tuned models for clinical tasks (e.g., EHR processing).
Domain-Specific Models	BioBERT, ClinicalBERT, Med-PaLM	Fine-tuned on biomedical corpora, specialized medical vocabulary	Significant improvements in medical text mining, entity recognition and question-answering tasks; tailored for medical domain nuances.
Advanced LLMs for Healthcare	GPT-4, Med-PaLM, BioGPT	Multimodal capabilities, advanced reasoning, large-scale deployment	Integration with clinical decision support, drug discovery and personalized medicine; capable of understanding complex, multi-sentence reasoning.

2.3 The Rise of Transformer Models

A significant advancement in NLP, and also in medical NLP, took place in 2017, with the launch of the transformer architecture (Vaswani et al., 2017). It enhanced text processing speed and capabilities compared to previous text processing systems e.g. RNNs and LSTMs that process text in a step by step fashion. It has a self-attention mechanism that enables the transformer to recognize words relationship in a sentence. Due to this, it has made it possible to develop very efficient and precise models that can process large healthcare data.

Nowadays, transformer-based models are the backbone of numerous state-of-the-art NLP systems including BERT, GPT, and some of their recent incarcerations. These are first trained on huge text collections, and then trained to perform particular tasks, such as question answering, text summarization, and language translation.The breaking point of BERT is its ability to identify the context of words in a very thorough manner which translated into the remarkable gains in language comprehension.

Transformer models in medicine such as BioBERT, ClinicalBERT and Med-PaLM were immersed in biomedical and clinical texts to identify the characteristics of medical language. These models are superior to the general-purpose language models since they were specifically adjusted for recognizing medical terms, clinical abbreviations and the typical uses of language with medical scenarios. The BioBERT was trained on enormous biomedical texts gathered from PubMed. So, it can perform biomedical text mining tasks like named entity recognition (NER) and document classification effectively (Denecke et al., 2024).

The need for domain-specific language models in the healthcare sector was possible due to ability of LLMs. Evolving from single-purpose models like GPT-3 that accommodated various data types from the internet. The model development and training of BioBERT and ClinicalBERT involved medical data only. The BioBERT was pre-trained on massive biomedical literature dataset like PubMed articles and gained deeper insights into the specifics of scientific publications and clinical terminology. ClinicalBERT was tuned to run efficiently with medical data focusing on electronic health records (EHRs) and radiology reports that contain very specific language and abbreviations (Vavekanand et al., 2026).

Med-PaLM is another example of medical-specific language model that can exhibit excellent results in medical question answering tasks. It is based on the GPT-3 architecture and was fine-tuned with medical question-answering data. It can better comprehend and respond to clinical queries posted by users. These domain-specific models are more trustworthy in clinical situations where incorrect interpretation of medical language might lead to fatal outcomes.

The emergence of these domain-specific models promoted building models trained on medical texts and mirroring the complexities of healthcare data. The advances of such models are to bring new breakthroughs in areas in personalized medicine, clinical decision support, drug discovery and public health monitoring effectively.

2.4 From Statistical Methods to Deep Learning: A New Era in Healthcare NLP

The development of language models in medicine from the initial rule-based systems to DL models created a significant change in the potential of AI in healthcare. The early rule based systems had difficulties in handling medical language complexities, contemporary LLMs are capable of analyzing and understanding complicated medical texts almost flawlessly. These models can facilitate the entire spectrum of healthcare operations from diagnostic decision support to automating medical documentation. They can reshape how healthcare professionals engage with data (Zhou et al., 2022).

Despite the advantages of these models, there are issues that requires serious consideration to adapt to healthcare domain. The data quality issues, the bias mitigation and the ability to interpret model outputs remains unaddressed. Obtaining strong and heterogeneous data, managing ethical issues related to the implementation of models and protecting patient safety are the key issues as LLMs continue to enter clinical practice. Further sections will clarify about the underlying architecture of LLMs, data preconditions necessary to deploy the technologies in medical contexts. The ethical and regulatory aspects that have to be followed when implementing the technologies in clinical practices are also discussed. In this revolutionary context, further development of LLMs will lead to the creation of a new paradigm in the healthcare delivery. Various milestones of NLP is depicted in Table 2.

Table 2. Milestones of NLP in medicine

Milestone	Model Used	Key Features and Advancements	Impact on Healthcare
Early Biomedical NLP Models	Traditional Rule-Based Systems	Human-crafted rules, simple text processing, limited to predefined vocabulary	Early attempts at medical decision support (e.g., for diagnosis assistance); lacked contextual understanding.
Introduction of Word Embeddings	Word2Vec, GloVe	Distributed representations of medical terms, context-dependent learning	Improved handling of synonyms and medical abbreviations; helped in semantic understanding in clinical texts like EHRs.
First Domain-Specific Model	BioBERT	Pretrained on PubMed and PMC datasets; fine-tuned for biomedical tasks	Revolutionized biomedical NLP by improving performance on tasks like named entity recognition (NER) and relation extraction.

continued on following page

Table 2. Continued

Milestone	Model Used	Key Features and Advancements	Impact on Healthcare
Clinical Text Understanding	ClinicalBERT	Fine-tuned BioBERT for clinical notes and electronic health records (EHRs)	Tailored for clinical environments, enabling better understanding of clinical terminology, patient records and medical coding.
Improved Question-Answering	Med-PaLM	Fine-tuned on medical question-answering tasks, based on GPT-3 architecture	Advanced understanding of clinical questions and answers; enhanced decision support for healthcare professionals.
Large-Scale Generalized Model	GPT-4	Large-scale transformer model, pre-trained on diverse and expansive medical data	Improved contextual understanding in medical tasks; capable of reasoning across complex multi-sentence clinical text.
Multimodal Biomedical Models	BioGPT	Multimodal capabilities (text, image and possibly genomic data), advanced reasoning	Integration of multiple data types, enhancing medical applications like radiology report interpretation and genomic analysis.

2.5 General-Purpose LLMs vs Domain-Specific LLMs

The emergence of LLMs has transformed the field of artificial intelligence, particularly in healthcare. Both general-purpose LLMs and domain-specific LLMs are used in healthcare applications, but they differ significantly in their design, training and performance. It is quite important to know such differences when choosing a model to address certain healthcare requirements. General purpose LLMs like GPT -4 are trained on general-purpose tasks. They rely on huge, broad data-books, internet, news and give them an opportunity to produce text, respond to questions and summarize data in numerous areas. They are experts in the work that depends on general knowledge of language such as content creation or chatbots. Their performance, however, reduces on areas that are specialized like healthcare. They can have difficulty in understanding medical terms, giving proper clinical counsel, and may make errors or hallucination and this is dangerous.

Specialized LLMs such as BioBERT, ClinicalBERT and Med-PaLM are acquired using specialized medical data. They are sensitive enough to pick up sensitive medical terminologies contained in clinical notes, research articles and patient records. The models are effective in recognizing named-entities, medical question answering, and clinical decision support. They are more qualified to be applied to the medical sphere, because they are able to better understand specialized terminology and relations within the context, and are therefore preferable to general models (Vavekanand et al., 2026).

LLMs are very flexible in general. They do not fail in most aspects- health care to entertainment and education. However, their implementation to a particular domain such as medicine needs extensive special data and a lot of computing resources. They may be optimised to health work, but not to the individual needs of medicine. Domain-specific LMs, in turn, are healthcare applications. Their excellence in work is seen in drug discovery, biomedical investigation, and electronic health record processing. These models are able to derive informative content out of medical literature and aid clinical decision-making at a high accuracy. However, they lack the versatility of general models and cannot perform other aspects due to specializing in particular medical activities (Savage et al., 2024).

General-purpose LLMs are ethically problematic in a number of ways. Their training on general internet information makes them repeat prejudices and fake facts. The fact that they are not interpretable also makes it difficult to trust their outputs by clinicians who may end up making wrong diagnoses or incorrect treatment recommendations. Healthcare is more suited to domain-specific LLM. They are taught through both filtered medical information that assists to minimize prejudices and greater accuracy in reading medical text. The models are also more consistent with healthcare rules, so they will not violate privacy protocols, including HIPAA and GDPR. General purpose vs domain specific LLM is presented in Table 3.

Table 3. Comparison of General purpose and Domain specific LLMs

Aspect	General-purpose LLMs	Domain-specific LLMs
Training Data	Trained on diverse, broad datasets (e.g., books, websites, news)	Trained on specialized medical data (e.g., clinical texts, biomedical literature, EHRs)
Versatility	Highly versatile, can handle tasks across various domains	Specialized for specific domains like healthcare and medicine
Performance in Healthcare	Struggles with medical terminology, abbreviations and nuanced clinical language	Excels in medical applications, understanding medical terminology and context
Use Cases	General tasks like text generation, summarization, question-answering	Medical-specific tasks such as clinical decision support, medical question answering, drug discovery
Flexibility	Adaptable to a wide range of tasks, but may require fine-tuning for specialized domains	Less flexible outside their domain, but performs exceptionally within healthcare tasks
Limitations	Misinterpretations and hallucinations, especially in medical contexts	Limited to healthcare-specific tasks, not suitable for general-purpose applications
Ethical Concerns	Risk of bias, misinformation and lack of interpretability	More focused on medical data, but still concerns about biases in training data

continued on following page

Table 3. Continued

Aspect	General-purpose LLMs	Domain-specific LLMs
Regulatory Compliance	May pose challenges in healthcare regulation (e.g., HIPAA compliance)	Better suited for compliance with healthcare regulations like HIPAA and GDPR
Applications in Healthcare	Can be used for patient communication, summarizing reports, or automating administrative tasks	Ideal for tasks like medical coding, EHR processing, biomedical research and clinical decision-making
Example Models	GPT-4, GPT-3, BERT	BioBERT, ClinicalBERT, Med-PaLM

3. ARCHITECTURE OF LARGE LANGUAGE MODELS

LLMs are the central component that determines the effectiveness of the approach in NLP tasks due to their design based on transformer architecture. These models have led to a significant change in various aspects especially in the medicine. The transformer architecture is the base of many LLMs which has shown effectiveness in handling the challenges in linguistics. This part gives a explanation of the main components of LLM architecture and its components like tokenization, embeddings, attention processes and the training processes as illustrated in Figure 2.

Figure 2. Architecture of LLMs in healthcare

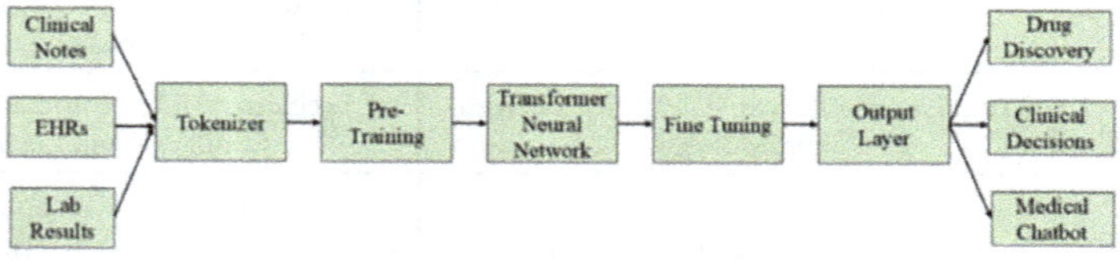

3.1 Transformer Architecture

Most of the modern LLMs are based on the transformer architecture. The models like RNNs process sequentially while the transformers process input sequences simultaneously. Self-attention mechanism makes this parallelism possible and systematically examines the relevance of each token in a sequence to all other tokens. This parallelization leads to faster training times and a better ability to capture long-range dependencies in textual data and makes the transformers useful in large scale NLP tasks.

Transformers are constructed with have encoder and decoder units. Models like BERT use only encoder while GPT consists of only decoder. The self-attention mechanism allows each token in the input sequence to attend to all the rest of the tokens. This does not consider the distance in position and allows the model to capture the intricate relationships and contextual information. This makes the model to work better on text generation, machine translation and summarization tasks.

3.2 Tokenization and Embeddings

The core of LLMs lies in tokenization that converts raw text into smaller units that can be processed by the model. Tokenization can be broken text into words, subwords or characters depending on the model requirements. The common popular techniques are BytesPair Encoding and WordPiece used to divide text into subword units. These methods enable the model to deal with unusual or unfamiliar words by splitting them into more familiar ones. Once it has been tokenized, every token is represented as a numerical vector which is an embedding (Ferreira et al., 2025).

Such high-dimensional vectors mock the meaning of the token, and they assist the model in grasping the relationship of words based on their context. The embeddings are trained during training and this way words with similar meanings are likely to enter the same area of the vector space. This narrowing down allows the model to work better with more complicated medical relationships, such as abbreviations and synonyms. (Ma et al., 2024).

3.3 Attention Mechanism

The self-attention mechanism is crucial for transformer-based LLMs. It allows the model to weigh the importance of each word in a sequence in relation to every other word. This is achieved by computing three vectors for each word namely the Query (Q), Key (K) and Value (V). The attention score is computed by taking the dot product of the Query and Key vectors, followed by a scaling operation and applying a softmax function to get the attention weights. These weights are then used to combine the Value vectors to produce a context-sensitive output for each word.

To further enhance the ability to capture different aspects of word relationships the transformers use multi-head attention. This allows multiple attention mechanisms to operate in parallel to focus on different parts of the sequence. The outputs from each attention head are concatenated and linearly transformed to provide a better understanding of the input data.

3.4 Pre-Training and Fine-Tuning

One of the key advantages of LLMs is their pretraining on large unlabelled datasets followed by fine-tuning for specific tasks. Pre-training typically involves unsupervised learning where the model learns to predict the next word in a sequence or to fill in masked words in a sentence.

After pre-training, the model is fine-tuned on a smaller task-specific dataset. This allows to adapt its general knowledge to healthcare specialized applications. This fine-tuning process is crucial for clinical decision support, drug discovery and biomedical research where domain-specific language and nuances need to be understood. For instance, models like BioBERT and ClinicalBERT are fine-tuned on medical corpora which enhances their ability to process clinical texts and biomedical literature.

3.5 Reinforcement Learning From Human Feedback (RLHF)

An emerging approach to improving LLMs involves Reinforcement Learning from Human Feedback (RLHF). In RLHF the models are fine-tuned by incorporating human feedback. This helps the model to improve the relevance and accuracy of its responses. This approach has been used to enhance models like GPT-3 and GPT-4 to make them capable of generating contextually appropriate and accurate answers (Abdellatif et al., 2023). RLHF can ensure that the model's predictions align with clinical best practices and ethical standards in healthcare applications.

3.6 Privacy-Preserving Techniques

The healthcare data is sensitive in nature. The privacy-preserving techniques are essential in the architecture of medical LLMs. Federated learning allows models to be trained on decentralized data from multiple institutions without sharing raw patient data. Only model updates are communicated to a central server ensuring that patient data remains private and secure. The techniques like differential privacy add noise to the training process to prevent the model from memorizing individual data points. This helps maintain privacy allowing the model to learn meaningful patterns from the data. Such methods are crucial in medical applications where data privacy is a significant concern.

3.7 Context in LLMs

Context is fundamental to understanding the meaning and generating coherent responses in LLMs. The transformer architecture is the core of most modern LLMs that employs a self-attention mechanism to capture context across long-range dependencies in text. Transformers, unlike other models like RNNs, use all the words at the same time, as opposed to processing input sequences word-by-word. As a system, parallel processing enables it to acquire word relationship irrespective of the sequence. In a medical context, understanding context is critical in deriving helpful and accurate inferences to clinical data. An example is the definition of the term diabetes: it can change radically based on the surrounding terms: insulin resistance or heart disease. The model is also good at intricate tasks such as clinical decision support and by the fact that it is also self-attentive it is able to detect these minor contextual variations. Thus, context is important to be included in order to enhance the precision of special fields.

3.8 Prompt Engineering

Prompt engineering refers to making, or creating, clear and specific instructions in order that the language models would generate intended results. Even though the large language models may be trained to complete a range of tasks, the clarity and detail of the prompt used are probably the primary determinants of the model quality. In the healthcare field, clearly defined prompts are particularly essential, as the definite request contributes to the model providing the correct and efficient response to the clinical queries (Patil et al., 2024). To illustrate, when a clinician queries an LLM concerning drug interactions, one of its prompts should be specific to drug-drug or patient-specific drug interactions and not should be generic drug facts. This narrowed down methodology minimizes ambiguity and maximizes clinical precision. Conversely, ill-constructed prompts may lead to erroneous or inappropriate information, which is dangerous in the medical setting (Wang et al., 2025).

Dynamic prompt engineering enables the models to change during a dialogue or activity. During a virtual clinical consultation, the prompts may be changed dynamically according to the medical history of a patient or their complaints and guarantee the relevance of the responses of the model to the current situation. This flexibility is critical in establishing good communication with the patients and the correct medical coding where specific answers are needed.

3.9 Retrieval Augmentation

RAG enhances the work of LLM by incorporating external knowledge. Although LLMs have good text-generation capabilities, they do not always have expertise to perform specific health-related tasks. The retrieval mechanisms enable LLAMs to retrieve the most recent domain-specific knowledge, which makes their responses more applicable and trustworthy (Abo El-Enen et al., 2025).

It is possible to query medical databases like PubMed or UpToDate with retrieval-augmented systems to get recent research articles, clinical trials, and treatment guidelines. This helps the model to present evidence-based responses that are more precise than those that are presented based on pre-trained knowledge. RAG and other models use retrieval and text generation to give accurate and contextual answers (Cui et al., 2026). As an example, a doctor or a nurse may question an LLM in case of knowing the latest findings on a given disease.. The LLM will be able to fetch recent publications or clinical trials to make sure that the response is reflective of the latest research depending on its own pre-trained knowledge. This method not only increases the accuracy but also guarantees that the model answers are consistent with the current medical standards.

4. DATA FOUNDATIONS IN MEDICAL LLMS

4.1 Types of Data: Clinical Text, EHRs, Radiology Reports, Biomedical Literature, and Patient Communications

Medical Large Language Models (LLMs) are built upon heterogeneous healthcare data sources that reflect the complexity of clinical practice as shown in Table 4.

- Clinical text refers to materials such as physician notes, discharge summaries, test reports and progress notes that provide a lot of reasoning and context but are frequently unstructured and with many abbreviations.
- Electronic Health Records (EHRs) include both structured elements and unstructured text. They are able to provide complete patient histories which are very important for temporal reasoning.
- Radiology reports focus on describing the findings and doctor's impressions through images that demand a precise interpretation of the diagnostic language and anatomical references used.
- Biomed literature like PubMed articles and clinical guidelines is mainly a source of evidence based on the latest scientific knowledge and terminologies of the field.
- Patient communications such as telehealth transcripts, symptom descriptions and chatbot interactions represent real world language variability and the way layperson express diseases.

Table 4. Types of data in LLM for heathcare

Data Type	Examples	Nature of Data	Role in LLM Training and Inference
Clinical Text	Physician notes, discharge summaries, progress notes, operative notes	Unstructured	Enables LLMs to learn clinical language patterns, reasoning workflows, and context-aware interpretation of patient conditions
Electronic Health Records (EHRs)	Structured and semi-structured hospital information systems	Structured and semi-structured	Supports factual grounding, temporal reasoning, patient trajectory modeling, and personalized clinical decision support
Radiology Reports	PACS systems, radiology information systems (RIS)	Semi-structured text	Trains LLMs to link textual findings with diagnostic reasoning and enables multimodal alignment with imaging data
Biomedical Literature	PubMed articles, clinical guidelines, systematic reviews, textbooks	Highly structured scientific text	Provides foundational medical knowledge, evidence-based reasoning, and supports knowledge-grounded generation
Patient Communications	Patient portals, emails, chat logs, telemedicine transcripts	Unstructured conversational text	Enables patient-centric language understanding, symptom extraction, triage assistance, and empathetic response generation

4.2 Data Preprocessing, Anonymization, and De-identification

Data preprocessing is an essential stage in the creation of trustworthy medical LLMs. Untreated healthcare data consists of noisy, inconsistent and of various types. Clinical notes have misspelled words, usage of short forms and incomplete sentences. The preprocessing is made up of different steps such as normalization, tokenization, sentence segmentation and removal of characters that don't add meaning. The structured EHR data should be made consistent between different hospital systems using different coding systems and documentation styles. The Protected Health Information (PHI) such as names, addresses, phone numbers, social security numbers, hospital IDs and biometric identifiers should be removed or covered before model training to secure the privacy of the data (Wiest et al., 2024). General preprocessing techniques include:

- **Rule-based de-identification:** Pattern matching using regular expressions to remove identifiers such as phone numbers or dates.
- **Machine learning-based NER models:** Detecting personal identifiers within free-text clinical notes.

- **Pseudonymization:** Replacing identifiable attributes with synthetic but consistent identifiers to preserve longitudinal relationships.
- **Data masking and hashing:** Encrypting sensitive fields while retaining referential integrity.

Apert from removing identifiers, anonymization must prevent re-identification through indirect attributes. Advanced techniques such as differential privacy introduce controlled noise into datasets to ensure that the individual patient records cannot be reverse engineered from model outputs. The preprocessing is not merely technical preparation it is an ethical safeguard ensuring privacy, fairness and reliability in medical AI systems.

4.3 Integration of Medical Ontologies and Terminologies

- In the medical field, LLMs have to interpret a highly specialized vocabulary. Standardized medical ontologies such as SNOMED CT, ICD, MeSH and UMLS are used and semantic consistency is preserved (Abdulnazar et al., 2024).
- Systematized Nomenclature of Medicine, Clinical Terms (SNOMED CT) is a clinical terminology with concepts for diseases, symptoms, procedures and anatomical parts. The hierarchical relationships enable models to realize that "myocardial infarction" is a subtype of "ischemic heart disease."
- International Classification of Diseases (ICD) is mainly utilized for billing, epidemiology and morbidity statistics. The mapping of free-text diagnoses to ICD codes opens up the possibility for automated medical coding and hospital analytics (Bikdeli et al., 2025).
- Medical Subject Headings (MeSH) is used for indexing biomedical articles in PubMed. In addition of MeSH terms, LLMs bridge the gap between research evidence and clinical practice (Roselló Atanet et al., 2025).
- The Unified Medical Language System serves as a meta-ontology linking vocabularies and providing concept identifiers. It promotes semantic interoperability between healthcare databases.

This process reduces ambiguity and improves factual consistency to enhances explainability. For example, when an LLM predicts "Type 2 Diabetes Mellitus," ontology alignment ensures it corresponds to a standardized SNOMED or ICD code to support traceability and auditability.

Table 5. Medical Ontologies and Terminologies for LLM Integration

Ontology	Description	Primary Use Case	Integration Benefit
SNOMED CT	Comprehensive clinical terminology	Clinical documentation & EHR mapping	Semantic hierarchy & interoperability
ICD	Global disease classification system	Billing, epidemiology	Standardized diagnostic coding
MeSH	Controlled vocabulary for biomedical indexing	Research literature retrieval	Enhanced evidence linking
UMLS	Meta-thesaurus integrating multiple ontologies	Cross-database mapping	Unified concept identification

Ontology-aware LLMs contribute to knowledge grounding and cuts down on hallucinations by limiting output to validated medical vocabularies as given in Table 5. Knowledge graphs derived from these ontologies also provide a notable boost to reasoning skills since they explicitly map the relationships between illnesses, medications and treatments. Incorporating structured medical terminologies changes LLMs from mere statistical models to ones capable of clinically reasoning with semantic knowledge (Liu et al., 2025).

4.4 Challenges: Data Imbalance, Multilingualism, and Domain-Specific Jargon

Data Imbalance

In many cases, medical data sets mainly include common diseases and neglect rare conditions that are far less common. Because of this imbalance, LLMs are inclined to diagnose the most common diseases and might even miss rare but serious conditions. In the same way, if the demographic imbalance exists the model may make biased decisions. The solutions include stratified sampling, fairness auditing and recruiting diverse patient populations for the training process.

Multilingualism

In a multilingual country like India, the healthcare data is available in various languages. In practice, the clinical documentation may be a mixture of English and local languages. A large number of medical LLMs are mostly trained on English texts that makes them not very suitable for other languages. To achieve fair deployment, it is essential to use multilingual embeddings, cross-lingual transfer learning and local corpora.

Domain-Specific Jargon

The clinical language heavily relies on abbreviations and words that have a meaning depending on the context (e.g. "CP" can stand for either chest pain or cerebral palsy). If LLMs are not equipped with the use of ontologies, they are likely to misunderstand such words. Regular updates with the help of domain-specific corpora and clinician-in-the-loop validation are a great way to preserve contextual correctness.

5. TRAINING AND OPTIMIZATION STRATEGIES

5.1 Pre-Training on General Text and Domain Adaptation Using Medical Corpora

Medical LLMs typically follow a two-stage learning strategy involving large-scale general pre-training followed by domain-specific adaptation. During general pre-training the transformer based architectures are exposed to massive corpora including books, web content and encyclopedic sources. The objective functions like masked language modeling (MLM) and causal language modeling (CLM) enable the model to learn grammar, semantic relationships, reasoning patterns and contextual dependencies. This stage equips the model with broad linguistic intelligence and general world knowledge (Kaiser & Wu, 2025).

The adaptation stage boosts the downstream performance of medical entity recognition, clinical summarization, ICD coding and medical question answering. Domain adaptation will reduce the rate of the hallucinated medical facts and improve the understanding of clinical subtleties by the model. Medical LLMs combine the general reasoning ability of large-scale linguistic pre-training with domain specific biomedical knowledge, to reach the domain specific accuracy necessary to be used safely in health care. (Kawas et al., 2025).

5.2 Instruction Tuning and Reinforcement Learning From Human Feedback (RLHF)

The AI alignment and safety of RLHF is enhanced through the model generating several possible solutions to a prompt. These responses are then checked and graded by medical personnel in terms of accuracy, clarity and safety. A model of rewards is constructed to be able to predict the preferences of the experts and the language model is trained to maximize that reward, to be sure that its outputs are based on expert judgment and are not simply a statistical trend (Frommeyer et al., 2025).

RLHF minimizes negative or untrue responses in healthcare. It reduces hallucinations and enhances the accuracy of facts and keeps answers within evidence-based guidelines. Another method through which RLHF can put ethical boundaries is to ensure that the model does not prescribe unapproved drugs or provide dangerous advice. With instruction tuning and expert guided learning, medical language models are made safer and more reliable and in close relationship with clinical best practice. (Banumathi et al., 2025).

5.3 Parameter-Efficient Fine-Tuning for Healthcare Deployment

Training LLMs on specific tasks consumes huge computational lobe and retraining billions of parameters. This is a problem in the healthcare environment where infrastructure is usually constrained and data privacy a priority. PEFT provides viable alternatives to parameter-efficient fine-tuning. They introduce very few new parameters and leave the majority of the old weights as they are (Zhang et al., 2025). Low-Rank Adaptation (LoRA) places low-rank matrices, which can be trained, into the attention layers of a transformer. With a small adjustment of the parameters, LoRA saves on memory and lowers the cost of computation. Consequently, the models can be stored locally, in various formats, e.g., to different EHR systems, medical specialties, or languages, without having to retrain the models. (Le et al., 2025).

5.4 Performance Evaluation Metrics: Accuracy, BLEU, ROUGE, Factuality, and Safety

Assessing medical LLMs, we are supposed to consider standard NLP measures and healthcare-specific safety measures. The most popular measure of classification tasks like disease prediction or the ICD code is accuracy. It calculates the percentage of the correct predictions, yet, it does not evaluate the quality of the text or the depth of arguments.

BLEU (Bilingual Evaluation Understudy) calculates the n-grams intersection between the text translations and reference text, which is appropriate in translation and structured reports generation. ROUGE (Recall-Oriented Understudy for Gisting Evaluation) uses the overlap of a summary with a gold-standard clinical summary to evaluate the summary. The measures come in handy when permitting documentation activities, which include discharge report summaries (Shool et al., 2025).

6. APPLICATIONS OF LLMS IN MEDICINE AND HEALTHCARE

6.1 Clinical Decision Support: Summarization, Diagnosis Assistance, and Guideline Interpretation

The clinical decision support systems are beginning to integrate LLMs to help doctors be more efficient and accurate in diagnostics. Doctors in bustling hospital settings have to go through a entire patient record, lab results and clinical guidelines within a short timeframe to make a decision. Summary tools powered by LLMs shorten the long clinical notes to give doctors organized information, revealing the main findings, medications, allergies and risk factors (Vrdoljak et al., 2025). The system for diagnosis support checks symptoms and lab results to propose a list of possible diagnosis. The module for guideline interpretation converts medical protocols into steps that can be followed and that suit the patients irrespective of the complication of the instructions. Such features help to lower the overload and allow the use of the latest medicine supported by evidence. These systems are merely assisting clinicians and should not be seen as replacements. The validation by humans is always necessary to avoid reliance on these systems and to lower the risks that come from incorrect inferences (Gaber et al., 2025). The main use cases and benefits of LLM-based clinical decision support are outlined in Table 6.

Table 6. Clinical Decision Support Applications of LLMs

Application Area	Function of LLM	Clinical Benefit	Example Use Case
Clinical Summarization	Condenses long EHR notes into key insights	Saves time, reduces cognitive load	ICU discharge summary generation
Diagnosis Assistance	Suggests differential diagnoses from symptoms and labs	Supports clinical reasoning	Early sepsis risk detection
Guideline Interpretation	Translates clinical protocols into patient-specific advice	Improves adherence to evidence-based care	Diabetes management plan generation
Risk Prediction	Identifies high-risk patients	Enables preventive care	Predicting readmission probability

6.2 Patient Interaction: Conversational AI for Symptom Checking and Telehealth

Conversational AI, which is a type of AI that uses large language models (LLMs) to provide patient interaction, has transformed patient interaction within digital health systems, providing 24/7 symptom monitoring services, pre-triage consultation, drug reminders and telehealth assistance. With an understanding of natural language, chatbots using LLM will be able to decode patient reports, e.g., chest tightness or persistent fatigue, and be able to convert them into easily understandable healthcare routes. They also have the benefit of assisting doctors in summarizing patient-reported histories in advance of virtual visits, which increases the efficiency of telemedicine. Moreover, the systems enhance access among rural dwellers and old people since the medical terms are simplified. They must clearly identify their limitations and must never make final diagnoses without clinical oversight (Jadhav & Bainalwar, 2026). Deployments that are directly facing patients require ethical protection, multilingual coverage and safety filter. Table 7 provides a summary of the key patient interaction applications.

Table 7. Patient Interaction Applications of LLMs

Application Area	Function of LLM	Patient Benefit	Example Use Case
Symptom Checker	Interprets patient-reported symptoms	Early triage guidance	COVID-like symptom screening
Telehealth Support	Summarizes patient inputs before consultation	Efficient virtual visits	Pre-consultation data summary
Medication Guidance	Provides reminders and instructions	Improves adherence	Daily insulin reminder chatbot
Multilingual Communication	Translates medical advice into local languages	Improved accessibility	Rural telemedicine assistance

6.3 Biomedical Research: Literature Mining, Drug Discovery, and Clinical Trial Matching

LLMs speed up the process of knowledge discovery by searching huge databases of biomedical literature. They derive gene-protein-disease-therapeutic relationships out of thousands of articles. The tools of summarization compile results of all the studies and assist the researcher in identifying trends and gaps. In drug discovery, the LLMs discover possible molecular targets and propose repurposing of currently available drugs through text analysis and structured datasets of biomedical information. To improve the efficiency of clinical trial recruitment, clinical trial matching systems rely on the use of LLMs to match patient records with the eligibility criteria of trial protocols. These applications save time and increase research productivity. It is still necessary to validate it against experimental and clinical data. Table 8 outlines the main applications of research.

Table 8. Biomedical Research Applications of LLMs

Application Area	Function of LLM	Research Benefit	Example Use Case
Literature Mining	Extracts insights from research articles	Faster evidence synthesis	Summarizing oncology trials
Drug Discovery	Identifies potential drug–disease links	Accelerates R&D	Drug repurposing analysis
Clinical Trial Matching	Maps patient data to eligibility criteria	Improved recruitment	Oncology patient–trial matching
Knowledge Graph Building	Links biomedical entities	Structured reasoning	Gene–disease association modeling

6.4 Documentation Automation: EHR Summarization and Report Generation

Healthcare practitioners waste a lot of time in documentation and it leads to burnout and loss of time to attend to patients. Large language models (LLM) can automatize such work by summarizing electronic health records, writing discharges, and writing formal clinical reports. The speech-to-text integration will enable automatic consultation transcription, and structural notes will be created to guarantee the use of a consistent vocabulary and reduce clerical overloads. Electronic coding software also contributes to proper billing by assigning diagnoses to standard codes. The automation increases the efficiency, but it is vital to make sure that it is properly validated, avoiding the mistakes of documentation. An overview of these applications related to documentation is given in Table 9.

Table 9. Documentation Automation Applications of LLMs

Application Area	Function of LLM	Operational Benefit	Example Use Case
EHR Summarization	Condenses patient history	Faster clinical review	Outpatient visit summary
Report Generation	Drafts radiology or pathology reports	Reduced administrative burden	CT scan interpretation draft
Speech-to-Text Documentation	Converts consultations to structured notes	Time-saving	Automated SOAP note creation
Coding Assistance	Suggests ICD codes	Billing accuracy	Automated diagnosis coding

6.5 Education and Training: Intelligent Tutoring and Knowledge Synthesis for Clinicians

LLMs are medical students and healthcare professional education helpers. They provide interactive descriptions of complicated concepts, model patient scenarios, and create practice questions which match licensing tests. The ability to synthesize their knowledge enables them to synthesize and summarize new guidelines and research findings fast. During clinical training, the LLM can be used to simulate cases of differential-diagnosis, providing learners with the practical experience of the reasoning ability. Individual tutoring is customized to the level of each learner (Vrdoljak et al., 2025). Although these benefits exist, the spread of old or wrong information on the internet should be monitored to ensure that the information shared by LLMs does not spread. Table. 10 contains the description of the educational applications.

Table 10. Educational Applications of LLMs in Healthcare

Application Area	Function of LLM	Educational Benefit	Example Use Case
Intelligent Tutoring	Explains medical concepts interactively	Personalized learning	Cardiology concept explanation
Case Simulation	Generates virtual patient scenarios	Clinical reasoning training	Differential diagnosis exercise
Knowledge Synthesis	Summarizes new guidelines	Continuous learning	Updated hypertension guideline summary
Exam Preparation	Generates practice MCQs	Licensing exam readiness	USMLE-style question generation

7. ETHICAL, PRIVACY AND REGULATORY CONSIDERATIONS

There is a variety of ethical, privacy and regulation concerns that exist when deploying large language models in healthcare. To achieve the advantages of the use of the LLMs and safeguard the rights of patients, safeguard transparency, and fulfill regulatory requirements is vital to address these issues.

7.1. Ethical Considerations

The ethical issues in healthcare LLM are concerned with prejudice, openness, and responsibility. Training data bias has the potential to create disparities in health, particularly when the underrepresented groups are overlooked. Open decision-making will allow clinical professionals to see how the model gets to a recommendation. The accountability implies that the users have the ability to follow the logic of the model. Informed consent is critical too; they should be aware when an LLM is participating in their treatment and the purpose of using their data. These problems are the main factors that should be addressed in order to make LLMs fair and trustworthy in the clinical environment (Palama, 2025).

7.2. Privacy Considerations

The privacy is one of the most important concerns in the field of healthcare, and LLMs are working with the most sensitive information about patients. It is most important to safeguard such data. Privacy-sensitive methods like federated learning and differential privacy ought to be employed by LLLMs, as a means of ensuring information remains confidential. Minimization of data used: it is important to access the data that is required to serve the purpose of the model. Strong anonymity should not allow re-identification. Such measures instill confidence in AI-based health systems.

7.3. Regulatory Considerations

The LLDs employed in the medical practice should adhere to the national and international standards. They are required to adhere to the HIPAA in the US, which ensures the privacy and safety of data. In Europe, GDPR rules apply. A large part of the LLMs can also be considered medical devices and be approved by agencies such as the FDA or EMA. The regulators check on safety and effectiveness. To launch the LLM, clinical trials or validation studies are required to demonstrate the compatibility of the LLM with health standards (Ojewale et al., 2026).

7. 4. Integrating the Ethical and Privacy Standards in Model Development

This should include ethics, privacy and regulatory provision in all levels of developing the LLM. The close collaboration with clinicians will make the model respond to actual clinical questions and adhere to the best practice guidelines. The audits and frequent reviews ensure that the system adheres to the ethics and law. The clarity of the reasoning behind the model leads to the creation of trust and allows users to evaluate the outputs, particularly in the high-stakes decisions.

8. CONCLUSION AND FUTURE DIRECTIONS

This chapter offers an in-depth discussion of the possibilities of the large language models (LLMs) in the healthcare field. It follows their development- of rule based systems to sophisticated transformer architectures and their increasing ability to process and comprehend medical data. The contextual reasoning and the capability of decoding complex medical terminology allows LLPs to be used in a wide variety of clinical applications, supporting decision-making as well as automating administrative processes, and are changing the nature of healthcare.

Having LLMs integrated into medical practices can assist physicians to diagnose more precisely, less paperwork, and improve the medical interaction with patients. The functionality of the models is not only based on the advancement of technologies but ethical standards, data management, and regulatory standards. To apply the use of LLMs in a responsible way, a consistent and continuous cooperation between clinicians, data scientists, and legislators is highly necessary to guarantee patient safety, decrease bias, and sustain transparent AI decisions.

The future of LLMs in the medical profession is bright, although challenges like data heterogeneity, biases, and patient privacy should be overcome. It is moving in the right direction and the emergence of new models providing multimodal integration and real-time flexibility will open up new possibilities of what can be accomplished by healthcare facilities.

To improve the multimodal integration, healthcare researchers should consider the ways to improve the data types including text, images, and signals, and provide the privacy provided by the federated learning. Explainability and interpretability in real-world clinical validation should be the priority of building clinician trust. It should be possible to identify biases in training data and provide a fair treatment of the patient groups. The adaption of LLDs to low-resource environments should also be used to expand LLDs, especially with edge AI solutions. All of these will help make the adoption of LLMs into the medical practice easy and will result in safer and more rewarding healthcare experiences.

REFERENCES

Abdellatif, A. A., Mhaisen, N., Mohamed, A., Erbad, A., & Guizani, M. (2023). Reinforcement learning for intelligent healthcare systems: A review of challenges, applications, and open research issues. *IEEE Internet of Things Journal*, *10*(24), 21982–22007. DOI: 10.1109/JIOT.2023.3288050

Abdulnazar, A., Roller, R., Schulz, S., & Kreuzthaler, M. (2024). Large language models for clinical text cleansing enhance medical concept normalization. *IEEE Access : Practical Innovations, Open Solutions*, *12*, 147981–147990. DOI: 10.1109/ACCESS.2024.3472500

Abo El-Enen, M., Saad, S., & Nazmy, T. (2025). A survey on retrieval-augmentation generation (RAG) models for healthcare applications. *Neural Computing & Applications*, *37*(33), 28191–28267. DOI: 10.1007/s00521-025-11666-9

Ahmad, H. F., Sajid, J., Rasool, R. U., & Malik, A. W. (2025). Beyond the hype: Exploring the impact, challenges, and potential of large language models in healthcare. *Cluster Computing*, •••, 28.

Akbar, S., Hayat, M., Tahir, M., Khan, S., & Alarfaj, F. K. (2022). cACP-DeepGram: Classification of anticancer peptides via deep neural network and skip-gram-based word embedding model. *Artificial Intelligence in Medicine*, *131*, 102349. DOI: 10.1016/j.artmed.2022.102349 PMID: 36100346

Alissa, K. A. (2025). A survey on privacy issues and mitigation strategies for LLMs in healthcare. *The Journal of Supercomputing*, *82*(1), 82. DOI: 10.1007/s11227-025-08146-1

Banumathi, K., Venkatesan, L., Benjamin, L. S., Vijayalakshmi, K., Satchi, N. S., & Satchi, N. S.IV. (2025). Reinforcement learning in personalized medicine: A comprehensive review of treatment optimization strategies. *Cureus*, *17*(4). PMID: 40406780

Bikdeli, B., Khairani, C. D., Bejjani, A., Lo, Y. C., Mahajan, S., Caraballo, C., Jimenez, J. V., Krishnathasan, D., Zarghami, M., Rashedi, S., Jimenez, D., Barco, S., Secemsky, E. A., Klok, F. A., Hunsaker, A. R., Aghayev, A., Muriel, A., Hussain, M. A., Appah-Sampong, A., & Krumholz, H. M. (2025). Validating International Classification of Diseases Code 10th Revision algorithms for accurate identification of pulmonary embolism. *Journal of Thrombosis and Haemostasis*, *23*(2), 556–564. DOI: 10.1016/j.jtha.2024.10.013 PMID: 39505153

Cui, L., Liu, Y., Ouyang, C., Yu, Y., Zhang, J., Wan, Y., & Yang, F. (2026). Bailicai: A domain-optimized retrieval-augmented generation framework for medical applications. *Big Data Mining and Analytics*, *9*(2), 376–392. DOI: 10.26599/BDMA.2024.9020097

Denecke, K., May, R., & Rivera-Romero, O. (2024). Transformer models in healthcare: A survey and thematic analysis of potentials, shortcomings and risks. *Journal of Medical Systems*, *48*(1), 23. DOI: 10.1007/s10916-024-02043-5 PMID: 38367119

Ferreira, J. C., Elvas, L. B., Correia, R., & Mascarenhas, M. (2025). Tokenization of electronic health records and healthcare data: Enhancing security and privacy while enabling usability. *Health and Technology*, *15*(6), 1011–1020. DOI: 10.1007/s12553-025-01012-3

Frommeyer, T. C., Gilbert, M. M., Fursmidt, R. M., Park, Y., Khouzam, J. P., Brittain, G. V., & Bihl, T. J. (2025, July). Reinforcement learning and its clinical applications within healthcare: A systematic review of precision medicine and dynamic treatment regimes. [). MDPI.]. *Health Care*, *13*(14), 1752. PMID: 40724777

Gaber, F., Shaik, M., Allega, F., Bilecz, A. J., Busch, F., Goon, K., & Akalin, A. (2025). Evaluating large language model workflows in clinical decision support for triage and referral and diagnosis. *npj. Digital Medicine*, *8*(1), 263. PMID: 40346344

Harshavardhan, H., Shetty, S., Shetty, R. P., & Shetty, P. U. (2025). Advancements in NLP: From Rule-Based Methods to Modern Language Models. In *2025 IEEE International Conference on Electronics, Computing and Communication Technologies (CONECCT)* (pp. 1-5). IEEE. DOI: 10.1109/CONECCT65861.2025.11306594

Jadhav, N. N., & Bainalwar, P. (2026). Remote Monitoring and Telehealth Solutions for Chronic Disease Care Integration of AI in Telemedicine for Continuous Patient Monitoring and Real-Time Interventions. *Artificial Intelligence and Machine Learning in Neurology*, *2*, 811–832. DOI: 10.1002/9781394389131.ch30

Kaiser, T., & Wu, D. (2025). Fine-Tuning Pre-trained Transformer-Based Models for Sentence-Level Medical Text Classification. In *2025 IEEE International conference on Medical Artificial Intelligence (MedAI)* (pp. 58-69). IEEE. DOI: 10.1109/MedAI67139.2025.00015

Kawas, M., Alkhatib, B., Omar, K., Tofelia, K., & Dashash, M. (2025). Using Medical Named Entity Recognition in Automatic ICD Prediction. *BioMed Research International*, *2025*(1), 6117755. DOI: 10.1155/bmri/6117755 PMID: 41031257

Le, T. D., Nguyen, T. T., Ha, V. N., Chatzinotas, S., Jouvet, P., & Noumeir, R. (2025). The impact of LoRA adapters on LLMs for clinical text classification under computational and data constraints. *IEEE Access : Practical Innovations, Open Solutions*, *13*, 109365–109377. DOI: 10.1109/ACCESS.2025.3582037

Liu, Z., Gan, C., Wang, J., Zhang, Y., Bo, Z., Sun, M., & Zhang, W. (2025, April). Ontotune: Ontology-driven self-training for aligning large language models. In *Proceedings of the ACM on Web Conference 2025* (pp. 119-133). DOI: 10.1145/3696410.3714816

Luo, Y., Li, W., Chen, C., Li, X., Liu, T., Niu, T., & Yuan, Y. (2025). LLM-Guided Decoupled Probabilistic Prompt for Continual Learning in Medical Image Diagnosis. *IEEE Transactions on Medical Imaging*, *44*(8), 3439–3450. DOI: 10.1109/TMI.2025.3566105 PMID: 40310742

Ma, Y., Kolla, S., Kaliraman, D., Nolan, V., Hu, Z., Guan, Z., . . . Shickel, B. (2024). Temporal cross-attention for dynamic embedding and tokenization of multimodal electronic health records. *arXiv preprint arXiv:2403.04012*.

Ojewale, V., Suresh, H., & Venkatasubramanian, S. (2026). Audit Trails for Accountability in Large Language Models. *arXiv preprint arXiv:2601.20727*.

Palama, V. (2025). A HIPAA-aware benchmark and evaluation harness for clinical LLMs to quantify hallucination, bias, and PHI leakage. *Well Testing Journal*, *34*(S3), 830–849.

. Panagoulias, D.P., Virvou, M.K., & Tsihrintzis, G.A. (2024). Evaluating LLM - Generated Multimodal Diagnosis from Medical Images and Symptom Analysis. *ArXiv, abs/2402.01730*.

Patil, R., Heston, T. F., & Bhuse, V. (2024). Prompt engineering in healthcare. *Electronics (Basel)*, *13*(15), 2961. DOI: 10.3390/electronics13152961

Qiu, J., Lam, K., Li, G., Acharya, A., Wong, T. Y., Darzi, A., Yuan, W., & Topol, E. J. (2024). LLM-based agentic systems in medicine and healthcare. *Nature Machine Intelligence*, *6*(12), 1418–1420. DOI: 10.1038/s42256-024-00944-1

Roselló Atanet, I., Tomova, M., Sieg, M., Sehy, V., Mäder, P., & März, M. (2025). Generating learning guides for medical education with LLMs and statistical analysis of test results. *BMC Medical Education*, *25*(1), 458. DOI: 10.1186/s12909-025-06978-2 PMID: 40158187

Savage, C. H., Park, H., Kwak, K., Smith, A. D., Rothenberg, S. A., Parekh, V. S., Doo, F. X., & Yi, P. H. (2024). General-purpose large language models versus a domain-specific natural language processing tool for label extraction from chest radiograph reports. *AJR. American Journal of Roentgenology*, *222*(4), 2330573. DOI: 10.2214/AJR.23.30573 PMID: 38230901

Shool, S., Adimi, S., Amleshi, R. S., Bitaraf, E., Golpira, R., & Tara, M. (2025). A systematic review of large language model (LLM) evaluations in clinical medicine. *BMC Medical Informatics and Decision Making*, *25*(1), 25. DOI: 10.1186/s12911-025-02954-4 PMID: 40055694

Shool, S., Adimi, S., Saboori Amleshi, R., Bitaraf, E., Golpira, R., & Tara, M. (2025). A systematic review of large language model (LLM) evaluations in clinical medicine. *BMC Medical Informatics and Decision Making*, *25*(1), 117. DOI: 10.1186/s12911-025-02954-4 PMID: 40055694

Uddin, J. (2025). Conversational AI in healthcare communication: Opportunities, risks, and implications for health equity. *Journal of Communication in Healthcare*, 1–4. DOI: 10.1080/17538068.2025.2594768 PMID: 41319058

Vaswani, A., Shazeer, N., Parmar, N., Uszkoreit, J., Jones, L., Gomez, A. N., & Polosukhin, I. (2017). Attention is all you need. *Advances in Neural Information Processing Systems*, 30.

Vavekanand, R., Ali Laghari, A., & Kumar, T. (2026). Applications and limitations of large language models to integrate medical context: A comprehensive review. *Iran Journal of Computer Science*, *9*(1), 12. DOI: 10.1007/s42044-025-00360-7

Vavekanand, R., Ali Laghari, A., & Kumar, T. (2026). Applications and limitations of large language models to integrate medical context: A comprehensive review. *Iran Journal of Computer Science*, *9*(1), 12. DOI: 10.1007/s42044-025-00360-7

Vrdoljak, J., Boban, Z., Vilović, M., Kumrić, M., & Božić, J. (2025, March). A review of large language models in medical education, clinical decision support, and healthcare administration. []). MDPI.]. *Health Care*, *13*(6), 603. PMID: 40150453

Vrdoljak, J., Boban, Z., Vilović, M., Kumrić, M., & Božić, J. (2025, March). A review of large language models in medical education, clinical decision support, and healthcare administration. []). MDPI.]. *Health Care*, *13*(6), 603. PMID: 40150453

Wang, J., Shi, E., Yu, S., Wu, Z., Hu, H., Ma, C., & Zhang, S. (2025). Prompt engineering for healthcare: Methodologies and applications. *Meta-Radiology*, 100190.

Wiest, I. C., Leßmann, M. E., Wolf, F., Ferber, D., Van Treeck, M., Zhu, J., . . . Kather, J. N. (2024). Anonymizing medical documents with local, privacy preserving large language models: The LLM-Anonymizer. medRxiv, 2024-06. DOI: 10.1101/2024.06.11.24308355

Zhang, D., Feng, T., Xue, L., Wang, Y., Dong, Y., & Tang, J. (2025). Parameter-efficient fine-tuning for foundation models. *arXiv preprint arXiv:2501.13787.*

Zhou, B., Yang, G., Shi, Z., & Ma, S. (2022). Natural language processing for smart healthcare. *IEEE Reviews in Biomedical Engineering*, *17*, 4–18. DOI: 10.1109/RBME.2022.3210270 PMID: 36170385

Zhou, Y., Liu, X., Ning, C., Zhang, X., & Wu, J. (2024). Reliable and Diverse Evaluation of LLM Medical Knowledge Mastery. *International Conference on Learning Representations.*

Chapter 2

Integrating Artificial Intelligence Into Healthcare:

Ethical Imperatives, Data Bias, and the Challenges of Clinical Implementation

Shubhangi Bajaj Bag
http://orcid.org/0009-0003-0274-2251
Amity University, Kolkata, India

Aayushi Goel
http://orcid.org/0000-0002-0561-8059
Symbiosis Law School, Symbiosis International (Deemed to be) University, Pune, India

Prashant Rahangdale
Symbiosis Law School, Symbiosis International (Deemed to be) University, Pune, India

Ekta Yadav
IILM University, Gurugram, India

ABSTRACT

Artificial Intelligence (AI) has become a groundbreaking technology in the field of medicine during the last decade, and the opportunities this specific area of application remain substantial as ANI may be used to automate the process of diagnosis, treatment, and disease prognosis. This paper explores the ethical issues surrounding

DOI: 10.4018/979-8-2600-2173-6.ch002

the application of AI as a decision- support system in medical diagnostics. Based on a qualitative research approach, the study aims to combine both the academic and semi-structured interviews with eight major healthcare stakeholders such as physicians, researchers, and IT specialists. The results indicate that the institutional approval of the AI integration is high; nevertheless, they also demonstrate several severe ethical contradictions that need to be resolved.

INTRODUCTION

With AI, the last ten years have established a paradigm shift in the clinical environment: it is not a hypothetical future anymore, but an effective tool that can be used to automate disease diagnosis, treatment, and prognosis (Xu et al., 2023). This technological innovation is not just an upgrade, but it marks a revolution in the field of medicine and suggests an opportunity to conduct intelligent decision support in screening patients, cancer therapeutic treatment, managing clinical trials, and developing a drug (Xu et al., 2023). Essentially, AI is a general concept that implies machines can reproduce human mental processes to re-create some complicated thoughts and acts (Hamet & Tremblay, 2017; Humerick, 2018). It is multidisciplinary and is applicable in robotics as well as in medical statistics and human biology, being able to combine the strength of the computer with the power of clinical intuition (Hamet & Tremblay, 2017). Medical AI is divided into two worlds, the virtual and the physical ones. The virtual branch applies the idea of deep learning informatics to operate, supervise health systems, oversee the electronic medical records, and include active advice to clinicians in treatment choices. On the other hand, the physical branch is defined using robotics to support the work of surgeons and aged individuals, as well as innovative nanorobots to deliver drugs (Hamet & Tremblay, 2017).

There is also a desire to handle large volumes of data extremely fast, which also forces the acceptance of AI into healthcare (Gupta & Kumar, 2023). This is not limited to protocol development, disease prevention, and real-time patient monitoring, where AI-based decision support has already proven significantly more effective than conventional approaches in frequencies of skin cancer detection and post-operative patient mortality (Gupta & Kumar, 2023). Nevertheless, the implementation of AI has been a complex process, regardless of these innovations, which is predetermined by the peculiarities of the healthcare industry. Despite AI having the ability to supplement human knowledge and improve the engagement between patients and healthcare providers, to implement it as a part of the trend, the collaboration between data scientists and experts in the medical sphere (radiologists) will be required on a fundamental level in the context of ensuring safety and efficiency (Carter et al., 2020; Le et al., 2019; Davenport and Kalakota, 2019). It is the growth-driven patent portfolio analysis that provides decision-makers with the experience they can see and feel how medical tech and diagnostics innovations are justified by the money (Zhang and Ming, 2023). Beyond the mechanical use, technology has some sort of influence on human perception and behavior. Like automobiles and telecommunication that qualitatively changed the geographical and social area, medical equipment fundamentally changes the mode of diagnosis and treatment (Verbeek, 2011). It is thus important to note that these tools have moral aspect; they are not inert tools but rather actors that affect the day-to-day practice in clinical practice and competition of values (Verbeek, 2011). We are of opinion that the objectives might have been made more specific. We now have made some adjustments to the last paragraph of the Introduction to reflect on the exact research problem and objectives that are going to direct this study.

LITERATURE REVIEW

Medical Diagnostics

Combination of machine learning and AI have also basically streamlined the decision-making within various fields and medical diagnostics have occupied the central place of enjoying the efficiencies. In medicine, medication can be used to reduce symptoms or cure underlying pathology, whereas diagnostics is the most important mechanism in determining a particular physiological condition or health impairment (Riis Hansen et al., 2022). The practicality of modern technology is great when specialists can make diagnostic conclusions based on synthesis of patient medical history through modern technology. When the diagnoses are correct, smart decision-support systems can make it possible to plan and implement specific medical interventions of patients with high precision. One of the most efficient approaches is the use of historical medication data to provide standardized diagnosis codes, namely, using machine learning models that are trained on general medical data (Riis Hansen et al., 2022). Although all automated diagnostic assignment systems are evident to be beneficial in clinical environments, the complexity of coding medical patient data is an issue that can be difficult to overcome (Riis Hansen et al., 2022). In particular, the difference in the quality of coding is common and it may lead to misunderstanding of medication profiles and therefore wrong diagnosis. As a result, strict accuracy of coding is a requirement leading to the highest functioning and effectiveness of such sophisticated diagnostic devices (Riis Hansen et al., 2022).

AI in Healthcare

Medical profession still has fundamental experiential basis, which is based on the passage of knowledge and skills through practice and clinical study. The common diagnosis procedure is a comparative analysis, in which a clinician compares the presenting symptoms of a patient to some internalized collection of pathological understanding and treatment history (Stone et al., 2022). Although practitioners continually improve their knowledge through the sheer number of patients and their interactions with the academic community, they are still limited through cognitive processes of data analysis and the number of clinical interactions they can have during a career. Conversely, AI can handle and analyse large volumes of information faster and more efficiently than the human brain is. These systems can be highlighted in that they can be used as the decision support mechanisms, both promoting productivity and clinical quality, and at the same time reducing the probability of errors in making diagnostic or therapeutic determinations. In the healthcare system, such decision-support systems are mostly concentrated in medication management, which enjoys extremely organized and centralized pharmaceutical data (Vinniva, 2018).

Existing study projects are actively increasing the presence of AI-based assistance in Sweden. As an example, one of the most prominent projects being carried out at Karolinska University Hospital applies deep learning algorithms to produce mammography images using clinical data, thus, detecting patients with a high-risk profile of malignancy (Vinnova, 2018). These health information systems are fundamental to a contemporary medicine where they help to enable the discovery of knowledge, automation, and advanced information acquisition (Peixoto et al., 2020). These systems can produce high-quality intuition using sophisticated analysis algorithms, which enhance the quality of the diagnosis made and simplify the process of decision-making of medical staff. Such intervention is of utmost importance in acute care units like the intensive care units. Such environments have numerous cases of clinical uncertainty and a large quantity of data produced by the differences in medical records and monitoring units will demand the intensive processing resources only available with AI (Peixoto et al., 2020).

The Importance of Ethics

Ethics basically involves choices of courses of life, ethical considerations and what is considered the good or what is the right course of action. Moralizing according to philosopher Claes Gustafsson is an archetypal human phenomenon; we continually assess the behavior of others in relation to moral behaviors. This framework is a critical pathfinder whenever making decisions, whose primary purpose is to foresee negative realities. Nevertheless, developing strong ethical thinking is not an individual pursuit but an operation that needs communal thinking and group discussion. In the medical field, such ethical frameworks have been progressively modified alongside the changes in the legal environment, but it should be said that health care laws are regionally bound (Varkey, 2020). Making a decision is the fundamental task of the doctor and it is controlled by an ethical requirement of promoting patient health, reducing harm, and preserving personal values (Varkey, 2020). The study of morality cannot therefore be done without clinical medicine. Some global norms, like the ban on killing, defense of the innocent, or the obligation to tell the truth are universal (Varkey, 2020). Though society gives the physicians the role, which is founded on trust and specialized knowledge, there is a tension that is inherent: the set professional standards are not always entirely in line with the overall moral expectations and can, in some cases, serve the interests of the medical field rather than that of the patient or even the population at large (Varkey, 2020).

Four core values, including beneficence, non-maleficence, autonomy, and justice, are the crucial instruments of navigation in healthcare (Varkey, 2020). Beneficence requires the practitioner to only do what is beneficial to the patient as a type of professional altruism. The principle of non-maleficence places the obligation of not causing harm as it means that clinical practices are not harmful to suffering. Autonomy implies that patients have adequate information to make self-determination, whereas justice implies the equal allocation of medical resources and equitable treatment in all patients (Varkey, 2020). The modern environment is marked by the development of AI-based decision-support tools that optimize these clinical decisions, and in most cases, show a level of predictability that is even greater than the professional one (Eisbach et al., 2023). Despite the clinically advanced developments made based on automated systems, deep-rooted issues still emerge in the sphere of legislatures and in the field of ethics when the information created by the algorithm has a direct impact on human beings. One of the main issues is the so-called issue of liability when it doubts the assignation of accountability when some mistakes or harm to the patient occur due to the use of intelligent decision-support systems (Varkey, 2020). There is still much uncertainty on which individuals will be morally and legally blameworthy when a system becomes too complex to be understood by a human being. This cooperation between humans and AI presents some additional complexity, including the concepts of underuse or overconfidence, which are related to the poor knowledge of predictive modeling.

As a result, they need to develop the so-called optimally adjusted trust, a thin line between functional dependency and suspicion (Eisbach et al., 2023). The fact that these systems are black boxes, which is also a complication, may compromise the treatment process and patients themselves (Zsidai et al., 2023). When a system is a black box, in that it is a device that produces conclusions without revealing its inner logic, then it is hard to give anything meaningful to the patients. Such a deficiency of transparency creates the possibility of a discrepancy between patient judgment and clinical advice thus deterrent to systemic trust building. This can be overcome through a strict element of risk-benefit analysis, usability, and technical interventions that would make algorithmic procedures more readable (Pedreschi et al., 2019). Major ethical challenges that practitioners encounter in medical settings involve incorrect decision-support system recommendations or hallucinations in highly specific medical settings. Such a system is painful to clinicians because complex calculations are difficult to understand to detect the existence of latent errors when a system represents the presence of a serious, asymptomatic pathology (Bertl et al., 2022). These situations compel doctors to maneuver themselves through complex ethical issues to decipher the logic in the system. Finally, the necessity to advance healthcare with the help of AI should be weighed against the basic ethical principles. It therefore calls on the need to develop effective ethical standards and regulatory measures that can make technology responsible and sustainable. Respect to patient autonomy, keeping integrity, and ensuring fairness are the three main principles that should be used in the development and deployment of medical AI (Castonguay et al., 2024). Even though the future of AI in technology in such a direction as the diagnostic sphere is well-documented in the current literature, and general principles of ethics (beneficence, non-maleficence and justice) are established, on-the-ground obstacles to actually deploying said systems into clinical practice are essential. This research gap addressed in this paper explores the ways medical stakeholders constructively negotiate the compromise between the efficiency of algorithms and ethical considerations, namely, transparency. The black box effect as well as the responsibility to assign liability in real-life medical situations.

Recent research highlights the importance of considering these ethical dilemmas in terms of going beyond theoretical frameworks to the implementation of practical and on-going mitigation measures. As an example, algorithmic bias alleviation is not a single algorithm but a life-long systematic auditing of training data and algorithms (Hasanzadeh et al., 2025). Moreover, the researchers speak of the urgent necessity to actively minimize the automation bias, i.e. clinicians can unconsciously rely on the assistance of automated solutions, by introducing organized risk evaluation (Abdelwanis et al., 2024). To guarantee that these technologies are safely and fairly incorporated into clinical workflows and do not contribute to the already existing disparities, it is necessary to establish clear, practical guidelines and protocols (Sun & Harris, 2024).

THEORETICAL FRAMEWORK

Technology Acceptance Model (TAM)

The use of the Technology Acceptance Model (TAM), initially theorized by Fred D. Davis would offer a sound theoretical framework on how to conduct analysis on the adoption of new technologies by the clinical setting. Technological systems which are specifically designed to provide certain responses to cognitive processing of practitioners are uniquely designed in the context of medical diagnostics. These reactions are mostly dictated by two determinant factors, i.e., perceived usefulness and perceived ease of use (Charness & Boot, 2016). These cognitive evaluations are synthesized to define the attitude of the user, which in turn determines his or her behavioral intention, that is the actual decision of adopting or rejecting the technological system. Although the TAM has received scholarly critiques, it is a key theoretical tool that can forecast the adoption of technology, especially in a diverse demographic population, including older adults (Charness & Boot, 2016). Through this model, one can work to close the gap between the technical design and subjective user experience, and make sure that the creation of AI-driven tools will not be incompatible with practical requirements of the medical professionals. The model is used as the main prism of the usability of AI, which is considered with regards to the ethical aspects and clinical decision support. The framework guides the qualitative inquiry formulation to have a more subtle perception of these dynamics as semi-structured interviews with the parties to the healthcare scenario. Figure 1 shows the TAM model. The goal will be to employ the main principles of the TAM to develop questions that investigate the perceived usefulness and availability of AI in diagnostics. This paradigm will permit conducting a thorough study of how medical providers are open to the adoption of intelligent systems and thus identify the key factors that enable or inhibit the effective adoption of AI in the healthcare industry.

Figure 1. The basic TAM (Rahimi et al., 2018)

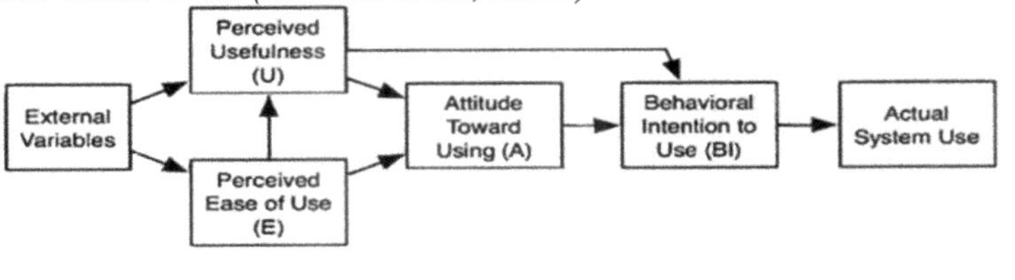

The Acceptance Model in a Healthcare Setting

TAM describes the concept of acceptance as the behavioral disposition or the mental readiness of an individual to use a particular technological innovation (Ward, 2013). Although it is considered a basic one, the use of this model in the practical context of the clinical field requires a complex adjustment of the model that takes into consideration the complexity of the sector. Unlike general systems, medical technologies are to be considered in terms of the sociotechnical approach that involves professional support, high-level training, and the integrity of the working process (Rahimi et al., 2018). Moreover, the adaptation of technology by the healthcare practitioners is largely dampened by organizational structures, culture, and individual emotional reactions (Ward, 2013). The results of empirical studies into the attitude of nursing personnel demonstrate that the perception of usability and ease of use are primary factors in defining intention to utilize healthcare information system (Pai & Huang, 2011). Likewise, studies involving physician opinion indicate that although TAM is the tool that can be used as a predictor it should be refined to make it more contextual to medical practice. The next petitions of academically based research ought to be thus focused on the mapping of clinician perceptions so that the model could mirror the particularities of the healthcare environment (Holden & Karsh, 2010). The acceptance of these technologies will continue to depend on the high rates of usability, the strong support in terms of technological aspects, and integration with existing clinical systems (Nguyen et al., 2020).

Information and communication technology (ICT) practices being transferred to healthcare organizations are often met with strong opposition, which requires an active adjustment of the TAM framework to adhere to the changing medical environments (Rahimi et al., 2018). This paper uses the model to discuss the analysis of qualitative interview data and investigates the change in medical practice and the ethical demands needed to implement AI to uphold ethical standards in this area. The emphasis is made on the fact that perceived usefulness and ease of use are direct determinants of AI-based decision support adoption, and, critical variables, including systemic trust and risk assessment, are incorporated. With the rate of AI expansion, ethical concerns become more urgent and affect user behavior and attitudes towards their work to a great extent (Gonçalves et al., 2023). These ethical dimensions should become an urgent need to be included in the study of technology acceptance. With the consideration necessarily added to the standard TAM model, it will be possible to examine the extent to which ethical judgment and belief of a practitioner in the technology can mediate their understanding of how useful the technology will ultimately become and how effortlessly it would operate. Although the four principles of medical ethics (beneficence, non-maleficence, autonomy, justice), are employed to contextualize the moral imperatives, TAM is directly used to examine the issues of acceptance and integration among the practitioners.

METHODOLOGY

Academic rigor dictates the qualitative methodological approach, namely, the employment of a case study as the means of interpreting complex meanings and analyzing human experiences along the systematic framework (Bourgeault et al., 2010). Primary data collection revolves around the qualitative research strategies that focus on the need to gather deep information that is obtained through direct observation, as well as semi-structured conversation (Oates et al., 2023). This type of methodology is the only one that best explains what the main ethical dilemmas of AI in the medical field are, which will enable us to compare the views of practitioners with the already existing scientific literature. Since the issues surrounding the integration of AI into the clinical setting have far-reaching ramifications, a fine-tuning sense of the difficulties that individuals in the healthcare industry encounter are necessary in the determination of systemic barriers that accompany the creation of intelligent decision-support. To move across the complex ethical reality of medical diagnostics, semi-structured interviews become the main tool of data collection. This style offers an overview of predetermined questions and the ability to move beyond them into an unprogrammed continuation, thus allowing the respondents to enlarge their thinking and provide a more detailed description of what happened to them in their professional life (Bryman & Bell, 2011; Bourgeault et al., 2010). Semi-structured approach is based on an exploratory conversation with participants unlike more rigid and structured formats because the sequence of themes may be adjusted to the flow of discourse, and rather subtle topics may be discussed in detail (Clark et al., 2021; Oates, 2023; Denscombe, 2018). This methodological laxity is especially important in instances where respondents are faced with issues of clinical or technical ambiguity because it enables the respondent to turn to the more familiar area of expertise yet still contributes to the overall range of views that must be gathered to enable good analysis. The participants were chosen based on the consideration of those who are currently active in the hospital system, both the public and the private sphere. Although given that professional qualification became a secondary approach, the prerequisite to be included was the demonstrative knowledge of clinical decision support, radiology, medical diagnostics, or strategic implementation of AI in healthcare. The study guarantees that practical experience of the deployment of intelligent systems is prioritized and as a result, used to determine the real need and challenges of the healthcare workforce as the data obtained will be genuine. This school of thought is central to creating a credible account of the existing technological change in the medical field. Table 1 shows the respondents who participated in the study.

Table 1. Summary of respondents

Respondent	Professional Role	Private/Public Sector	Interview Duration
Respondent A	AI Specialist in Medical Diagnostics	Private	45 minutes
Respondent B	Researcher in Digitalization & AI in Healthcare	Public	42 minutes
Respondent C	Researcher in Digitalization & AI in Healthcare	Public	36 minutes
Respondent D	Physician – involved in R&D of diagnostic techniques/tools	Public	28 minutes
Respondent E	Technical Expert in Healthcare Technology	Private	48 minutes
Respondent F	Researcher in AI Technology for Medical Diagnostics	Private	39 minutes
Respondent G	Physician – expertise in Radiology	Public	32 minutes
Respondent H	IT Specialist in Healthcare	Public	47 minutes

The study assumes rigor of methodology based on a qualitative framework, through which semi-structured interviews will be conducted to earn subtle insights on the side of healthcare professionals. The interview guide was formulated based on the principles of Deniscombe (2018) and allowed adhering to the flow of themes and at the same time provide enough flexibility to discuss any emergent knowledge. The investigation started with the general contextual based open-ended questions and then transitioned into explicit applications of the TAM which is based on the use of AI and the ethical and epistemological issues related to it. The resultant data will give that granular insight into professional attitude towards technological adoption to the clinical sphere. Purposive sampling was employed in the recruitment process, which was triggered by formal electronic communication with the study objectives, the right to be anonymous, and participation as voluntary (Oates, 2023). Another phenomenon was that of snowballing an effect where one initial respondent assisted in opening to a wider professional network and this promoted the effectiveness of the search. Interviews were revealed through digital platforms (via Zoom and Google meet) to allow the timetable of the clinicians (lasting 25 to 50 minutes). To preserve data integrity, the audio recordings were videotaped with direct permission, which allowed engaging in verbatim communication and reflecting on it subsequently and reducing the possibility of missing important information.

To have a more critical review, the transcription phase included the transformation of the oral discourse into written text (Denscombe, 2018). There was a complied edited transcription approach where disfluencies and noise sounds were removed to make the communication more accurate without affecting the initial meaning or situation. The transcription was initiated immediately after every session to ensure that the record remained accurate. This made it possible to identify important themes in real-time and facilitated an iterative process of the inquiry. Thematic method of data analysis was conducted subsequently to make sense of the huge amount of textual data received. The first round of coding was used to pick the pertinent sections, e.g., Data privacy concerns, User acceptance of AI, etc. The synthesis of these sections was conducted to produce major themes. As an example, the codes on accountability and transparency fell under the title: Ethical dilemma and accountability in AI to help in medical diagnosis. These themes were subsequently analyzed in relation to the existing theoretical frameworks to analyze whether the results support or refute the currently existing scholarly literature or not. The research used must be scholarly and valid and reliable. Internal validity was sought through a match between the interview questions and the theoretical themes that were set to be explored, whereas the external validity or transferability considered the relevance of these results in the greater context of the healthcare sector. Even though technological advancement is mostly homogeneous, it is agreed that various departments might be at different levels of implementation. Digital flexibility of respondents enhances reliability by removing environmental stress and facilitating natural responses.

Three overarching principles are needed when respecting the ethics of research, including the right to privacy, informed consent, and the need to be faithfully represented. Informed consent was obtained using written agreements and by verbal confirmation where the participants were in full knowledge of the purpose of the study. Anonymized identifiers and immediate deletion of audio files after the process of transcription served to provide privacy. Moreover, the necessity of proper reproducing means that information is shown in as full and unbiased a form as possible, which will be met by careful transcription and instant post-interview notation. There are certain strengths and significant weaknesses associated with the methodology as exposed in a critical review. The first limitation is that the sample size is quite small, which limits the external validity of the study and the applicability of its findings (Jacobsen, 2017). Moreover, as efficient, digital interviewing can be a lot more one-sided than face-to-face interaction. Nevertheless, the semi-structured interviews used contributed to a high level of internal validity due to the possibility of discussing the topic in depth and flexibly. Future studies will need to consider a mixed-methodology study and a bigger sample of respondents to further develop the knowledge of AI adoption in healthcare facilities.

Although the sample size (eight people) is quite limited, it is acceptable and typical when the study is based on a qualitative case study with a high level of specialization of specialists. Since the purposive sample included people with direct experience in the strategic implementation of AI, clinical research, and medical diagnostics, interviews provided deep, granular information. This enabled the study to attain adequate thematic richness and content saturation to effectively map the fundamental ethical and practical dimensions of AI integration, by placing greater emphasis on the quality and usefulness of the data, rather than statistical generalization.

RESULTS

The analysis below was based on transcribed and coded data of the interviews through which thematic patterns were identified to support or dispel the available literature. In accordance with the methodology of sorting and argumentation, which was presented by (Bourgeault et al., 2010), critical elements of the respondent testimony were chosen to respond to the key questions of the research. In this process, preservation of integrity of the respondents was paramount, respondents were well informed on their rights and their identities as far as their institutional affiliations were considered to be anonymous. To uphold the rigour and consistency of the analysis, the analysis will incorporate scholarly excerpts to enable it to lead to the analysis of the raw empirical information to theoretical interpretation.

Progress and Challenges of AI in Medical Diagnostics: A Multifaceted Survey

The impact of technology can be felt in all spheres of modern life, however, the AI in medical diagnostics should not be viewed as the tool that is neutral. In line with the discussion found by Peter-Paul Verbeek regarding the ethical aspect of technology, AI is regarded as an agent that actively influences the process of clinical decision and human behavior. The review of the respondents reveals that despite the possibility of AI providing fast and accurate diagnostic outcomes with the assistance of the processing of medical images, its use presupposes when an ethical system is developed. This framework should deal with data security, just sharing of the health facility resources, and maintenance of human skills during the growth of automations. The use of AI in practice has a great range of variations in terms of socioeconomic settings. According to Respondent B and his associates, *"by making the use of digital microscopes in hospitals in isolated locations standard, and through AI to preview the sample and facilitate the work of doctors, we can access a larger population of people. We have produced some microscope prototypes using other mobile industry components to save money. Also, we have trained several AI algorithms to detect several diseases in the digital specimen."* Nonetheless, Respondent C remarks that systemic issues such as a drastic lack of pathologists and the cost-prohibitive nature of laboratory facilities usually stand in the way of these solutions successfully being implemented. Nevertheless, with these obstacles, it is proposed that a possible direction toward lowering costs and training algorithms that detect pathologies in digital samples is achieved through the development of prototypes using the mobile-industry components. Moreover, the secondary gain of the high-income countries is the alleviation of professional burdens, as well as the delay in diagnoses, which is shortened by such innovations.

Having a common set of guidelines that will be adopted by various stakeholders is a widespread agreement on the need for standardized frameworks to enable the exchange of data on a regional system and ensure that AI is integrated consistently. The general popularity of such projects can be explained, in part, by the fact that the whole nature of algorithmic processing is the ability to operate tirelessly and be biased by feelings, the factors that, traditionally, affect human decision-making. Respondent E emphasizes that such initiatives can be successful only when multi-disciplinary teams are gathered to make sure that intelligent decision support will help to minimize the manual data gathering and equalize data analysis on patients. Considering the clinical value of those tools, Respondent A sees the predictive capability of AI as an important resource to manage the health of the population, as seen in the Covid-19 pandemic. In the professional sphere of radiology, Respondent G affirms the growth of AI applications that intend to improve the work process and diagnostic accuracy. However, a certain level of hesitation can also be outlined here, where Respondent F and H doubt the ability of AI to act without the radiologists whereas Respondent E proposes complete validation and testing before it can be used in the scale. This is a poignant individual to weigh the technological opportunity with the technical and ethical limitations of the healthcare sector especially in terms of user acceptance and responsible management of decision-support systems.

The Way Forward for AI In Medical Diagnostics

AI is a complex, cross-functional field, which has integrated the effort of computer science, philosophy, psychology, and mathematics. In these areas, different dimensions are pursued: computer science is aimed at building computational units that can act intelligently, and philosophy asks the question of the nature of intelligent behavior concerning mechanical systems (Dignum, 2019). Also, psychology allows understanding the interaction between a human and a system, and mathematical relations and engineering offer the necessary systems of algorithms and their implementation (Dignum, 2019). There is empirical data in the form of surveys of stakeholders; it has been shown on a continuum of views about the role of AI in medical diagnostics. Following the TAM construct of perceived usefulness, Respondent E categorically believes in the usefulness of the technology as long as there is strict implementation and subsequent extensive tests done on the practice.. On the contrary, Respondent F assumes that the overall effect of AI on radiologic performance is yet to be fully clarified, and the substantial developmental milestones must be achieved, before tangible positive results are achieved.

As far as the operational effect on the field of radiology is concerned, one can observe that Respondents A, B, C, and F agree on the point that AI can become more effective in clinical work and make it simpler to conduct complex medical tests with the help of it. AI can reduce the inter-observer variation in healthcare by acting as a powerful decision support instrument or as a second opinion of diagnosis, which facilitates healthcare delivery. Nevertheless, the latest technological versions are not placed to essentially scare away human skills, as Respondent A comments. Constant professionalization is mandatory to maximize workflow integration. In line with the TAM framework, Respondents G and H emphasize that a key factor of successful integration is perceived ease of use: AI must be used as a problem-solving tool, which will not introduce an extra mental burden to the medical professional. Although overall positive attitude to healthcare AI is voiced by Respondents G, H, and E, there are still serious technical and systemic issues. Respondent E emphasizes the frustration of developing specialized tools that take long and clinical risks of false-positive outcomes. In the end, the effective implementation of such technologies will be based on the proper regulation of the social aspect and the establishment of the favorable institutional environment. Leaders of feedback loops that help improve the process repeatedly are perceived to exert a critical effect on the sustainability of AI tools in the long run. Altogether, these observations have created a subtle image of AI in the diagnostics field, between the technological advance and the need to overcome the long-standing ethical and practical challenges to have a sustainable version of healthcare integration.

Ethical Challenges and Division of Responsibilities in AI For Medical Diagnostics

AI, being multidisciplinary, requires holistic approach to understand how intelligence and technology meet to reconfigure society. The deeper the functionality of these systems resembles the human cognitive process, the greater the ethical issues, most of which concern the question of responsibility, require a strict solution (Dignum, 2019). Based on the clinical practice experience, the introduction of AI into medical diagnostics is accompanied by intense ethical concerns, with the threat of algorithmic bias being the key one. This kind of bias takes place when training data and algorithm designs choose one type of decision-making over the other, which may lead to unfair treatment of patients. Therefore, defining the area of strict separation of labor and responsibility between human actors and automatic machines is a highly urgent task. The main obstacle that prevents successful integration of these technologies is the gap of transparency. As stated by Respondent C, minimal knowledge about the functionality of AI between users tends to develop uncertainty and systemic distrust. Respondent D goes on to state further that an answer to this skepticism would be drastic receptiveness to the specific problem-solving abilities of the technology. To reduce these anxieties, the institutional systems will be required to engage in a candid debate and avail an all-inclusive access to information to ensure that clinicians have a sensible view of the gains as well as the inherent constraints of the program.

The issue of legal and moral responsibility is a critical issue. In as much as the physician who authorizes a diagnosis is the main party of responsibility, there is an inertia that developers, system administrators and institutional players have a joint responsibility about the ethical operation of the AI system. Aiming to ensure representational integrity and overcome bias, Respondents A and F suggest implementing proactive measures, such as the routine audit of datasets and algorithms, and greater openness of automated decision-making procedures. The safety of patients is a controversial question of the professional population. According to some stakeholders, AI is an opportunity that can be used to improve medical care; however, other stakeholders are concerned about the quality of data and the possibility of technological gaps becoming a factor that undermines patient health. This would require a set of constant reviews to track the effect of AI on safety measures and reduce clinical risks. Nonetheless, Respondent B, E and H have hope that trust will grow longitudinally as the users become more experienced and change of heart occurs. After all, the shift to ethical and sustainable healthcare AI relies on the inclusion of ethical concerns at all developmental phases and a permanently enduring cooperation of researchers, clinicians, and tech giving out solutions.

Sharing Experiences and Collaboration: Keys to Successful AI Implementation

The effective application of AI requires a multi-disciplinary combination of expertise, since the field is too complex to be viewed without knowledge in machine learning, natural language processing, pattern recognition, and expert systems (Dignum, 2019). What is necessary to appreciate is the fact that these systems are not only becoming more sophisticated in terms of computational intelligence, but their associated flaws and limitations. It therefore follows that an effective implementation plan demands strong investment towards longitudinal training in the fields of computer science, philosophy and medicine to see to it that such technologies are implemented effectively as well as in an ethically responsible manner. According to empirical data of the interviews conducted with the stakeholders, there are critical ethical tensions, namely, the risk of algorithmic bias that proliferated. It is a phenomenon where the choice of training datasets may affect clinical decision making and instigate the advent of unfair patient outcomes. This has brought about the need to come up with clear guidelines that will outline the scope of responsibility between human actors and automated agents. Respondent C notes that there are enormous differences in the number of specialists who are technologically literate, which indicates that although some small number of experts can fully master the knowledge, the general clinical population needs more educational assistance to address the ethical risk and the complexity of working with AI.

The present participation is not that coverage; although as Respondent B notes, academic conferences and workshops are available, there are no mandatory institutional expectations of mastering AI. Development of understanding may take place in the laboratory setting or clinical practice as explained by many practitioners like Respondents D and G in which learning-by-doing may develop. Respondent G describes this process as parallel to the establishment of a professional connection with a cohort- a process of probing at systematic strong and weak areas. On the other hand, Respondents E and H would oppose compulsory technical training of radiologists stating that much attention paid to the technological background may divert the major clinical responsibilities. Finally, successful implementation of AI depends on the creation of professional comfort and the increase of the overall educational level to be more observed in terms of the practical issues detection and correction. Although the overall attitude of the healthcare professional community is favorable, with references to the greater accuracy of diagnosis and the decrease in workloads, it is mixed with omnipresent concerns about the issue of liability, biases, and patient safety. To maintain the user trust, it is also necessary to ensure that ethical considerations are not included as auxiliary, but they are part of the very lifecycle of AI development and implementation to be provided through the continuous interdisciplinary effort.

ANALYSIS

AI (AI) has become a disruptive component of the medical sphere in the last ten years, namely, its ability to automatize and optimize the diagnostic process (Xu et al., 2023). Focusing on stakeholder discourse, AI is not a technical fix to the clinical dilemma, but it, on one hand, triggers a systemic change making it an obligatory aspect to consider a strategy of sustainable integration. One option would be the incorporation of mobile microscopy which can be combined with cloud-based AI because it offers a paradigm shift of more sophisticated diagnostics that can be more accessible and affordable. But the fulfillment of this potential is often hindered by the fact that there is often great shortage of pathologists, and the cost of laboratory infrastructure is prohibitive. The complex solution comprises the development of low-cost AI models and the implementation of efficient training programs that will help to raise the technical level of medical workers is needed to overcome these obstacles. In addition, public-private associations are crucial in terms of achieving the necessary funding of innovation. To make AI an effective part of the overall global health, technology developers, clinicians, and policymakers should come together to make sure that such solutions are affordable and on a global scale, especially in those that have lower access to quality services. Among the major stipulations of the ethical execution of these systems is the fact that there must be a critical balance between the achievements of its algorithms and human control. Although AI can be considered a great element of diagnostic accuracy and efficacy of criticism, it is important to consider it a support mechanism, not an alternative to the experience of a human being (Xu et al., 2023). These distinctions play a vital role in the continuation of a person-centered, emphatic clinical support. The balance between AI and human intervention, according to both Varkey (2020) and Xu et al. (2023) is of the utmost importance.

The most significant factor which affects the well-being of the patients is the proper prevailing of human intuition and machine processing. The use of AI in diagnostics simplifies the process of identifying a disease at an earlier stage and offers unprecedented possibilities of individual medicine based on patient characteristics. By good juggernauting along these technical and ethical borderlands, the medical fraternity can maximize with the technology without letting it run amok into the hands of unscrupulous knowledge and medical negligence. The strategic partnership surrounding the field of AI will prove highly beneficial to the enhancement of patient outcomes as well as alleviating the economic and physical strain that today's healthcare systems are put under. However, a rigid trade-off of the clinical opinion of a human and the algorithmic treatment is without compromise. This balance is not only the motif of functional effectiveness in the field of diagnostics and treatment, but also the primary element of the conservation of the whole, patient-centered care. In order to preserve this synergy, it is essential to create all-inclusive guidelines, i.e. specific training, standardized practice and solid ethical framework. Applying to the empirical evidence given by the stakeholders, the introduction of AI poses a serious technical and ethical challenge, as it may result in possible data breaches, not to mention the intrinsic complexity of decoding the convoluted algorithmic decision making. This type of risk requires the establishment of strong security measures and increased degree of transparency to protect the well-being and privacy of the patients. Since Respondent E notes, although AI has the potential to revolutionize medical practice to some extent by decreasing professional workload and enhancing access to care, it also adds additional layers of complexity to the practice. Dualism requires a paradigm shift in the modern model of healthcare delivery.

Therefore, the integration of effective security measures that guarantee management of data is compulsory within the dynamism of legal and ethical laws in the present era. Moreover, the methodologies should be created in such a way that AI decision-making process could be explained to clinicians and patients. That would include the strict testing of the systems to identify algorithmic biases or mistakes and the lifelong learning of medical personnel on how to interpret the results of AI. The consideration of the ethical dimension is an essential part rather than a biased element as it has a direct impact on the integrity of the patient-clinician relationship as often supported by Castonguay et al. (2024). The implementation of the TAM demonstrates the excessive intricacy and volatility of implementing AI into the clinical setting. Although the traditional determinants of perceived usefulness and the ease of use are crucial elements in institutional acceptance, the introduction of ethical aspects like trust, integrity, and accountability is the final determinant of the acceptance of these technologies among the practitioners. These ethical dilemmas will keep growing as AI keeps on a state of omnipresence in the medical industry as Gonçalves et al. (2023) point out. The use of the TAM in the medical field requires a complex restructuring to fit the complex socio-technical systems of healthcare. It will be clear that the conventional model will have to be extended to include institutional support, intense pedagogical training, and smooth consideration into the well-established clinical processes. This is justified by the role played by scholars such as Pai & Huang (2011) and Holden and Karsh (2010), who both suggest that to stay within the context of the healthcare setting, this model should be carefully adjusted to its particulars. This broadened approach to heuristics can be used to gain a better insight into the consistently disparate reaction that present themselves within healthcare professionals when dealing with technological innovation.

In-depth interviews can be used to understand the perceptions of AI in a substantial degree of heterogeneity. The most important factors when determining adoption are the perceived utility and ease of use, but organizational, cultural, and emotional factors have a significant impact on the process of acceptance. Respondents G and H show that they firmly believe in AI because it can maximize the efficiency of the workflow; however, Respondent E says that he is rather doubtful about the effect that AI has on clinical performance and cognitive workload. Such results imply that technology acceptance is doubling an interpersonal and institutional process as it is the technical functionality. Moreover, the thematic analysis can reveal that it is an absolute need, that some form of technological implementations shall be carried out that will comply with the professional and personal ethics of the end-user. It requires consistent communication between software developers, clinicians, and ethical consultants to make sure that AI implementation is responsible and effective. A mastery of technical aspects and ethics are dual in terms of the impact of AI to manage the latter. According to the empirical data, the different levels of acceptability of the staff will require a customized strategy of adoption, which is sensitive to the specifics of the needs of the specific clinical setting. The pillars of beneficence, non-maleficence, autonomy, and justice, which are the fundamental ethical principles of this study, are backed by Varkey (2020). These concepts give the much-needed outline on which to assess the transforming roles of the physician during the era of algorithmic decision-support. One of the major ethical dilemmas is the liability attribution. Since the decisions made by AI can become too complex and humankind can possibly not understand them anymore, strict areas of jurisdiction need to be formulated to explain the boundaries between the contributions of machines and human beings. In line with that, the articles by Eisbach et al. (2023) and Zsidai et al. (2023) note that the most significant interventions to prevent professional skepticism and ensure the integrity of the patient-clinician relationship are transparency and user education. Assigning legal and moral responsibility to algorithmic decision-making is a very tricky requirement.

Even though the responsibility of diagnosis approval in the system is mainly issued by the attending physician, it is becoming more apparent that the liability lies jointly in the hands of the various actors in the system lifecycle. Constant monitoring and active correction of the bias is necessary to prevent inequality of care, as the choice of training data and architecture peculiar to any specific algorithm are likely to accidentally cause discriminatory clinical results (A & F). Enhancement of systemic trust depends on this moral vigilance, as practitioners will become more experienced and knowledgeable, this trust in the reliability of the technology will grow. The ideological division in the professional language of AI in radiology is quite noticeable. On the one hand, there is a reserved mistrust which is also shown by the example of Respondents E and H who are against the implementation of mandatory training on technical aspects because they believe that it can reduce the focus on clinical responsibilities. In his turn, Respondent A claims that the only possible way towards the successful and responsible use of these tools is thorough education. The wider belief of Respondents B, C, D, F, and G, however, on the need to engage in lifelong learning. Adequate pedagogical models should support the technical, ethical, and clinical aspects of AI to equip radiologists with the changing need of newer healthcare settings.

Experiential learning and teamwork are often viewed as motivating factors toward effective learning in this field. Respondents C and F like to stress pedagogical merits of the laboratory experience and direct involvement in the research project whereas D and G point at the significance of sharing inner knowledge. This learning laboratory can empower professionals to bridge the functional knowledge gap that is likely to blur the practical impacts of AI on radiological decisions. This candor is not just a technical desideratum, but an ethical one. Clinicians must be able to perceive all the potential dangers to make informed and responsible decisions. AI practices and applications in the medical field can be ethically viable, and therefore, it will require a sustainable commitment to interdisciplinary education. This kind of training should include some theory and practice to bring medical and technical together. To steer the social implications of these technologies in every corner of the world, an all-inclusive discussion to include medical practitioners, researchers, patients and legal experts is needed. Through increasing the scope of the stakeholders, the healthcare system may have a chance to make advances in AI development controlled in a fair and ethically sound manner.

DISCUSSION

The ethical ambiguity of the ethical problems related to AI (AI) and its application as a clinical decision-support tool and its institutional normalisation provided the proper context to insist on a kind of moral restraint over technological utility, i.e. strictness. The main question that the discussed topic is dictated by is how the ethical dilemma can be alleviated and what is the contribution of constant professional training to ensuring responsible deployment. According to the results of the qualitative data analysis of the interviews and the academic materials, the ethical obstacles concern primarily accountability, transparency, and distributive justice. Therefore, there is need to establish effective accountability mechanisms and universal guidelines that can be established to establish systemic trust between these automated systems. Lifelong learning is the key mechanism that can be used to make sure that medical professionals use AI effectively and in an ethical way. This element of pedagogy not only deals with technical knowledge but also a very cognizant recognition of the ethical limitations, as well as the risks that novel technology can involve. The practitioners underline the importance of having a thorough understanding of what an AI system is capable of, as a condition to develop quality clinical decisions and preserve the patient-clinician relationship. Even though the degree of acceptance of professional people interviewed showed a positive trend towards the implementation of AI, the willingness to use such technology is conditioned by the effective resolution of the ethical dilemmas and the survival of the competence training.

Table 2. Thematic Synthesis: Mapping Ethical Imperatives to TAM Constructs

TAM Construct	Associated Ethical Theme	Primary Practitioner Concern (Interview Data)	Proposed Mitigation Strategy
Perceived Usefulness	Beneficence & Distributive Justice	AI can increase diagnostic speed, but high costs and lack of infrastructure may worsen health disparities (e.g., mobile microscopy challenges).	Develop low-cost AI models and secure public-private funding to ensure equitable access.
Perceived Ease of Use	Autonomy & Transparency (The 'Black Box')	The systems are opaque and complex, and this brings about uncertainty. Clinicians have no easy way of explaining AI-driven diagnoses to patients.	Require transparent algorithmic auditing and incorporate explainable AI interfaces to use in clinical settings.
Attitude Toward Using	Non-Maleficence & Automation Bias	The possible danger of being too dependent on algorithms and the potential of continuing the transmission of biased training data with the result of harming patients.	Implement continuous AI literacy programs and routine bias checks on local datasets.
Behavioral Intention	Accountability & Liability	Confusion over who is legally and morally responsible (developer, hospital, or physician) if an AI diagnostic error occurs.	Establish clear institutional guidelines, AI ethics review boards, and shared liability frameworks.

Artifacts used in technology are not morally neutral, but they do have embedded values which actively influence clinical outcomes. In line with the theories of Verbeek, AI systems may strengthen the systematic imbalances in case they are based on discriminatory datasets which will result in misguided and discriminatory care. This supports the points by Dignum (2019), who states that the development of AI should be based on a strong sense of social responsibility. Empirical evidence has shown that the values latent in AI algorithms affect clinical judgement, and that there is need to adopt a multi-pronged method to responsible implementation, involving use of standardized diagnostic procedures and interdisciplinary collaboration between medicine, ethics, computer science and law. To overcome these ethical risks in practice, it is proposed to develop uniform principles of data collection and algorithmic analysis. Moreover, establishing forums of interdisciplinary discourse will also see AI systems being technically sustainable and ethically defensible. Nevertheless, they are just restricted to a limited number of samples due to the demographic and geographic settings of the current study. More research in the scientific community would involve diversified cultural and technological conditions and study the effects of the AI integration over time in the attempt to comprehend the dynamism in the relationship between medical practitioners, patients, and the new technologies.

CONCLUSION

The ethical dilemmas that must be resolved when using AI (AI) as a clinical assistive technology are optimistically subject to the sound conception of the overlapping of the technological effectiveness and the ethical responsibility. The central aspect of this question is establishing the way responsibility is shared when the algorithmic outputs become uninterpretable to humans. IDAO: It is due to the very nature of an opaque AI system which requires an introduction of clear ethical standards and regulatory provisions that will serve to make the technical architecture and the medical practitioner responsible in the context of transparency in the diagnostic process. Information security and strengthening security measures are a secondary, but no less important, obstacle. Because information about patients is incredibly sensitive, a systemic trust can only be established if tight security measures are enforced to curtail any unauthorized violations. This custodianship transparency is the key to AI absorption institutional and social legitimacy. Moreover, the reduction of algorithmic bias must be undertaken to avoid the perpetuation of the current health inequities. The training datasets and algorithmic logic should be systemically audited, and it should be guaranteed that AI-based care must not be discriminatory and unequal. TAM is a major controller of success in the implementation of these technologies since it has perceived usefulness and ease of use as the major determinants of integration among the users. Nevertheless, technical functionality is not sufficient, as it is highlighted by practitioners that the key to linking technological potential and ethical practice lies in continuous education. Such pedagogical obligation should not stop at the technical literacy but is to be informed with an insight into the ethical aspects of AI, and hence, mitigating the risk of clinical error and making sure that the technology is being applied in a way acceptable by the professional standards. These results are in line with theoretically relevant works of Verbeek (2019) and Dignum (2019) that state that technology is always values loaded and must be socially responsible in its application. The longitudinal effects of AI, incorporation of patients in the development of the AI system, and the establishment of finer ethical principles should be the primary focus of scholarly investigation in the future. The only feasible way to interdisciplinary relationship between developers, clinicians, and ethical advisors is a long-term cooperation that leads to an environment of medical diagnostics that provides benefits to patients without undermining professionalism. The quantitative validation of these systems should be a part of the research in the future.

REFERENCES

Abdelwanis, M., Alarafati, H. K., Tammam, M. M. S., & Simsekler, M. C. E. (2024). Exploring the risks of automation bias in healthcare artificial intelligence applications: A Bowtie analysis. *Journal of Safety Science and Resilience = An Quan Ke Xue Yu Ren Xing (Ying Wen)*, *5*(4), 460–469. DOI: 10.1016/j.jnlssr.2024.06.001

Bertl, M., Ross, P., & Draheim, D. (2022). A survey on AI and decision support systems in psychiatry - Uncovering a dilemma. *Expert Systems with Applications*, *202*, 117464. Advance online publication. DOI: 10.1016/j.eswa.2022.117464

Bourgeault, I., Dingwall, R., & de Vries, R. (2010). *The SAGE handbook of qualitative methods in health research*. SAGE. DOI: 10.4135/9781446268247

Bryman, A., & Bell, E. (2011). *Business research methods* (3rd ed.). OUP Oxford.

Carter, S. M., Rogers, W., Than Win, K., Frazer, H., Richards, B., & Houssami, N. (2020). The ethical, legal and social implications of using artificial intelligence systems in breast cancer care. *The Breast : Official Journal of the European Society of Mastology*, *49*, 25–32. DOI: 10.1016/j.breast.2019.10.001 PMID: 31677530

Castonguay, A., Wagner, G., Motulsky, A., & Paré, G. (2024). AI maturity in health care: An overview of 10 OECD countries. *Health Policy (Amsterdam)*, *140*, 104938. Advance online publication. DOI: 10.1016/j.healthpol.2023.104938 PMID: 38157771

Charness, N., & Boot, W. R. (2016). Technology, gaming, and social networking. In *Handbook of the psychology of aging* (8th ed., pp. 389–407). Academic Press., DOI: 10.1016/B978-0-12-411469-2.00020-0

Clark, T., Foster, L., Bryman, A., & Sloan, L. (2021). *Bryman's social research methods*. Oxford University Press.

Davenport, T., & Kalakota, R. (2019). The potential for artificial intelligence in healthcare. *Future Healthcare Journal*, *6*(2), 94–98. DOI: 10.7861/futurehosp.6-2-94 PMID: 31363513

Denscombe, M. (2018). *Forskningshandboken* (4th ed.). Studentlitteratur.

Dignum, V. (2019). *Responsible artificial intelligence: How to develop and use AI in a responsible way*. Springer. DOI: 10.1007/978-3-030-30371-6

Eisbach, S., Langer, M., & Hertel, G. (2023). Optimizing human-AI collaboration: Effects of motivation and accuracy information in AI-supported decision-making. *Computers in Human Behavior: Artificial Humans*, *1*(2), 100015. Advance online publication. DOI: 10.1016/j.chbah.2023.100015

Gonçalves, A. R., Pinto, D. C., Rita, P., & Pires, T. (2023). Artificial intelligence and its ethical implications for marketing. *Emerging Science Journal*, *7*(2), 313–327. DOI: 10.28991/ESJ-2023-07-02-01

Gupta, N. S., & Kumar, P. (2023). Perspective of artificial intelligence in healthcare data management: A journey towards precision medicine. *Computers in Biology and Medicine*, *162*, 107051. Advance online publication. DOI: 10.1016/j.compbiomed.2023.107051 PMID: 37271113

Hamet, P., & Tremblay, J. (2017). Artificial intelligence in medicine. *Metabolism: Clinical and Experimental*, *69*, S36–S40. DOI: 10.1016/j.metabol.2017.01.011 PMID: 28126242

Hasanzadeh, F., Josephson, C. B., Waters, G., Adedinsewo, D., Azizi, Z., & White, J. A. (2025). Bias recognition and mitigation strategies in artificial intelligence healthcare applications. *npj. Digital Medicine*, *8*(1), 154. Advance online publication. DOI: 10.1038/s41746-025-01503-7 PMID: 40069303

Holden, R. J., & Karsh, B. T. (2010). The Technology Acceptance Model: Its past and its future in health care. *Journal of Biomedical Informatics*, *43*(1), 159–172. DOI: 10.1016/j.jbi.2009.07.002 PMID: 19615467

Humerick, M. (2018). Taking AI personally: How the E.U. must learn to balance the interest of personal data privacy & artificial intelligence. *Santa Clara High-Technology Law Journal*, *34*(4), 393–418. https://digitalcommons.law.scu.edu/chtlj/vol34/iss4/2

Le, E., Wang, Y., Huang, Y., Hickman, S., & Gilbert, F. J. (2019). Artificial intelligence in breast imaging. *Clinical Radiology*, *74*(5), 357–366. DOI: 10.1016/j.crad.2019.02.006 PMID: 30898381

Oates, B. J., Griffiths, M., & McLean, R. (2023). *Researching information systems and computing* (2nd ed.). SAGE Publications Ltd.

Pai, F. Y., & Huang, K. I. (2011). Applying the Technology Acceptance Model to the introduction of healthcare information systems. *Technological Forecasting and Social Change*, *78*(4), 650–660. DOI: 10.1016/j.techfore.2010.11.007

Pedreschi, D., Giannotti, F., Guidotti, R., Monreale, A., Ruggieri, S., & Turini, F. (2019). Meaningful explanations of black box AI decision systems. *Proceedings of the AAAI Conference on Artificial Intelligence*, *33*(1), 9780–9784. DOI: 10.1609/aaai.v33i01.33019780

Peixoto, H., Guimarães, T., & Santos, M. F. (2020). A new architecture for intelligent clinical decision support for intensive medicine. *Procedia Computer Science*, *170*, 1035–1040. DOI: 10.1016/j.procs.2020.03.077

Rahimi, B., Nadri, H., Lotfnezhad Afshar, H., & Timpka, T. (2018). A systematic review of the Technology Acceptance Model in health informatics. *Applied Clinical Informatics*, *9*(3), 604–634. DOI: 10.1055/s-0038-1668091 PMID: 30112741

Riis Hansen, E., Sagi, T., Hose, K., Lip, G., Bjerregaard Larsen, T., & Skjøth, F. (2022). Assigning diagnosis codes using medication history. *Artificial Intelligence in Medicine*, *128*, 102307. Advance online publication. DOI: 10.1016/j.artmed.2022.102307 PMID: 35534145

Stone, P., Brooks, R., Brynjolfsson, E., Calo, R., Etzioni, O., Hager, G., Hirschberg, J., Kalyanakrishnan, S., Kamar, E., Kraus, S., Leyton-Brown, K., Parkes, D., Press, W., Saxenian, A., Shah, J., Tambe, M., & Teller, A. (2022). *Artificial intelligence and life in 2030: The one hundred year study on artificial intelligence*. Stanford University. https://doi.org//arXiv.2211.06318DOI: 10.48550

Sun, C., & Harris, S. L. (2024). Reducing bias in healthcare artificial intelligence: A white paper. *Health Informatics Journal*, *30*(4), 14604582241291410. Advance online publication. DOI: 10.1177/14604582241291410 PMID: 39541598

Varkey, B. (2020). Principles of clinical ethics and their application to practice. *Medical Principles and Practice : International Journal of the Kuwait University, Health Science Centre*, *30*(1), 17–28. DOI: 10.1159/000509119 PMID: 32498071

Verbeek, P. P. (2011). *Moralizing technology: Understanding and designing the morality of things*. The University of Chicago Press. DOI: 10.7208/chicago/9780226852904.001.0001

Vinnova. (2018). *Artificiell intelligens i svenskt näringsliv och samhälle - Analys av utveckling och potential* (Report No. 2018:08). Vinnova - Sveriges innovationsmyndighet.

Ward, R. (2013). The application of technology acceptance and diffusion of innovation models in healthcare informatics. *Health Policy and Technology*, *2*(4), 222–228. DOI: 10.1016/j.hlpt.2013.07.002

Xu, N., Yang, D., Arikawa, K., & Bai, C. (2023). Application of artificial intelligence in modern medicine. *Clinical eHealth, 6*, 130–137. https://doi.org/DOI: 10.1016/j.ceh.2023.09.001

Zhang, B., & Ming, C. (2023). A patent portfolio value analysis based on intuitionistic fuzzy sets: An empirical analysis of artificial intelligence for healthcare. *Journal of Open Innovation*, *9*(3), 100124. Advance online publication. DOI: 10.1016/j.joitmc.2023.100124

Zsidai, B., Hilkert, A. S., Kaarre, J., Narup, E., Senorski, E. H., Grassi, A., Ley, C., Longo, U. G., Herbst, E., Hirschmann, M. T., Kopf, S., Seil, R., Tischer, T., Samuelsson, K., & Feldt, R. (2023). A practical guide to the implementation of AI in orthopaedic research—Part 1: Opportunities in clinical application and overcoming existing challenges. *Journal of Experimental Orthopaedics*, *10*(1), 117. Advance online publication. DOI: 10.1186/s40634-023-00683-z PMID: 37968370

ADDITIONAL READING

Abdelwanis, M., Alarafati, H. K., Tammam, M. M. S., & Simsekler, M. C. E. (2024). Exploring the risks of automation bias in healthcare artificial intelligence applications: A Bowtie analysis. *Journal of Safety Science and Resilience = An Quan Ke Xue Yu Ren Xing (Ying Wen)*, *5*(4), 460–469. DOI: 10.1016/j.jnlssr.2024.06.001

Ferrara, E. (2023). Fairness and Bias in Artificial Intelligence: A Brief Survey of Sources, Impacts, and Mitigation Strategies. *Sci*, *6*(1), 3. Advance online publication. DOI: 10.3390/sci6010003

Hasanzadeh, F., Josephson, C. B., Waters, G., Adedinsewo, D., Azizi, Z., & White, J. A. (2025). Bias recognition and mitigation strategies in artificial intelligence healthcare applications. *NPJ Digital Medicine*, *8*(1), 154. DOI: 10.1038/s41746-025-01503-7 PMID: 40069303

Norori, N., Hu, Q., Aellen, F. M., Faraci, F. D., & Tzovara, A. (2021). Addressing bias in big data and AI for health care: A call for open science. *Patterns (New York, N.Y.)*, *2*(10), 100347. DOI: 10.1016/j.patter.2021.100347 PMID: 34693373

Sun, C., & Harris, S. L. (2024). Reducing bias in healthcare artificial intelligence: A white paper. *Health Informatics Journal*, *30*(4), 14604582241291410. DOI: 10.1177/14604582241291410 PMID: 39541598

Vorisek, C. N., Stellmach, C., Mayer, P. J., Klopfenstein, S. A. I., Bures, D. M., Diehl, A., Henningsen, M., Ritter, K., & Thun, S. (2023). Artificial Intelligence Bias in Health Care: Web-Based Survey. *Journal of Medical Internet Research*, *25*, e41089. DOI: 10.2196/41089 PMID: 37347528

KEY TERMS AND DEFINITIONS

Algorithmic Bias: Systematic errors of an AI system that occur due to bias training data or broken mathematics model, which may contribute to unfair treatment of patients. It requires ongoing observation to make sure that medical AI does not promote the status quo of social or demographical differences.

Black Box Effect: The fact that the decision-making process in an AI system is not transparent or visible to the user and gives the output without providing them with a clear rationale. This introduces very daunting ethical challenges of transparency and trust or explanation of a diagnosis by clinicians.

Cardsinal Principles of Medico-Ethical: The principles that entail the underscoring of beneficence, non-maleficence, autonomy, and justice that govern clinical practice. These values would be associated with determining whether AI applications advance the well-being of a patient without infringing on their own self-determination and equitable resources distribution.

Human-in-the-Loop (HITL): An interaction model in which AI decision support is taught with human professional remaining supreme and in charge. This makes the effectiveness of automation proportional to the clinical intuition and responsibility.

Liability Dilemma: The medical and ethical grey area of who is at fault, the doctor, the developer, or the organization, when a decision that is based on AI causes harm to the patient. There should be clear lines of jurisdiction to control accountability with systems becoming more autonomous.

Socio-Technical Systems: A complex organizational design methodology that acknowledges the interplay of people and technology at the workplace. It underlines that acceptance of AI is both a technical and a complex question, which is heavily shaped by institutional culture and relationships between humans.

Technology Acceptance Model (TAM): An effective approach based on a theoretical framework being useful to predict the adoption by the users of new technology depending on how they will rate the usefulness and convenience of technology based on perceptions. Of interest in this study, it is the main prism that determines the reaction of healthcare professionals to the implementation of AI.

Chapter 3

Principles and Applications of LLMs in Healthcare:

Methods, Models, Data Privacy, New Medical Treatments, and Challenges

Updesh Kumar Jaiswal
http://orcid.org/0009-0002-1572-8275
School of Engineering and Technology, Vivekananda Institute of Professional Studies - Technical Campus, India

Amrita Bhatnagar
Noida Institute of Engineering and Technology, Greater Noida, India

Jaishree Jain
http://orcid.org/0000-0003-0173-7664
Ajay Kumar Garg Engineering College, Ghaziabad, India

Harnit Saini
http://orcid.org/0009-0007-3103-9070
Ajay Kumar Garg Engineering College, Ghaziabad, India

Vikas
http://orcid.org/0000-0002-5432-5156
School of Engineering and Technology, Vivekananda Institute of Professional Studies - Technical Campus, India

Shashank Sahu
Ajay Kumar Garg Engineering College, Ghaziabad, India

Kriti Mishra
Ajay Kumar Garg Engineering College, Ghaziabad, India

ABSTRACT

Large Language Models (LLMs) are improving patient care and clinical research, with a significant role in transforming the healthcare industry. LLMs are improving

DOI: 10.4018/979-8-2600-2173-6.ch003

healthcare providers' capacity to deliver effective patient care by providing good-quality medicine and clinical safety. LLMs examine patient information, medical research, and related protocols. LLMs provide immediate insights for diagnosis, treatment strategies, medicine, and observation, enhancing patient care results, clinical safety, minimizing mistakes, and increasing satisfaction in healthcare. In this chapter, we deal with how LLMs can improve the speed of medical research by using large datasets from medical trials and scientific publications. Using LLMs, it will be easy to find out complete patient treatment and health histories. LLMs ensure a thorough understanding of the patient's condition before treatment. LLMs analyze data from various sources for better patient insights. This research ends with discussing the role of LLMs in discovering new treatments and comprehending disease mechanisms.

1. INTRODUCTION

Extremely big Deep Learning models that have been pre-trained using massive amounts of data are known as large language models (LLMs) (Ahmed et al., 2023; Chen et al., 2024). The transformer is a group of neural networks that consists of an encoder and a decoder with self-attention capabilities. The encoder and decoder extract meanings from a text sequence by understanding the relationships between words and phrases (Ahammad et al., 2024). LLMs are remarkably flexible. A model may do a wide range of tasks, including answering questions, summarizing papers, understanding languages, and completing sentences (Yujia & Jan, 2024; Desbordes et al., 2024). LLMs have the ability to alter both the creation of information and how users utilize search engines and virtual assistants. Copywriting, knowledge base response, text classification, code production, and text generation are just a few of the numerous useful uses for LLMs. Transformer-based neural networks are massive. These networks consist of multiple layers and nodes. Each node in a layer has a bias and a weight, and they are all connected to each other. Figure 1 shows the working of LLM.

Figure 1. Working of LLM

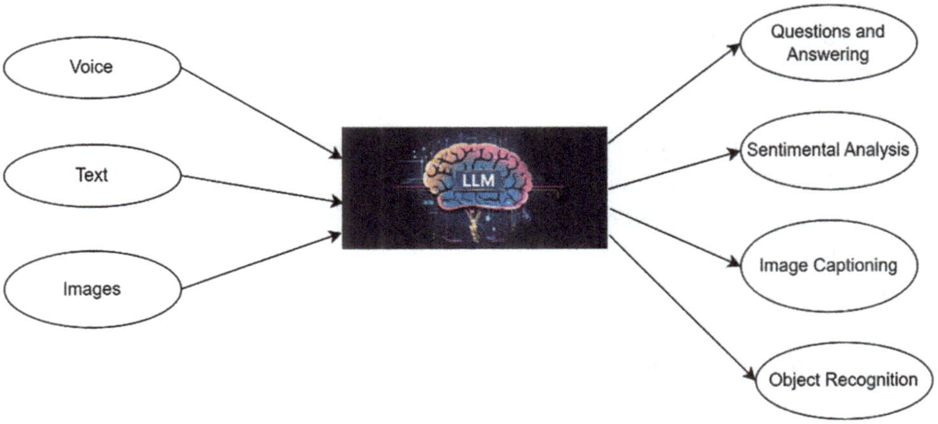

LLMs are extremely valuable in medical field because of their capacity to process and synthesize enormous amounts of patient information, medical literature, and the constantly growing corpus of clinical research (Artsi et al., 2025). Healthcare data are by their very nature varied, complicated, and even overwhelming. LLMs help healthcare workers who are overwhelmed by information by acting as a potent force multiplier.

2. BACKGROUND

Medical care is required during the pandemic, but diagnosing common illnesses is challenging in today's world. By identifying mild symptoms, modern Artificial Intelligence (AI) systems with natural language processing capabilities enable humans to identify early disease indicators, resulting in less expensive AI diagnostic results. Before performing Multinomial Naïve Bayes classification, the model's symptom processing starts with text pre-processing and Count Vectorizer vectorization. With the help of this method, the initial disease diagnosis system expands its range and enhances the effectiveness of the diagnostics process. Research indicates that AI systems that run on the Natural Language Processing (NLP) include the work of healthcare diagnostics and the development of medical institutions access. The advances in AI are useful to the medical systems because they facilitate early detection of the disease, reducing health risks, improving patient outcomes, and minimizing mortality (Shool et al., 2025; Shammi et al., 2025). Using the insights of millions of unstructured data (doctor notes and electronic health records), reducing clinician burnout by automating documentation, speeding up drug discovery, assisting with clinical decisions based on predictive models, and improving patient care by improving patient analysis and communication, AI and NLP are turning healthcare into data-driven, productive processes (Shad et al., 2025; Nivethitha et al., 2025). In order to create reliable and efficient AI models, data collection and augmentation are essential. They should be done carefully to address biases and data privacy issues while guaranteeing that the collected data are representative, balanced, and varied. When gathering and enhancing data for AI models, a number of issues should be taken into account. Limited data access, annotation is expensive, processing many types of data and patient data security are the most common issues in medical AI research (Liu et al., 2025). A shortage in data, especially in uncommon circumstances, is a considerable problem in the medical field of AI. The robust model training requires sufficient data, but in some exceptional situations, entire datasets are often unavailable. Moreover, with more common cases, it is rather difficult to access medical records because of strict privacy regulations. Such challenges are compounded by the fact that the process of the real-world dataset creation is also resource-intensive, involving data collection, data cleaning, and data annotation.

3. CORE ARCHITECTURE OF LLMS

The key component of an LLM is the Transformer model, as shown in Figure 2, which consists of stacked self-attention and feed-forward network layers. Text to numbers is achieved with the help of Token Embeddings and Positional Encoding and processed contextually to predict outputs (Lysyi, 2025).

Figure 2. LLM Architecture

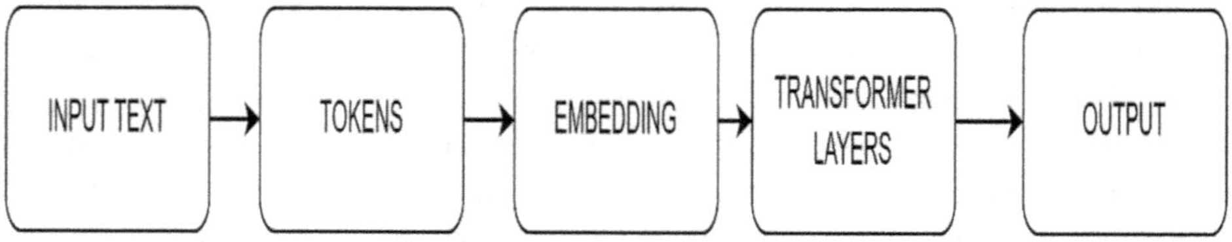

It is the stable training that is guaranteed by residual connections and normalization. These blocks, which may be Decoder-only (GPT) or Encoder-Decoder based, act as the engine, and long-range relationships are dealt with by these blocks to gain an understanding of subtle language meaning.

4. LLMS IN MEDICAL FIELD

Neural networks that learn to anticipate words in a sequence are known as large language models. They can produce meaningful language that mimics human reasoning because they work on patterns rather than rules. One of the most famous users, ChatGPT, has been optimized through the reinforcement learning of the human feedback. Findings of this approach are within the acceptable medical and conversational standards. Its understanding of structured and unstructured data is an opportunity to improve the processing and presentation of information in nephrology. With nephrology, the conventional data systems can be fragmented. Renal function tests of a patient can be stored in one database but imaging, pathology reports and clinical notes are located elsewhere. LLMs can combine these streams by cohesively transforming unprocessed text into a story. As an example, a model can give an account of the history of chronic kidney disease in a patient, including such important milestones as changes in drugs or periods of glomerular filtration rate decline. The produced summary would provide important information succinctly, but it would not take the place of medical judgment. LLMs minimizing oversight and saving clinicians' time.

Thorough assessments of FM/LLM-based medical AI have been published in the Nature publication series. FMs are therefore used as building blocks for language models, while LLMs are the outcome of optimizing and scaling up FMs (Xu et al., 2024). The key differences between the two are their sizes and capacities. The models that are known to be the most versatile and generalized are called foundation models that are typically trained on a large amount of text data. In contrast, language models are also explicitly scaled-up versions, which demonstrate very high performance in a particular task but retain the overall language understanding that the foundation models have.

In this review, we focus on medical AI that is powered by FM/LLM. We propose a paradigm of categorizing them into three by the specificity of task and modality.

(1) Disease-specific models: Disease-specific models are special-purpose models that target some medical activity or medical situation and specialize their functionality to address that medical situation or activity (Sun et al., 2023; Bhatnagar & Singh, 2024).
(2) General-domain models: These models are flexible to most types of activities and applications in the medical profession and have proven to be widely applicable in various fields of clinical medicine (Griot et al., 2024)
(3) Multi-modal models: The models also use the data of different modalities, including clinical text, medical images, and other forms of data, to enhance the general understanding of the health conditions of patients and assist in making

accurate diagnoses, specific treatments, and well-informed decisions (Cascella et al., 2024).

4.1 Disease-Specific Models

These disease-specific models exhibit remarkable adaptability and reliably produce extraordinary results in a variety of clinical activities, including those using multicenter datasets (Madzime & Nyirenda, 2024). The use of multi-modal datasets has significantly increased recently. This method enables a comprehensive examination of many facets of an illness, leading to better diagnosis, more precise forecasts, and a greater comprehension of the underlying mechanisms.

4.2 General-Domain Models

In order to overcome the shortcomings of specialized models and cover a variety of clinical applications, including grounded radiological reports, augmented procedures, and decision assistance, universal medical AI models are presently under development. ChatGPT has proven its ability to identify both common and uncommon medical diseases by utilizing its vast dataset of 45 terabytes of text data and 175 billion parameters. LLMs and universal segmentation models for medical imaging analysis were the two main areas of concentration for international efforts to create universal medical AI models by the end of 2023. Researchers from Google Research and DeepMind used instruction fine-tuning to create the Med-PaLM, a specific medical language model, in a work that was published in Nature. A refined version of SAM called MedSAM was trained on a sizable dataset that included over a million image-mask pairs from ten distinct imaging modalities and over thirty different cancer types (Maurya et al., 2025). Table 1 shows the difference of these two models.

Table 1. Difference between General Domain Models and Disease Specific Model

General Domain Models	Disease Specific model
1. Training done on large dataset.	Trained on specific dataset.
2. Can be used in multiple domains like health and education.	Focused on specific condition.
3. High Flexibility and adaptability.	Higher Accuracy & precision in specific domain.
4. Deep clinical Accuracy not provided.	Not useful in outside the domain area.
5. Higher risk of hallucination in specific medical contexts.	Required high quality labeled data.

4.3 Multi-Modal Models

This multi-modal medical AI tackles the major problem of the scarcity of publicly labeled medical pictures and performs better than earlier contrastive language-image pre-trained models. LLMs use substantial pre-training on biomedical text and data to represent clinical knowledge, which is then refined for particular medical applications and improved by integration with knowledge graphs (Singhal et al., 2022).

5. APPLICATION OF LLMS IN MEDICAL FIELD

AI, especially LLMs, has been widely incorporated into various medical specialties, from wearable-based patient monitoring in cardiology to sophisticated imaging analysis in radiology, among many other uses. Neurological illnesses represent considerable challenges to healthcare systems and sometimes necessitate a lengthy and unpredictable diagnosis process.

5.1 Multimodal Imaging and Virtual Assistance

Multimodal visual language models have great potential to improve medical imaging analysis by combining textual and visual data. Multimodal visual language models are very promising to enhance the analysis of medical imaging since they can combine text and visual data. These models can help radiologists to find the abnormalities in medical images at an early stage and produce improved and more complete diagnostic interpretations which will ultimately lead to the improved accuracy and effectiveness of the medical imaging diagnostic processes (Khader et al., 2024). These models can help in the process of radiologists to diagnose a medical image at an early phase and create more accurate and exhaustive diagnostic interpretations that will ultimately improve the accuracy and the quality of medical imaging diagnostic tests (Zhang et al., 2025).

Such models can assist the radiologists to identify abnormality in the medical images in the early stages and develop more effective and more detailed diagnostic interpretation which ultimately will be used to enhance accuracy and efficiency of the diagnostic processes by medical imaging diagnostic procedures (Khader et al., 2024).This kind of models may assist radiologists to recognize a medical image at a tender age and generate superior and comprehensive diagnostic explanations that will eventually enhance quality and precision of medical imaging diagnostic procedures (Zhang et al., 2025).

Massive LLMs do incredibly well at being able to properly analyze and summarize medical literature in bulk. Ultimately, this ability fosters evidence-based and high-quality healthcare services as it assists researchers and clinicians to remain abreast with new developments and evidence-based practices. The ability to keep abreast of the latest developments is also imperative within a fast-developing field such as healthcare.

5.2 Drug Discovery

Because of their capacity to process complex molecular structures, discover compounds with pharmacological potential, and forecast the safety and efficacy profiles of drug candidates, big language models are having a huge influence on drug discovery (Guo et al., 2025). Chemical language models have shown a major breakthrough in the area of de novo drug creation.

5.3 Automated Medical Report Synthesis From Imaging Data

Automated production of medical reports based on pictures is needed to allow pathologists and radiologists to carry out their time-intensive and error-prone tasks in a more efficient way. This new field at the intersection of AI and healthcare aims to enhance the precision of healthcare professionals less experienced in their field, and ease the burden on more experienced professionals. The combination of AI with medical imaging simplifies the automatic generation of reports, which contain relevant normal findings, abnormal data, and patient history. In the case of single-sentence reports, the first efforts made employed neural networks that were data-driven, consisted of convolutional and recurrent models; they did not succeed in capturing the complexity of real-life medical cases.

5.4 Clinical Decision Support and Administrative Tasks Assistance

LLMs are becoming important resources that health personnel should consider whenever making decisions (Gaber et al., 2025). By analyzing a large volume of medical data, LMs are able to produce evidence-based advice which enhances the overall, treatment-related, and diagnostic accuracy of the patient (Saeidnia, 2024).

Although kidney illness sometimes stays undiagnosed until its advanced stages, early detection is essential. Laboratory abnormalities may be mild, and symptoms are nonspecific. By examining longitudinal patient data, LLMs can help identify illness tendencies early on. Consistent reports of increased creatinine or proteinuria in patient records could be flagged by a model, highlighting those who need further care. By doing this, it serves as a system of support for doctors, making sure that little but significant patterns are not missed.

5.5 Medical Dialog Summarization

Medical Dialogue Summarization (MDS) applications apply the methods of artificial intelligence (AI) known as Large Language Models (LLMs) such as GPT-3 to automatically generate brief Electronic Health Records (EHRs) based on doctor-patient conversations, therefore lessening physician work and enhancing documentation (Madzime & Nyirenda, 2024). This is usually done by removing vital information (goals, history, and symptoms) into the format of SOAP notes just to mention a few. Sophisticated methods like two-stage models and specialized prompt engineering have been developed in response to several challenges, including managing long talks, ensuring factual accuracy (faithfulness, avoiding hallucinations), and accurately understanding medical nuances like negations.

5.6 EHRs, Clinical Letters and Medical Note Generation

Despite gathering a lot of data, electronic health record systems frequently struggle to display it in an understandable manner. Finding information across several pages of records might take a lot of time for doctors. LLMs are able to reorganize this information into readable stories. A nephrologist looking at a patient file may be presented with the model with a summary: at present how well the kidneys are working, how well the patient adheres to medications, blood pressure measurements of the patient, and recent imaging. Such systems would also find inconsistencies or omissions in documentation.

As an example, the model could dictate that the doctor should perform relevant tests when a note indicates having new edema and fail to enclose the results of subsequent laboratory tests. They are helpful functions that can be used to guarantee the presence of consistency and completeness but does not imply the absolute autonomy is required. Doctors can dictate notes during a consultation and paired with speech recognition technologies, ChatGPT may enable doctors to do so. The model would convert speech into structured text by automatically adding relevant codes and phrases in it. This role liberates additional time to work with patients because it reduces the administrative burden.

EHRs are central to the operation of modern healthcare systems, and are designed to enhance efficiency in operations and optimization of clinical processes. But it is actually the quality of this colossal bulk of data that dictates whether it is useful or not. A robust data quality assessment (DQA) system, therefore, is a key requirement but a major challenge in ensuring the data reliability and maximum use of EHRs to improve patient outcomes.

In every evaluation criterion, LLM-DQR performed better. The GPT implementation outperformed CIM-DQR, achieving total coverage rates of 97.1% on the PIC dataset and 99.6% on the MIMIC-IV dataset. For complicated dimensions, performance was especially good: CIM-DQR achieved 0% coverage, while Consistency rules achieved 100% coverage on both datasets. When compared to manual methods, construction time was cut by more than ten times. Furthermore, LLM-DQR produced 89 additional, expert-validated rules on the PIC dataset.

5.7 Medical Education and Language Translation

The LLMs have been applied in a variety of medical education and language translation scenarios. These include the creation of multiple-choice questions, the assessment of medical tests, educational programs in pharmacogenomics and rehabilitation, applications in licensing exams like the USMLE and the JMLE, and the simplification of complex medical imaging reports to improve healthcare education (Abd-Alrazaq et al., 2023).

5.8 Clinical Health Reasoning and Diagnostic Reasoning

While diagnostic reasoning is a key component specifically focused on identifying the patient's illness by generating and refining differential diagnoses from patient cues, history, and exams using both analytical (slow) and intuitive (fast) thinking to reach a conclusion for treatment, clinical reasoning is the broad cognitive process of healthcare professionals making decisions, encompassing data collection, problem-solving, and care planning.

5.9 Medical Product Safety Monitoring and Disease Diagnosis

LLMs find their use in healthcare, primarily as an effective tool in the hands of human specialists, to observe the safety of medical products (pharmacovigilance) and diagnose diseases. They are efficient at handling extensive amounts of data, but as they may contain errors, and have to be confirmed by the human, they are currently under the control of humans.

5.10 Integrated Application of LLMs in Medical System

The integration of LLMs to other applications and systems within the health care systems is gradually becoming a major concern as the medical technology continues to change. This intersect has given health care providers the potent tools through which they can manage, analyze and utilize huge volumes of health care data. The implementation of LLM, including ChatGPT, into the health care frameworks could transform the provision of health care (Jung, 2025).

LLMs can enhance clinical decision-making and the accuracy of diagnosis by analyzing large volumes of medical data to identify the relevant information and prescribe the potential diagnosis of the given symptoms. Second, they are able to process and generate language in an effective way to support medical professionals summarize medical literature, support research, and also enhance patient-provider communication. The rapid uptake of easily available LLMs by the medical community, such as ChatGPT, indicates that the medical fraternity has the awareness of how it can transform the delivery of healthcare.

The general level of healthcare delivery can be improved because LLMs are able to offer individualized diagnoses and treatment suggestions based on the assessment and synthesis of patient medical information. Moreover, the LLMs are needed to enhance the doctor-patient interactions. They are in a position to give more customized medical guidance by applying NLP technology to comprehend the requirements and interests of patients better. This enhances the overall effectiveness of the medical procedures besides the pleasure of the patients. There can be no doubt that the LLMs can enhance the digital health care processes. It is projected that in future, LLM will expand in the healthcare industry as a result of more empirical research and technological advances.

5.11 Multimodal LLMs in Real-World Medical Scenarios

The multimodal LLMs are reshaping the medical industry as it has the potential to process and create various forms of data including text, photos, audio, and videos. The integration of the numerous types of data makes the LLMs able to make more detailed and more precise predictions and it does not mean that the possibilities were not heard before. It is of great significance to develop the multimodal LLMs to be in a position to comprehend the way they operate. This is because the multimodal LLMs have the ability to process, understand and generate different kinds of data at high accuracy which is the main factor that drives the prediction potential of the multimodal LLM models.

One of them is that such models have the ability to produce more accurate and detailed diagnoses in the medical profession by integrating textual details on the patients record with the imaging data on the computed tomography, x-rays, and magnetic resonance imaging (MRI).

Further, the comprehension of the model can be enhanced through the integration of sound information about the patients during the interview, or video information about the medical procedure, that will result in more precise and individualized propositions of the treatment plans. Multimodal LLMs would have the opportunity to take into account all the advantages of a variety of data, which are frequently required to create complicated diagnoses and treatment plan and fully get to know the condition of a patient.

The importance of the LLM in medical imaging is increasing. In the case of an MRI scan or a computed tomography, say of a patient, an LLM can easily analyze and synthesize the image with the textual medical history of a patient and make more detailed and comprehensive diagnostic conclusions. Moreover, LLMs will be able to detect and outline essential areas in medical images automatically, which will provide researchers with accurate references and enable them to identify potential issues. Learning more, based on the data on the picture studied, the LLM can give automated image reports that give preliminary interpretations and treatment recommendations, which can significantly enhance the efficacy and accuracy of medical diagnosis and treatments.

6. METHODOLOGY OF USING LLMS IN HEALTHCARE SYSTEMS

The methodology of utilizing LLMs in the healthcare system is illustrated in Figure 3. Firstly, we need to collect or acquire the dataset. Large and varied datasets, including clinical records, medical literature, healthcare guidelines, and domain-specific knowledge resources, are necessary for medical LLMs. For this research data is collected from clinicaltrial.gov. Clinicaltrial.gov is a public online database which is managed by U.S National Library of medicine which is freely available to researchers, doctors and patients. These trials are used by researchers and medical professionals to monitor current research & examine the evidence before publishing.

After the data acquisition pretraining of the model done. Models construct representations of medical language that capture semantic linkages, clinical reasoning patterns, and domain-specific knowledge structures by learning to anticipate tokens in context through pre-training.

Next step is fine tuning, The act of adjusting a pre-trained model to a particular job by further training it on a smaller, domain-specific dataset is known as fine-tuning. Without requiring a large dataset or costly processing resources, it enhances the model's capabilities and increases its accuracy in specific tasks.

After the finetuning we require prompt engineering. Because it immediately affects the accuracy, relevance, and quality of generative AI outputs, prompt engineering is essential. The In-context learning (ICL) approach is an intriguing method of using LLMs after training. The model learns to handle a new task during inference by being given a prompt, which includes task examples, without any gradient change. This includes content creation, sentiment analysis, speech synthesis, and translation. By incorporating pertinent examples or guidelines into their prompts, healthcare providers can tailor model behavior for certain clinical settings, patient demographics, or medical specializations.

Figure 3. Methodology of using LLM in medical field

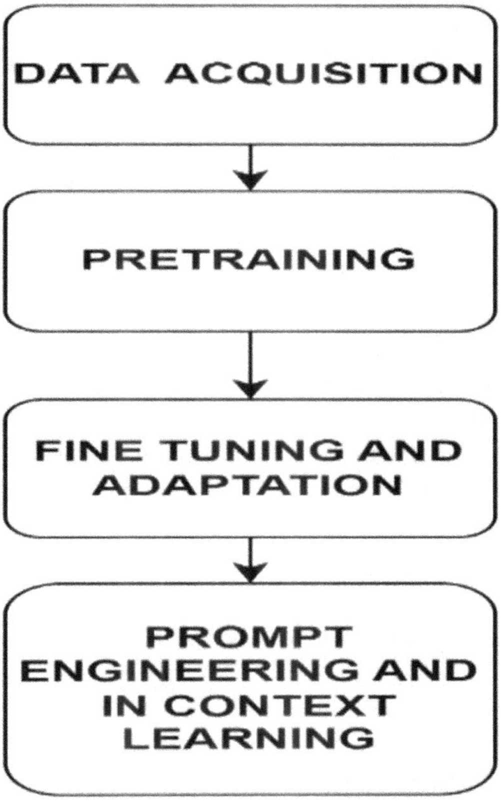

7. DATA PRIVACY, SECURITY, AND PATIENT CONFIDENTIALITY IN LLMS FOR HEALTHCARE

Patient data is the basis of smart healthcare whether it is sensitive personal, financial, medical or research data. Today people are not only to be taken care of, but also their data should be secure. This data should be stored in order to humanize healthcare. Nonetheless, frequent cyberattacks pose a range of risks to health businesses, such as operational risks when essential services are destroyed, the risk of losses due to ransom threat, and reputational losses due to breaches of information. When dealing with LLMs, the same strategy may be used in order to avoid leakage of sensitive information and ease compliance.

7.1 De-Identifying Sensitive Data for LLMs

De-identified data is swapped with tokens as part of the data collection process, and these tokens are passed along and stored within traditional application systems like databases and various logging systems.

7.2 Multi-Party Model Training

When an LLM generates a response, vault-generated deterministic tokens can be detokenized as the answer is given to the user, replacing these tokens with the original sensitive data pieces or masked data, according on the access control policies. Each company has fine-grained access control over the data kept in the data privacy vault since only authorized individuals are allowed to detokenize the sensitive data. This lets both companies in the joint venture share a de-identified dataset while retaining data governance for PII and other sensitive data that are isolated in their respective vaults. A data privacy vault gives us effective data privacy and protection across our infrastructure and systems, and throughout the entire lifecycle of LLMs.

8. LLM BIASES AND HALLUCINATIONS

Following methods are used to remove the LLM hallucination issues.

8.1 Improved Training Data

The sources of knowledge are important to LLMs. LLMs can learn from trustworthy sources by using high-quality, fact-checked data that incorporates a variety of viewpoints. Improved training lessens factual errors or innate biases that cause hallucinations.

8.2 Fact-Checking Mechanisms

A number of methods for including fact-checking into LLM response production enable models to instantly compare input to reliable sources, hence lowering the possibility of hallucinations.

8.3 Context Expansion

LLMs can produce more targeted and pertinent answers when given additional details about the topic or prompt's context. This setting reduces the possibility of inaccurate or foolish answers.

8.4 Uncertainty Quantification

By assessing the accuracy of their answers, LLMs can be taught to evaluate themselves. Users can utilize this information to spot comments that might not be trustworthy.

8.5 Regularization Techniques

Overfitting can be lessened by using LLM strategies like dropout or early ending during training. These techniques improve LLMs' ability to generalize and prevent them from depending just on patterns they have committed to memory from the training set.

9. NEW TREATMENTS IN MEDICAL FIELD USING LLMS

The following are the new treatment possibilities provided by the LLMs.

9.1 LLMS in Surgery

MedGPT's training on surgical records to produce preoperative, operation, and discharge summaries is one example of how LLMs have recently attracted interest in surgical contexts for automating note-taking and clinical recording. In addition to saving time, this enhances the quality of surgeons' records3. Additionally, LLMs have the potential to be used as intelligent chatbots for patient education, follow-up care, and remote supervision, promoting patient understanding and engagement, as well as to extract important data from patient records to help surgical decision-making. Clinical risk in using LLMs are wrong drug dosage and incorrect surgical steps.

9.2 LLMs for Mental Health

In order to fill therapeutic and research gaps in mental health care, LLMs present interesting applications (Philippe et al., 2021). LLMs have the potential to improve mental health care's efficiency, accessibility, and personalization. However, present solutions frequently ignore crucial contextual and design elements that affect acceptance and results in the real world (Higgins et al., 2023). The review emphasizes that the self-attention mechanism—a crucial part of LLMs—is insufficient on its own. To appropriately integrate LLMs into mental health care ecosystems, future research must go beyond technical viability to examine integrated care models, user experience, and longitudinal treatment outcomes. Clinical risk in using LLMs are suggesting inappropriate coping strategies and misinterpreting symptoms of serious order.

9.3 Stroke Diagnosis Using LLM

Neuroradiology big data research depends on labeled datasets, which are frequently manually retrieved from images in a labor-intensive and time-consuming process (Aggarwal et al., 2023). The sharing of medical photographs is restricted due to security concerns, even as AI advances automated analysis. An alternative is provided by radiology reports, although these need to be manually labeled. AI-assisted labeling might be useful, however LLM models have specific development for neuroimaging and diagnose a stroke with high accuracy. Clinical risk in using LLMs are lack of imaging interpretation imaging and misclassify the type of stroke.

9.4 LLMs for Structured Data Extraction From Radiology Reports

Building large-scale datasets that are used to train and assess medical AI models requires the extraction of structured labels from free-text radiological reports. LLMs can be used successfully for this purpose (Gupta et al., 2025).

9.5 A Smart Manual and Active Assistant for CT Imaging Workflows Based on LLMs

In order to operate scanners properly and efficiently, technologists doing medical imaging exams should ideally possess both profound clinical knowledge and technical expertise. However, despite a steady increase in patient numbers, there remains a dearth of highly qualified workers in radiology. As a result, intelligent support is required to simplify process modifications and lessen human labor. In order to help clinical personnel with Computed Tomography (CT) protocol and postprocessing setup, this work introduces an LLM- based chatbot that integrates clinical data particular to each patient and equipment. Clinical risk in using LLMs are may suggest nonurgent and generic responses.

9.6 LLMs for Self-Care

Everybody has challenges in their daily life, which can cause unpleasant feelings and have an impact on their wellbeing. We use conscious and unconscious coping and emotion management techniques, like actively confronting or repressing unpleasant thoughts, to deal with such challenges. This can entail a variety of methods, including using digital tools and taking walks or conversations with friends (Nazi & Peng, 2024). People are using technology more and more for self-care, including, more lately, using conversational interfaces powered by LLMs to ask for assistance. Clinical risk in using LLMs are unsafe medicine can be advised and suggest incorrect dose.

9.7 Drug Reaction Management Using LLMs

Adverse drug events (ADEs) are caused by medication errors, which present serious concerns to patient safety. An estimated 237 million such errors are made in England each year, of which about 66 million may be clinically important. These accidents result in 1708 deaths, 181,626 bed days, and an annual cost to the National Health System (NHS) of almost £98.5 million. Similar to this, prescription and administration errors have a significant economic impact in the US, where they are estimated to cost $20 billion a year.

CDSSs have come in handy in enhancing patient safety and minimizing medication errors. These technologies assist in venting potential ADEs through providing evidence-based guidance and notifications to the healthcare personnel. The conventional CDSSs however, have several disadvantages. They tend to be based on rule-based algorithms and previously fixed datasets which might overlook the nuances of particular cases of patients or the latest developments of clinical medicine. To illustrate, these systems would issue warnings to a drug with potential cross-reactions being prescribed without considering the complex clinical situations as documented in medical notes, e.g., prior patient-specific tolerance, distinguishing between true allergies and benign side effects, or risk-benefit analysis of a situation. Clinical risk in using LLMs for drug reaction management are misidentification of adverse drug reaction and inaccurate severity management.

9.8 Kidney Transplantation and Postoperative Care

Kidney transplantation requires close attention and interdisciplinary cooperation. LLMs can reduce the time spent on this process by collecting pre-transplant tests, summarizing donor compatibility reports, and immunosuppressants adherence. They are able to identify the signs of graft dysfunction at an early stage during follow-up through test reports and clinical notes. ChatGPT can be utilized to assist patients with communication to explain the side effects of medications, describe the necessity of post-transplant-diagnostic, and remind the patient to draw blood or visit the clinic. This contact is highly helpful in regions where there is a shortage of transplant specialists. As an example, a patient who is far away may discuss the importance of not taking particular over-the-counter drugs or use a model to understand how creatinine levels may vary (Tahavvori et al., 2025). Clinical risk in using LLMs in kidney transplantation is errors in Immunosuppressive Management.

9.9 Alzheimer Detection

The most common form of dementia is the Alzheimer disease (AD). It is characterized by mental impairment, forgetfulness and deviant behavior. Through in-depth analysis and integration of a number of data sources such as clinical data, neuroimaging and genetic data, LLMs have a greater potential of early and more precise diagnosis of AD, detecting subtle cognitive characteristics which Conventional approaches may overlook. Fine-grained linguistic analysis is also provided by LLDs, which is more accurate in diagnosing language-related cognitive impairment. Clinical risk in using LLMs are unnecessary testing and costs a, social stigma and labeling.

9.10 Multiple Sclerosis

The central nervous system (CNS) is affected by multiple sclerosis (MS), an acquired autoimmune disease that primarily affects young individuals. The neurodegenerative disease multiple sclerosis causes axonal degeneration and demyelination in the central nervous system.

Similar to other neurological disorders, LLMs have promise for precise diagnosis and appropriate management of MS, hence supporting doctors in clinical evaluation. Clinical risk in using LLMs misinterprets nonspecific symptoms like (fatique, symtoms) and provide generic output without proper differential diagnosis.

9.11 Parkinson's Disease

LLMs can analyse massive amounts of data and include useful feedback in the form of near real-time insights, which allows development of a consistent ontology of Parkinson disease PD monitoring. Moreover, LLMs are effective at managing the practice of PD, as it personalizes the patient with his or her requirements and adjusts the dosage and frequency of medicines. Clinical risk in using LLMs are, miss early sign and provide delayed and inappropriate advice.

9.12 Diagnostic Support in Oral Diseases

The diagnosis of dental disorders is often performed with the help of clinical examination and interpretation of the text data, such as case notes, patient history, and test results. In the diagnosis process, LLMs can be used to compile and contextualize the information, although the radiographs and histology slides are not analyzed. When assessing a patient with the chronic toothache, a dentist might apply ChatGPT to review the alternative diagnoses that may correspond to the symptoms and medical history of the patient. The model could include the list of similarities between pain related to sinus, periapical abscess and chronic pulpitis before rendering the overview of the key differences and the treatment choices. This type of support makes professional judgment stronger instead of replacing it as professional judgment, by facilitating critical thinking. LLMs have the ability to relate dental information with possible underlying conditions to present systemic manifestations of oral disease, including oral signs of diabetes or anemia. This is because the ability to cross-reference the information of the dentistry and medical spheres allows specialists to treat the patients more holistically. Clinical risks in using LLMs misclassify benign lesions as malignant and early sign of cancer.

9.13 Antimicrobial Stewardship and Rational Therapy

Antimicrobial resistance continues to be a major worldwide concern. Antibiotic abuse and misuse hasten the emergence of resistant strains. By ensuring that the diagnosis, culture results, and selected antibiotics are compatible, LLMs can aid in the promotion of sensible medication. LLMs can create case-based exercises to teach junior physicians or students how to choose antibiotics. They are able to talk about possible connections and describe pharmacological mechanisms. Clinical risk is LLMs can recommend broad spectrum antibiotics unnecessarily and choose ineffective drugs for specific pathogens.

9.14 Dialysis Management

Dialysis is a process that consumes a lot of data. Each of the sessions provides us with the data concerning the disappearance of biochemical results, the speed of blood flow, and the volumes of ultrafiltration. Browsing and interpreting such information of all patients may be a lengthy process. LLMs could analyze and summarize these daily data and point out any possible change that may need medical care. They may, as an example, determine regular cases of hypotension or low clearance rates, which would lead to a change of thought regarding the dialysis prescription. ChatGPT may be a readily available companion to people undergoing home dialysis. It will help them interpret machine readings, remember about hygienic procedures and guide them through set ups. These characteristics are capable of increasing compliance and reducing fear. Moreover, a conversational style of a model stimulates patients to engage in self-care as learning becomes less formal and engaging (Jaiswal et al., 2023).

9.15 Management of Epilepsy

A persistent brain condition that can strike at any age is epilepsy. It has a number of causes and is typified by seizures that can take many different shapes (Goel et al., 2025). Early and precise epilepsy diagnosis is possible thanks to LLMs' ability to extract clinical data from a variety of text sources, including patient reports and medical records. Furthermore, LLMs enable professionals build and fine-tune an LLM that provides a novel way to retrieve seizure frequency data from electronic health records, giving clinicians more precise information about how frequently patients have seizures.

customized therapy regimens based on the state of each patient and the disorder's stage by examining the copious amounts of clinical data that are already accessible. Clinical risk in using LLMs Misinterpret symptoms such as fainting or psychological episodes and Confuse seizures with conditions like Syncope or Psychogenic non-epileptic seizures.

10. CHALLENGES OF LLMS IN HEALTHCARE AND MEDICAL FIELD

As LLMs get more sophisticated, they are more likely to produce offensive or dangerous information, like such as racial hate speech, hallucinations, and spam. Additionally, these models could generate answers that seem reasonable but are erroneous or ludicrous.

10.1 Data Security and Privacy Preserving

Private and demographic information about patient records may unintentionally be disclosed in medical reports. Achieving the best possible medical results can be easier than protecting patient privacy and following data security laws.

10.2 Incorrectness and Risk of Inaccurate Information

After being trained on vast amounts of online data, LLMs show significant promise in carrying out a wide range of tasks that normally need human capabilities. However, this training could unintentionally incorporate biased and false information, which could have serious negative effects such producing false or inaccurate information (Wang & Zhang, 2024).

10.3 Fairness and Bias

Institutions in wealthy, English-speaking nations usually provide the training data for LLMs, which may significantly reduce the representativeness of perspectives from other parts of the world. In high-income nations, this may result in biases in the mechanistic theories of health and illness. For instance, doctors in Africa may concentrate on treatment models that are exclusive to high-income nations when using LLMs to create diabetes treatment programs. Structural bias and unfair treatment may result from the disparity between the model's output and the diagnosis of experienced medical experts. Therefore, when creating models and algorithms, it is crucial to recognize any risks and deviations that could impact physicians, patients, and healthcare professionals. One drawback of LLMs is that discriminating results may be sustained even after the model has been recalibrated if biased data is used for training (Gallegos et al., 2024).

10.4 Transparency, Explainability, and Accountability

Smart healthcare relies heavily on the interpretability and explainability of AI models employed in clinical risk prediction and medical imaging analysis. Clinical suggestion validation may be hampered by a lack of explainability and transparency. In order to improve the decision-making process, good governance places a strong emphasis on interpretable frameworks and continuing or continuous explainability. Clinicians must comprehend how medical disorders are caused as well as the models and techniques used to aid in decision-making. Explainability must be taken into account, along with the possibility for AI applications to function autonomously and any unforeseen repercussions. Ensuring data security, privacy, and secrecy can improve the reliability of AI models (Jain & Jaiswal, 2025).

10.5 Cost and Potential Human Resource

Generative AI LLM has serious operational and economic challenges to its deployment in medical and healthcare settings. The expensive nature of these models, requiring both complex processing hardware such as GPUs or TPUs and an effective data management structure to ensure reliable and secure model execution is a major obstacle. The expense of having these systems is augmented with the complexity of managing systems, larger storage capacity and updating at a high rate. The lack of skilled employees is also problematic. The collaboration of LLMs within health care requires personnel with high AI competence and who have a strong knowledge base in their fields. These specialists are already scarce, although such a duality of skills is required to interpret the results of LLM correctly and apply them to a clinical situation. This specialist workforce that is required to make its widespread usage makes it difficult and also creates extra training requirements on the current healthcare staff. Such models can also significantly boost the productivity and reduce the amount of effort, yet they can also lead to the restructuring of existing job factors. Due to disruptions that may affect the workforce, there is a need to plan strategically and up-skill to minimize the risk of losing a job. In order to reap all the benefits of AI-based products in the smart healthcare sector and to avoid taking away the employment opportunities, it is absolutely crucial to maintain the balance between the technical innovations and the prudent staffing control.

11. CONCLUSION

ChatGPT and other large language models have great potential to revolutionize the treatment of autoimmune disorders. They are useful allies for both patients and clinicians because to their ability to comprehend language, process information, and provide coherent communication. They improve efficiency and accessibility across several aspects of care by helping with diagnosis, treatment planning, documentation, research, and education. Although there are still issues with privacy, bias, and accuracy, these problems can be lessened with appropriate integration and supervision. LLMs will become more integrated into healthcare systems as technology advances, enhancing rather than displacing human skill. These technologies provide a means of bringing clarity to communication and structure to complicated, long-term problems like autoimmune disorders, where language, data, and emotion interact. They could contribute to redefining the practice of individualized, knowledgeable, and compassionate clinical medicine with continued development and responsible application. Additionally, by addressing issues with justice, accountability, privacy, and robustness, the article has emphasized the critical significance of the reliable and secure deployment of medical LLMs. It has brought attention to the necessity of thorough assessment, ethical issues, and the creation of legal frameworks. In order to assist the appropriate expansion of medical LLMs, the review has identified promising future research topics, including as algorithmic breakthroughs, market reforms, and policy developments. Before the models can be used in clinical settings, these recommendations usually concentrate on validating them through rigorous clinical studies to make sure they fulfill certain safety, effectiveness, and ethical standards. On the other hand, LLMs have enormous growth potential in the medical field. By combining virtual and augmented reality, they can improve patient experiences, provide thorough medical advice through multimodal research, and use theory of mind to humanize doctor-patient interactions. We expect significant increases in the processing speed and accuracy of LLMs due to continuous developments in algorithms and computer capacity.

12. FUTURE DIRECTION

In order to increase diagnostic accuracy, we advise future research to concentrate on the creation of multimodal LLMs that integrate text, imaging, and other medical data. Oncology, radiology, medical imaging, cardiology, and other domains may benefit from domain-specific models that are adapted to their particular requirements. Additionally, human-AI hybrid systems that allow physicians to monitor or engage with LLM outputs could reduce hallucinations and increase clinical trust. Furthermore, in order to ensure safe and successful integration into healthcare systems, research on the ethical issues surrounding LLMs—particularly with regard to data privacy and bias—will be essential. Better benchmarking norms and regulations specific to medical LLMs are also essential in order to ensure safe, equitable and repeatable implementation in care settings. However, in order to make the most out of the revolutionary potential of the use of the LLPs, their effective application will be determined by the ability to eliminate these challenges. Lawmakers, AI researchers, and medical practitioners have to work together to exploit these models completely and still ensure patient safety and ethical standards are observed.

REFERENCES

Abd-Alrazaq, A., AlSaad, R., Alhuwail, D., Ahmed, A., Healy, P., Latifi, S., Aziz, S., Damseh, R., Alrazak, S., & Sheikh, J. (2023). Large language models in medical education: Opportunities, challenges, and future directions. *JMIR Medical Education, 9*, e48291. Advance online publication. DOI: 10.2196/48291 PMID: 37261894

Aggarwal, K., Manso Jimeno, M., Ravi, K. S., Gonzalez, G., & Geethanath, S. (2023). Developing and deploying deep learning models in brain magnetic resonance imaging: A review. *NMR in Biomedicine, 36*(12), e5014. DOI: 10.1002/nbm.5014 PMID: 37539775

Ahammad, S. H., Kalangi, R. R., Nagendram, S., Inthiyaz, S., Priya, P. P., Faragallah, O. S., Mohammad, A., Eid, M. M. A., & Rashed, A. N. Z. (2024). Improved neural machine translation using natural language processing (NLP). *Multimedia Tools and Applications, 83*(13), 39335–39348. DOI: 10.1007/s11042-023-17207-7

Ahmed, S., Nielsen, I. E., Tripathi, A., Siddiqui, S., Ramachandran, R. P., & Rasool, G. (2023). Transformers in time-series analysis: A tutorial. *Circuits, Systems, and Signal Processing, 42*(12), 7433–7466. DOI: 10.1007/s00034-023-02454-8

Artsi, Y., Sorin, V., Glicksberg, B., Korfiatis, P., Nadkarni, G., & Klang, E. (2025). Large language models in real-world clinical workflows: A systematic review of applications and implementation. *Frontiers in Digital Health, 7*, 1659134. Advance online publication. DOI: 10.3389/fdgth.2025.1659134 PMID: 41098649

Bhatnagar, A., & Singh, K. (2024). Hypertension detection system using machine learning. In *Prediction in medicine: The impact of machine learning on healthcare* (p. 95). https://doi.org/DOI: 10.2174/9789815305128124010009

Cascella, M., Semeraro, F., Montomoli, J., Bellini, V., Piazza, O., & Bignami, E. (2024). The breakthrough of large language models release for medical applications: 1-year timeline and perspectives. *Journal of Medical Systems, 48*(1), 22. Advance online publication. DOI: 10.1007/s10916-024-02045-3 PMID: 38366043

Chen, Z., Lin, M., Wang, Z., Zang, M., & Bai, Y. (2024). PreparedLLM: Effective pre-pretraining framework for domain-specific large language models. *Big Earth Data, 8*(4), 649–672. DOI: 10.1080/20964471.2024.2396159

Desbordes, T., King, J., & Dehaene, S. (2024). Tracking the neural codes for words and phrases during semantic composition, working-memory storage, and retrieval. *Cell Reports, 43*(3), 113847. DOI: 10.1016/j.celrep.2024.113847 PMID: 38412098

Gaber, F., Shaik, M., Allega, F., Bilecz, A., Busch, F., Goon, K., Franke, V., & Akalin, A. (2025). Evaluating large language model workflows in clinical decision support for triage and referral and diagnosis. *NPJ Digital Medicine*, *8*(1), 263. Advance online publication. DOI: 10.1038/s41746-025-01684-1 PMID: 40346344

Gallegos, I. O., Rossi, R. A., Barrow, J., Tanjim, M. M., Kim, S., Dernoncourt, F., & Ahmed, N. K. (2024). Bias and fairness in large language models: A survey. *Computational Linguistics*, *50*(3), 1097–1179. DOI: 10.1162/coli_a_00524

Goel, R., Jaiswal, U. K., Singh, P., Yadav, S. P., & Upadhyay, P. (2025). Deep learning for early brain tumor detection: A Keras-Based approach using MRI and CT imaging. In *Demystifying the role of natural Language processing (NLP) in mental health* (pp. 145-180). IGI Global Scientific Publishing. DOI: 10.4018/979-8-3693-4203-9.ch009

Griot, M., Hemptinne, C., Vanderdonckt, J., & Yüksel, D. (2024). Impact of high-quality, mixed-domain data on the performance of medical language models. *Journal of the American Medical Informatics Association : JAMIA*, *31*(9), 1875–1883. Advance online publication. DOI: 10.1093/jamia/ocae120 PMID: 38781312

Guo, H., Xing, X., Zhou, Y., Jiang, W., Chen, X., Wang, T., Jiang, Z., Wang, Y., Hou, J., Jiang, Y., & Xu, J. (2025). A survey of large language model for drug research and development. *IEEE Access : Practical Innovations, Open Solutions*, *13*, 51110–51129. DOI: 10.1109/ACCESS.2025.3552256

Gupta, G. K., Singh, A., Manikandan, S. V., & Ehtesham, A. (2025). Digital diagnostics: The potential of large language models in recognizing symptoms of common illnesses. *AI*, *6*(1), 13. DOI: 10.3390/ai6010013

Higgins, O., Short, B., Chalup, S., & Wilson, R. (2023). Artificial intelligence (AI) and machine learning (ML) based decision support systems in mental health: An integrative review. *International Journal of Mental Health Nursing*, *32*(4), 966–978. Advance online publication. DOI: 10.1111/inm.13114 PMID: 36744684

Jain, J., & Jaiswal, U. K. (2025). Revolutionizing Medicine: The Impact of Artificial Intelligence in Healthcare. In *Generative Intelligence in Healthcare* (pp. 176-209). CRC Press.

Jaiswal, U. K., Chauhan, A., & Gupta, R. (2023). Brain Tumor Recognition Leveraging Machine Learning and CNN. In *International Conference on Artificial-Business Analytics, Quantum and Machine Learning* (pp. 53-65). Singapore: Springer Nature Singapore.

Jung, K. H. (2025). Large language models in medicine: Clinical applications, technical challenges, and ethical considerations. *Healthcare Informatics Research*, *31*(2), 114–124. DOI: 10.4258/hir.2025.31.2.114 PMID: 40384063

Khader, F., Müller-Franzes, G., Wang, T., Han, T., Arasteh, S., Haarburger, C., Stegmaier, J., Bressem, K., Kuhl, C., Nebelung, S., Kather, J., & Truhn, D. (2024). Multimodal deep learning for integrating chest radiographs and clinical parameters: A case for transformers. *Radiology*, *309*(1), e230806. DOI: 10.1148/radiol.230806 PMID: 37787671

Liu, J., Cen, X., Yi, C., Wang, F., Ding, J., Cheng, J., Wu, Q., Gai, B., Zhou, Y., He, R., Gao, F., & Li, Y. (2025). Challenges in AI-driven biomedical multimodal data fusion and analysis. *Genomics, Proteomics & Bioinformatics*, *23*(1), qzaf011. Advance online publication. DOI: 10.1093/gpbjnl/qzaf011 PMID: 40036568

. Lysyi, P. (2025). Principles of large language models (LLM). *Journal of Numerical and Applied Mathematics*. https://doi.org/DOI: 10.17721/2706-9699.2025.1.06

Madzime, R., & Nyirenda, C. (2024). Enhanced electronic health records text summarization using large language models. *arXiv*. https://doi.org//arxiv.2410.09628DOI: 10.48550

Maurya, S., Asudani, D. S., Jain, J., Jaiswal, U. K., Jain, E., & Malviya, K. (2025). Evaluating the effectiveness of regression algorithms in predicting cancer progression. In *Parul University International Conference on Engineering and Technology 2025 (PiCET 2025)* (Vol. 2025, pp. 1367-1373). IET. DOI: 10.1049/icp.2025.1593

Nazi, Z. A., & Peng, W. (2024). Large language models in healthcare and medical domain: A review. *Informatics (MDPI)*, *11*(3), 57. DOI: 10.3390/informatics11030057

Nivethitha, V., Daniel, R., Surya, B., & Logeswari, G. (2025). Empowering public health: Leveraging AI for early detection, treatment, and disease prevention in communities—A scoping review. *Journal of Postgraduate Medicine*, *71*(2), 74–81. DOI: 10.4103/jpgm.jpgm_634_24 PMID: 40488301

Philippe, T., Sikder, N., Jackson, A., Koblanski, M., Liow, E., Pilarinos, A., & Vasarhelyi, K. (2021). Digital health interventions for delivery of mental health care: Systematic and comprehensive meta-review. *JMIR Mental Health*, *9*(5), e35159. Advance online publication. DOI: 10.2196/35159 PMID: 35551058

Saeidnia, H. R. (2024). Foundations of artificial intelligence in healthcare. *Decision Making*, *1*(2), 5.

Shad, R., Klinton, B., & Potter, K. (2025). *The role of artificial intelligence in early disease detection: A review of current applications*. FMDB Transactions on Sustainable Health Science Letters., DOI: 10.69888/FTSHSL.2025.000361

Shammi, S., Ghosh, P., Sutradhar, A., Shamrat, F., Moni, M., & Oliveira, T. (2025). Advances in artificial intelligence and blockchain technologies for early detection of human diseases. *IEEE Transactions on Computational Social Systems*, *12*(1), 210–237. DOI: 10.1109/TCSS.2024.3449748

Shool, S., Adimi, S., Amleshi, R., Bitaraf, E., Golpira, R., & Tara, M. (2025). A systematic review of large language model (LLM) evaluations in clinical medicine. *BMC Medical Informatics and Decision Making*, *25*(1), 117. Advance online publication. DOI: 10.1186/s12911-025-02954-4 PMID: 40055694

Singhal, K., Azizi, S., Tu, T., Mahdavi, S., Wei, J., Chung, H., Scales, N., Tanwani, A., Cole-Lewis, H., Pfohl, S., Payne, P., Seneviratne, M., Gamble, P., Kelly, C., Scharli, N., Chowdhery, A., Mansfield, P., Arcas, B., Webster, D., & Natarajan, V. (2022). Large language models encode clinical knowledge. *Nature*, *620*(7972), 172–180. DOI: 10.1038/s41586-023-06291-2 PMID: 37438534

Sun, Z., Wong, Y., & Yeong, C. (2023). Patient-specific 3D-printed low-cost models in medical education and clinical practice. *Micromachines*, *14*(2), 464. Advance online publication. DOI: 10.3390/mi14020464 PMID: 36838164

Tahavvori, A., Chelan, R. J., Aminoleslami, S., Moghadam, O. F., Haghighi, L., Abdian, Y., & Moradi, D. (2025). Large language models and ChatGPT in medical sciences: Foundations, capabilities, and challenges. *Kindle*, *5*(1), 1–222.

Wang, D., & Zhang, S. (2024). Large language models in medical and healthcare fields: Applications, advances, and challenges. *Artificial Intelligence Review*, *57*(11), 299. DOI: 10.1007/s10462-024-10921-0

Xu, M., Cai, D., Yin, W., Wang, S., Jin, X., & Liu, X. (2024). Resource-efficient algorithms and systems of foundation models: A survey. *ACM Computing Surveys*, *57*(5), 1–39. DOI: 10.1145/3706418

Zhang, H., Qi, Y., Xu, H., & Lv, R. (2025). Multimodal deep learning method based on multiple spectra for lung cancer early diagnosis. *Spectrochimica Acta. Part A: Molecular and Biomolecular Spectroscopy*, *346*, 126932. DOI: 10.1016/j.saa.2025.126932 PMID: 40957203

Chapter 4
Navigating Trust and Acceptance:
Exploring Healthcare Professionals' Perspectives on AI-Assisted Diagnostic Tools

Shubhangi Bajaj Bag
http://orcid.org/0009-0003-0274-2251
Amity University, Kolkata, India

Pooja Kumari
University of Petroleum and Energy Studies, Dehradun, India

Annirudh Vashishtha
University of Petroleum and Energy Studies, Dehradun, India

Manisha Madhav
University of Petroleum and Energy Studies, Dehradun, India

ABSTRACT

The sudden spike in Artificial Intelligence (AI) attention has prompted investigations of its uses in healthcare domain, specifically in medical imaging and diagnostics. In this chapter, a qualitative case study explores the level of trust healthcare providers have in diagnostic artificial intelligence systems and the factor behind this case is described. The study provides essential preconditions of achieving clinical confidence in the form of the interviews with the participants working in various clinical positions and experience levels. The results demonstrate that the degree of trust depends on personal experience, but the high level of trust is usually provided

DOI: 10.4018/979-8-2600-2173-6.ch004

under the condition of the meeting of some certain conditions. The main assumptions of such findings lie in the fact that AI is not a substitute tool to human judgment, but a decision stressor.

INTRODUCTION

The digital revolution has basically reorganized the paradigms in the world, and it affects even simple day to day activities as well as complex professional activities. AI is a future game changer, but it can have far-reaching influences with various industries such as product development, manufacturing, and healthcare being some of these spheres (Dlamini et.al., 2020). Although wearable technology and algorithmic marketing are methods of introducing AI to the personal world, there is the crushing inevitability that both will be needed in the future to replace humans in many areas (Adabi & Berada 2018; Bajene 2020). However, this integration requires even a more critical study of ethical principles and privacy safeguards (Lockey 2021). The effective implementation of these technologies is thus based on the development of strong trust on the developers and even on the algorithm frameworks themselves. The concept of AI is defined by the simulation of human cognitive processes, that is, learning and problem-solving, in computational systems aimed at doing what only the human mind could be. (Pesapani, Codari & Sardanelli 2018; Glikson & Woolley 2020). Being more efficient than the biological mind in processing information, AI makes it possible to achieve optimized results and cut down on human labor (Glikson & Woolley 2020, Lamb et.al., 2022; Ericksson et.al., 2018). Though the discourse of futuristic type often focuses on the so-called General AI, which can perform all activities as good as humans do and even better, this possibility is hypothetical and is unlikely to become a reality until the 2040s (Glikson & Woolley 2020; Băjenesc 2020). The existing applications can be limited to Narrow AI that means specific tasks, using learning protocols, but without explicit programming (Băjenesc 2020). These systems also are further divided into automated AI, which automatically replaces human work, and augmented AI, which can be used as a decision-support mechanism to optimize human performance (Lockey et.al., 2021).

The re-emergence of AI in the clinical environment and especially in radiology can be seen because of the inability to make new progress following the late 20th-century stagnation due to the high false-positive rates in the initial image analysis (Ericksson et.al., 2018; Chan, Samala & Hadjiiski 2019; Lamb et.al., 2022). The modern reality is characterized by the astute rise in the volume of data due to advanced modalities in the form of CT, MRI, and PET scans, accompanied by the shortage of qualified radiologists around the world (Ericksson et.al., 2018; Lamb et.al., 2022). Therefore, the AI-based diagnostic systems capable of working with these large volumes of data in a better way and faster are in high demand (Dlamini et.al., 2020; Gille, Jobin & Ienca 2020). Newer versions of these systems are based on deep learning, which is a variation on representation learning but involves the use of multi-layered neural networks to autodetect and abstract data patterns, thus being able to make medical interventions earlier and more accurate (Chan, Samala & Hadjiiski 2019; Bera et al., 2019). Algorithms can be trained on large datasets to perform multiple layers of data and achieve intricate mathematical representations that possess the ability to extract information with a high degree of accuracy and variability (Chan, Samala & Hadjiiski 2019; Ericksson et.al., 2018). Since the deep learning approaches can be used without explicit guidance, the human resources needed to develop them are significantly less compared to the efforts of historical computational models (Ericksson et.al., 2018). The main aim is to incorporate them into clinical practices- triage and the early screenings, in order to maximize the efficiency of the system (Asan, Bayrak & Choudhury 2020; Dlamini 2020). Although such algorithms, synthesized thousands of historical data, can detect oncological risks more precisely than a human practitioner (Gao et. al., 2019), in fact, empirical studies indicate that, AI and human expertise work together in the most effective way to diagnose (Dlamini et.al., 2020).

In addition to technical reliability and statistical accuracy, the implementation of the diagnostic AI should be successful because healthcare professionals are also required to be willing to adopt the technology (Lamb et.al., 2022). Although the earlier versions of the Technology Acceptance Model have mainly paid attention to technical utility, recent studies posit that trust is an important predictor of acceptance in the clinical context (Glikson & Woolley 2020; Gille, Jobin & Ienca 2020). Trust is a relative, complex concept, but it is interdisciplinary and there are two key elements that are the positive expectations about the results and readiness to accept the vulnerability (Lockey et.al. 2021, McKnight et.al. 2011, Fulmer & Gelfand 2012, Mayer, Davis & Schoorman 1995; Jacovi et.al., 2021). In this model, trust can only prevail once the party that places the trust thinks there is a risk of losing it (Fulmer & Gelfand 2012). Human-machine trust is psychologically different compared to interpersonal trust (Andras et al., 2018). Such a belief in a machine is associated with a unique vulnerability; since autonomous systems do not possess intentionality and structured communication, users disproportionately focus on performance (Adabi & Berrada 2018; Lockey 2021). Therefore, the tolerance of the error in the algorithms is much lower than that of humans (Malle & Ullman 2021; LaRosa & Danks 2018). Although AI is expected to provide faster diagnoses and minimize the administrative load (Dlamini et.al., 2020; Miller & Brown 2018), it relies on the acceptance of its users (Gille, Jobin & Ienca 2020). Due to the stakes of the healthcare sector, where the consequences of care safety are unconditional, the perception of trust is much tighter than in other industries but by no means (LaRosa & Danks 2018; Sunarti

2020). The existing study aims at bridging the gap in knowledge regarding how healthcare professionals view those tools, including whether the AI system requires functioning as an independent decision-maker or a supportive system (Chan, Samala & Hadjiiski 2019; Lamb et.al. 2022). The two major questions examined as a part of this inquiry are the degree to which professionals are trusting AI-based diagnostic tools and the precise factors that determine this trust. Such attitudes are the key ingredient to grasp because the alleged benefits of AI will only be theoretical unless the practitioners have a level of confidence that they can apply them in their day-to-day practice as clinicians.

THEORETICAL FRAMEWORK

Furthermore, trust is subjectively bound up in conceptualization which makes its definition impossible. The present analysis utilizes a well-known interdisciplinary framework in which trust is based on two main pillars, which include, first, the ability to maintain a positive expectation, and second, a corresponding willingness to be vulnerable (Lockey et.al., 2021; McKnight et.al., 2011; Fulmer and Gelfand 2012; Mayer, Davis & Schoorman 1995; Jacovi et.al., 2021). The positive expectations are considerations about how the party of trust will behave; this is most importantly pegged by empirical fact to tell between functional trust and blind trust or just hope (Lockey et.al. 2021; Fulmer & Gelfand 2012). On the contrary, vulnerability acceptance perceives the uncertainties and the deficiencies that can be inherent in the party of trust (Fulmer & Gelfand 2012). Since only situations entailing the risk of loss or injury can be considered as having trust as a variable, the aspect of risk is an invariable part of this exchange (Fulmer & Gelfand 2012; McKnight et.al., 2011).

Trust in the clinical setting is a conclusive factor when using AI. Although the motivation behind the integration of AI is that of systemic value, its high likelihood to cause harm to patients through algorithmic error and jeopardizing data security remains a high risk. In the same way that a clinician can experience a lapse in judgment thus making a misdiagnosis, an AI diagnostic system can also give false forecasts (Sunarti et.al., 2020). Nevertheless, trust in AI is not like interpersonal or classical machine trust (Andras et al., 2018; Adabi & Berrada 2018; Malle & Ullman 2021). Technical systems are non-intentional, which fundamentally changes the attitudes to honesty and goodwill (Asan, Bayrak & Choudhury 2021). Moreover, the AI does not interact with people as well as human interaction does, and its communication barriers are unique and make it more difficult to establish a common language (Lockey et.al., 2021).

The quality of interpersonal trust is frequently fostered in the form of social interaction, but the trust in AI is practically performance-based (Malle & Ullman

2021). As a result, the positive expectations in relation to an AI system are elicited through the documented records of accuracy and predictability, without any element of social flair (Lockey et.al., 2021). This result-focused dependence creates two-sided risks of overconfidence and distrust. Overconfidence occurs when a user mistakenly believes the AI to be more correct than him or her and might end up abusing the system (Okamura & Yamada 2020). Meanwhile, lack of trust is the situation when a human user does not appreciate the quality of a superior AI system (Okamura & Yamada 2020). The goal is not, in other words, to maximize trust but to reach an optimal level of trust- a state of calibration, where the users of the system, through rigorous training and systemic knowledge, depend on the system at the point of its actual capabilities (Asan, Bayrak & Choudhury 2021; Malle & Ullman 2021; Okamura & Yamada 2020). Moreover, the design of human-AI interaction, such as a friendly user interface and integration of workflows, plays a key role in building trust.

FACTORS THAT INFLUENCE TRUST IN AI

The cognition of clinician trust would also need to consider the cognitive heuristics that affect decision-making within highly automated settings. One of the key issues is automation bias, a cognitive bias according to which medical workers can overuse or even refer to automated diagnostic advice even in the case of opposing clinical facts (Abdelwanis et al., 2024). Technical accuracy alone does not resolve this cognitive risk and needs active and structured risk assessments and human-AI interface designed in such a way that it fosters critical involvement over passive acceptance (Abdelwanis et al., 2024). As a way of avoiding under-trust (skepticism) and over-trust (complacency) within a clinical context, it is necessary to acknowledge these psychological trust frameworks (Hasanzadeh et al., 2025).

Transparency and Explainability

The synthesis presented below outlines the key players of trust towards AI in the clinical sphere, with six different types of influence being identified. Among the main terms of the discussion sphere are transparency and explainability, which is a vital aspect in all AI applications (Gille, Jobin & Ienca 2020; Lockey et.al.2021; Burrell 2016). Algorithms that do not give a distinguishable explanation of their results are classified as "black boxes" this is metaphoric meaning that the learning and reasoning mechanisms of certain models are hard to understand (Adabi & Berrada 2018; Burrell 2016; Gille, Jobin & Ienca 2020). Although these black box algorithms are often linked to high efficiency and quality of deep learning, they also give rise to major issues of accountability and transparency (Gille, Jobin & Ienca 2020). The creation of explicability in machine learning is thus a primary requirement that the user must determine to authenticate and entrust a source of computations (Andras et al., 2018; Lockey et.al., 2021; Burrell 2016, Glikson & Woolley 2020).

Precision and Reliability

The lack of transparency is especially acute in medical analysis because, when making clinical decisions, a variety of variables of backgrounds must be taken into consideration. Practitioners need to be equipped to be sure that every relevant aspect is considered to get the right diagnosis (Lockey et.al., 2021; Adadi & Berrada 2018; Glickson & Woolley 2020). In addition, the pillars of trust are represented by technical precision and reliability (Lockey et.al., 2020). Due to the lack of human goodness and goodwill in AI systems, their accuracy and performance become the main measures according to which they are assessed (Malle & Ullman 2021; LaRosa & Danks 2018). Miscarriage of results does not only worsen the user experience; it ushers biases and inequalities, which present direct risks to patient safety. There is thus empirical evidence pointing at a positive correlation between the corruption of reliability, and the following loss of user confidence (Lockey et.al., 2021). It is critical to draw the line between trust and reliability because the latter is not necessarily associated with the former (Gille, Jobin & Ienca 2020). The difficulty of trustworthiness is further heightened due to the evolving nature of AI; as these systems keep encountering new data over time, their behaviours change, although their functionality does not (Asan, Bayrak & Choudhury 2021; Glikson & Woolley 2020). This volatility in behavioral products over time is a special dilemma in the healthcare industry where consistency and foreseeability are most important to the professionalism & security of patients.

Automation vs Augmentation

This difference between automated and augmented systems is instrumental in clinical integration of technology. Manifested in automated AI, there are major risks involved, where it is demonstrated that such systems may lead to overconfidence, especially among the lower-experienced users (Lockey et.al. 2021; Lysaght et.al. 2019). In the high-risk clinical setting, there is an urgent reason to be concerned about how automation will divert the basic doctor patient relationship (Lockey et.al., 2021). This fear is supported by qualitative data in which medical workers were found to fear the loss of patient rapport of the system, whether it is used as an autonomous decision-maker or an augmented support mechanism (Buck et.al., 2022). Human professionals will still be the best in requiring and producing contextual conditions and social signals- components of care that are highly hard to calculate using algorithms (Lysaght et.al., 2019). As a result, the current agreement stipulates that AI is to serve as a supplement, but not as a substitute for the risk evaluation of a dying specialist (Lockey et.al., 2021; Lysaght et.al., 2019). This will maintain the human-centric aspect of human medicine and take advantage of the computational capabilities of technology.

Data Security and Privacy

The problem of data security and privacy is one of the rare AI challenges mainly due to the high costs associated with training, and using these systems require large quantities of data (Lockey et.al., 2021). Research in this niche is newly emerging, and perceived loss of privacy and sharing of information without the consent of the user has been observed to be an inhibitor to user trust (Buck et.al., 2022; Lockey et.al., 2021; Sunarti et.al., 2021). When it comes to the medical industry, one should assume that any personal data can possibly be identified so the strong protection regulations and disclosure of the source of training data should be guaranteed (Hamid 2016). The fear of data leaks or abuse also shapes clinical attitudes greatly and affects the entire receptivity to AI significantly (Buck et.al., 2022). On the contrary, a high availability of patient information with security, standardization, and thus, transparency, and consequently, trust may promote the latter (Asan, Bayrak & Choudhury 2021).

Lack of Knowledge

This difference between automated and augmented systems is instrumental in clinical integration of technology. Manifested in automated AI, there are major risks involved, where it is demonstrated that such systems may lead to overconfidence, especially among the lower-experienced users (Lockey et.al., 2021, Lysaght et.al., 2019). In the high-risk clinical setting, there is an urgent reason to be concerned about how automation will divert the basic doctor patient relationship (Lockey et.al., 2021). This fear is supported by qualitative data in which medical workers were found to fear the loss of patient rapport of the system, whether it is used as an autonomous decision-maker or an augmented support mechanism (Buck et.al., 2022). Human professionals will still be the best in requiring and producing contextual conditions and social signals- components of care that are highly hard to calculate using algorithms (Lysaght et.al., 2019). As a result, the current agreement stipulates that AI is to serve as a supplement, but not as a substitute to the risk evaluation of a dying specialist (Lockey et.al., 2021; Lysaght et.al., 2019). This will maintain the human-centric aspect of human medicine and take advantage of the computational capabilities of technology.

Working Conditions

The problem of data security and privacy is one of the rare AI challenges mainly due to the high costs associated with training, and using these systems require large quantities of data (Lockey et.al., 2021). Research in this niche is newly emerging, and perceived loss of privacy and sharing of information without the consent of the user has been observed to be an inhibitor to user trust (Buck et.al., 2022; Lockey et.al., 2021; Sunarti et.al., 2021). When it comes to the medical industry, one should assume that any personal data can possibly be identified so the strong protection regulations and disclosure of the source of training data should be guaranteed (Hamid 2016). The fear of data leaks or abuse also shapes clinical attitudes greatly and affects the entire receptivity to AI significantly (Buck et.al., 2022). On the contrary, a high availability of patient information with security, standardization, and thus, transparency, and consequently, trust may promote the latter (Asan, Bayrak & Choudhury 2021).

METHODOLOGY

In the investigation of the degree of trust related to AI-assisted diagnosis systems, I would use a qualitative case study methodology. It is a specific methodology used especially to outline the subjective experience and reality of individuals in their natural setting and in which depth of interpretation is given precedence over statistical extrapolation (Saldana 2013). With the application of a descriptive and interpretivist paradigm of research, we will observe information systems in a larger social context of surroundings that we know that reality is no longer a singular objective truth but as a creation influenced by the factors of the social environment and individual opinions (Oates 2006; Checkland & Holwell 1998; Heron 1996). These methods enabled data collection by using semi-structured interviews, which enable one to explore complex feelings in detail and descriptive characteristics that cannot be answered in questionnaire (Oates 2006). Such interviews had a guiding topicish context instead of exact questions, and the respondents could elaborate on the relevant issues (Oates 2006). The choice of participants was based on the purposive sampling method to allow inclusion of participants with certain knowledge in the field of imaging and diagnostics in the healthcare system. The last group comprised eight professionals such as radiology doctors, hospital physicists and researchers. To be ethically sound, we followed ethical principles of informed consent, anonymity, and confidentiality and gave the participants an option to withdraw at any point (Oates 2006; Saldana 2013).

Table 1. Phases of the Qualitative Research Methodology

Phase	Key Activities & Details
Phase 1: Research Design	• Qualitative Case Study Approach • Formulation of Semi-Structured Interview Guide based on TAM
Phase 2: Participant Recruitment	• Purposive & Snowball Sampling • Selection of Specialized Healthcare Stakeholders (n=8)
Phase 3: Data Collection	• Semi-Structured Interviews via Digital Platforms (Zoom/Google Meet) • Duration: 25–50 minutes per session
Phase 4: Data Processing	• Audio Recording (with explicit informed consent) • Verbatim Transcription & Anonymization of Identifiers
Phase 5: Data Analysis	• Thematic Analysis & First-Round Coding • Synthesis of Major Ethical Themes mapped to TAM Constructs

Interpretation of the uncoded audio files was conducted after following a strict two-cycle coding procedure by means of MAXQDA software (Saldana 2013). During the initial cycle, I used the attribute coding to position backgrounds of the participants, structural coding to extract the parts that would respond to research questions, and descriptive coding to overlay general themes (Saldana 2013; Oates 2006). Pattern and focused coding that constituted the second cycle included reorganising the data based on its themes to form connections between the empirical results and the already known theories of trust (Saldana 2013). Our method was an abductive method that collates both deductive literature-based themes and inductive themes growing out of the data per se, and we over-exploited the interpretative value of the few empirical data available (Josephson & Josephson 1994; Oates 2006). Lastly, I need to agree that this qualitative approach has methodological weaknesses. The sample size is limited, which presupposes that the findings cannot be generalized to the whole healthcare industry because transcription and analysis are time-consuming processes (Oates 2006). Moreover, I acknowledge the possibility of respondent bias and subjective interest in a researcher. To reduce risk aspects, we anonymized all data, adopted open-ended questions to make it objective, and completed cross-checks as the data was being transcribed to achieve maximum reliability (Oates 2006).

Table 2. Background information about the participants

Respondent	Profession / Current Role	Professional Experience
Respondent 1 (R1)	Acting Operations Manager, specialized in breast cancer	30 years in breast cancer care
Respondent 2 (R2)	Radiography Nurse (Radiographer)	34 years in medical imaging
Respondent 3 (R3)	Researcher in AI for medical applications	19 years in AI
Respondent 4 (R4)	Researcher in medical epidemiology and biostatistics	10–12 years in medical applications
Respondent 5 (R5)	Radiologist and Professor of Radiology	25 years as a physician; 20 in radiology
Respondent 6 (R6)	Radiologist	5 years as a physician
Respondent 7 (R7)	Hospital Physicist	10–12 years in MRI and X-ray
Respondent 8 (R8)	Hospital Physicist	25 years in radiology

EMPIRICISM

Transparency and Explainability

Utilizing structural coding, I have been able to identify 251 segments that were related directly to the main research question. The following discussion is a synthesis of these results on the six theoretical themes identified in the literature review above and supports two emergent categories defined through abductive reasoning: the human factor and legal aspects. To be clear and precise in academics, verbatim accounts have been shortened through the elimination of colloquialism, without distorting the original intent and the technical background. The discussion on the issues of transparency and explainability shows the subtle conflict between the practical and theoretical meaning. Although explainable AI (XAI) is also often touted, the nature of the user limits the usefulness of the explanation due to the underlying knowledge in the user, which, as noted by R3, in fact leads to more confusion if the clinician is not sufficiently technically or otherwise prepared. R3 states that, "*People postulating that transparency is good enough since black boxes are bad, clarified AI or XAI is phenomenal where you can interrogate this black box, why did you do this and that? The issue is that such explanations worsen the situation when there is the lack of basic prerequisites in the person.*" The same thing can be said about

R4, which affirms that the concept of explainability is a key aspect of institutional trust, holding that the capability of a system to provide a logical explanation that is, the ability to identify a set of causal variables that lead to a given output is the key to achieving clinical buy-in. R4 states that, "*Can the system tell me that I get this result because of this, this and this it is like a logic reasoning that can be connected and this is one doctors can purchase. Yes, but it will certainly raise confidence, I believe that there is no mistaking it.*" This implies that a doctor will have to buy the result, which will require the algorithm to mimic some sort of deductive reasoning that is common to medical practice. In terms of manufacturing and operation, trust can be developed through transparency on the way forward with development. R5 points out that software developers should reveal themselves and demonstrate that they have some hidden tricks to gain the trust of decided professionals. This delving requirement is reiterated by R7, who finds the black box model of delivery, where all that is known about it is its inputs and outputs, to be a major adoption obstacle. R7 states, "*But I as well sense that this manufacturer enters our premises and says to us: we this AI product is a black box good []. You only get what you give in and not to get more.*" Since there is no observability of the algorithmic reasoning mechanism, a physicist or clinician cannot rely on the data that will be provided to them under any circumstances. Moreover, R6 argues that a system with graded measures of inaccuracy and not binary results is more useful to the clinical process, specifically in patient prioritization, than one with binary outcomes because more complex human-mediated decision-making can be facilitated.

Precision and Reliability

The professional opinion on the criteria of AI performance demonstrates that there is a particular attention to accuracy and managing algorithmic uncertainty. Specialty practitioners, e.g., R1, note that AI approaches have often been found to perform better in velocity and precision than the average clinician, especially in the field of pathology and radiology. Moreover, AI can be viewed as a method of clinical standardization; R4 is of the opinion that such systems decrease the variation of diagnostics in practitioners thus improving the overall quality of care. R4 states that, "*When these systems are brought into reality, they will be exposed to what they are actually untrained to deal with, examples, which they have never heard of, types of patients, which they have never experienced before and then there must be the ability to allow AI systems to say, I do not know what this is, you must tell me.*" Nevertheless, the first stage of deployment is established as a crucial phase of trust development. Professional peer conversation is likely to trigger a steep decline in the reputation of the system as minor technical fallibility on the launch phase leads to the possible triggering of a rapid decline in the reputation of the technology, claiming its social life to be as crucial as its mathematical precision. Another common necessity of the introduction of clinical trust is uncertainty detection or a self-report in an out-of-distribution manner. R4 states that, "*I believe that such kind of straightforward errors, when they are committed on a huge scale initially when an AI system is introduced to a clinic, I believe the latter may become notorious quite fast and doctors may talk about it amongst themselves.*" Systems should be endowed with meta-cognitive ability to detect when they have reached patient profiles or data types that are still within their training parameter, in which case they should be alerted by humans that an intervention is required. This idea of the algorithm requesting assistance is reflected on R5, who proposes that one should decide based on the level of trust the system must have offered on a case-by-case basis. R5 states that, "*I believe that at least in the first run, it is essential to be very certain what the algorithm does and debug, verify that you know it works, and that you receive some form of indication of how much uncertainty the algorithm is should aid in an impressive manner. That they require assistance as required.*" Clinicians will be able to balance their trust in the system by observing algorithm outputs relative to human knowledge at the initial phases of the implementation process. Although this has potential benefits, a certain degree of caution is still observed in terms of maturity of the technology. R8 holds to the position that AI in the healthcare field is at an early phase of growth, with a gap between the potential of technology and the functionality to date. According to this attitude, although the course of AI is encouraging, its modern situation may not be as ready as it needs to be to ensure a continuous range of accuracy and performance to allow clinical trust in full.

Automation vs Augmentation

The concept of introducing AI into the clinical setting is envisioned as an add-on utility rather than a functionality to be used in lieu of human professionals. The views of professionals, including the ones of R2, indicate that even though AI is a useful tool, serious distrust of the shift toward autonomous decision-making systems is still in place. This feeling is in line with a more general slowness when it comes to giving diagnostic control over non-human beings. The contemporary clinical discussion insists that AI is to be used as a diagnostic aid only. Technology can best be said to be an AI-enhanced framework or a so-called clinical-decision-support system as R3 suggests, which becomes more useful over time by learning longitudinally. R3 states that, "*Instead, they will add AI-augmented or that they have a good clinical decision support system which has learned and becomes more useful with time.*" The main advantage of such systems is that repeating data analysis in large volumes can be performed with a high degree of accuracy that is not influenced by fatigue, which is a considerable advantage compared to human thinking in repetitive operations.

However, physician as the ultimate authority is a vital compulsion to the integrity of the ethical and clinical profession. AI implementation is the double-redundancy of a safety net, which would give clinicians one more level of certainty as they seed in the complicated spectrum of diagnosis. As per R4, the overall evolution that AI will need to be able to perform without human control is far. R4 states that. "*I believe that long enough it will be a sort of second security measure, an additional. security system within healthcare. I believe that it is still a long distance before these systems are prepared to make their own decisions without the interference of doctors in the same process since the challenges are too many.*" According to the existing consensus, there are complex multifactorial issues that, at the long-term perspective, will still demand the presence of medical professionals in the decision-making process, which can only preserve AI as a supportive mechanism of a security system but not its agent.

Data Security and Integrity

The digitization of the healthcare industry presents an increased level of system vulnerability. Since R2 notes, the increase in digital platforms will spread the area of technical failure or exploitation by default and will generate an equivalent number of clinical weak points. This vulnerability of architecture requires careful integration, whereby the incorporation of new technologies would not jeopardize the core stability of the medical infrastructure. The main limitation of the development of medical AI is the lack of access to high-fidelity data, which can be used to train algorithms. R5 mentions that one of the biggest friction points between the AI developers and the medical industry is that such actions are predominantly controlled by strict legal regulations and privacy laws. R5 states that, "*A reason why this requires data to be shared would be to train all these systems, and many restrictions exist, such that you cannot simply share medical records or images.*" Since medical records and diagnostic imagery require strict confidentiality measures, the uninterrupted nature of information exchange, which is essential to the process of training all these systems, is often hampered by such legal requirements. The reality-based use of AI is further complicated by the fact that the clinical setting is a high stakes setting. R7, being a hospital physicist, mentions that healthcare is one of the most difficult areas to apply AI, as it directly influences human life. R7 states that, "*That everyone is training on and training on something limited and homogeneous, but healthcare works with. different groups of patients.*" One of the important issues is the homogenous property of existing training data: to developers, a limited, homogeneous data is used, whereas real healthcare concerns the heterogeneous group of patients whose biological and demographic issues are not necessarily reflected in existing models. With these challenges aside, the shift to so-called big data has the potential to greatly improve clinical efficiency. R8 hypothesizes that with bigger and more representative datasets being available on a systemic scale, AI will be able to make much more accurate diagnostics. R8 states that, "*This big data in the medical and that entire thing, I think that once it begins to be deployed in large quantities and when you arrive, I think we will have far more precise diagnostics and time to examine what is severe*." These systems will help reduce time and expertise spent in the medical field by automating the routine analytical work and enabling practitioners to devote more of their attention to the most urgent cases.

Lack of Knowledge

The mental aspect between clinical practice and algorithmic integration is based on a subtle interpretation of the functional transparency. A general unawareness of what one does not know often destroys trust. As R1 implies, the logistics of trust are intertwined with a base understanding of AI workings, but most of the practitioners are unaware of the impact of their technical weaknesses. Such ignorance is a system threat to the degree that the effectiveness of such tools relies on whether the user can differentiate between their proper use. In the realm of radiography, the scope of practice, tiring technical knowledge might not be a requirement, but the understanding of the inherent constraints is crucial. R2 underlines the main goal of a X-ray nurse to find out possible pitfalls and avoid the overconfidence of autonomous system. R3 agrees with this warning saying that there is a strategy gap in determining where AI can genuinely contribute clinical value. It is currently common to observe institutional hype of the implementation process rather than an expression of practical need and develop systems that may not statistically provide significant advantages to patient outcomes. The explainability demands a minimum of technical literacy among the medical practitioners. R4 claims that although physicians do not need a granular cognition of the algorithmic architecture, a physician needs to be aware of the strengths and weaknesses of the systems used. R4 states that, "*It is very important, and I would believe it will cause such an immense impact on the healthcare of the future and that is why I believe awareness should be elevated at the undergraduate level among doctors as well. The fact they have courses where AI systems are taught and it is apparently obvious that they do not need to possess that knowledge of the process directly, but they need to know the nature of an AI system and its advantages and disadvantages and the way they can make good use of them. I think that is important*." This training would then preferably start at the undergraduate age, where the awareness would be grown on how to apply AI in a good way. The medical profession is at the mercy of the two extremes of overconfidence and excessive suspicion without this pedagogic underpinning. This educational vacuum leads to systemic distrust as in most cases. R5 assumes that blind trust and reflexive skepticism may be fixed by means of in-service training and interdisciplinary cooperation. R5 states that, "*Perhaps I do not need to know the finer details of how the system is organized but I have a feeling of the pitfalls, and what the constraints of what the system is, I think.*" It would be especially pertinent in the case of specialists such as R6 whose poor experiences with poorly integrated systems emphasize the importance of having a sense of what the pitfalls are. In the case of physicists of hospitals such as R7, the inability of physicians to have even the most basic technical training becomes an enormous obstacle as it tends to lead to the lack of trust in the effectiveness of the technology, which promotes the adoption of AI in high-stakes healthcare setting.

Working Conditions

The concept of professional incorporation of AI in clinical settings presupposes that the notion of practitioner autonomy and practice effectiveness should be considered in a very strict manner. As R2 testifies, there is a major ontological issue of the decline in specialized clinical competencies. According to this participant, when a task that involves diagnoses or a procedure is given to the automated systems in excess, there is a risk of instigating professional deskilling and resultant decrease in intellectual stimulation to the extent of making clinical practice a monotony. These sentiments highlight the conflict between algorithmic performance and maintaining human skills. Contrarily, R6 focuses on the practical pragmatics necessary to ensure the effective implementation of AI, stating that these systems should be used first as initiators of the smooth clinical process. The systemic workload can be reduced by using AI to do triage and prioritize the cases, which theoretically can allow practitioners to dedicate their limited time resources to higher-priority interventions. R6, however, notes that introduction of "technological friction" should be avoided where new systems are viewed as new administrative burdens instead of facilitating devices. R6 states that, "*I was not keen on it because it was the time when I had much to do. I did not feel that it was beneficial to me at that moment but instead it was an added burden since the program was very new.*" The prior experience of the participant is a key case study: at the time when psychic load was enormous, the presentation of a nascent AI program was thrown out since it could not produce immediate utility. Making the system less mature served to turn the technology into an additional assignment, which is the next indicator that the perceived value of AI is closely intertwined with the ability to fit the technology into the range of existing professional pressures.

The Human Factor

The development of the concept of trust in medical AI will require a comparative study of the error rates of anthropogenic and algorithmic diagnostic agents. R3 suggests that the logic behind the hypocrisy of putting AI under stricter scrutiny than human practitioners is that once such a system can exhibit an equivalent level of mean error to a physician, it deserves an equal degree of trust. According to this view, the focus on parity-based models of trust should have as its secondary effect that it is the frequency of the error, rather than its source, whether biological or computational. The sociological fact of making mistakes is however an important obstacle to implementation. R4 points to an existent significant psychological imbalance in the way society responds to errors, pointing out that social disposition towards forgiving computational errors is significantly worse than it is with human errors. R4 states that, "*This concerns the fact that individual scandals may have quite a significant influence since there may be AI systems that surely contribute value to patients in the healthcare sector at the population level. But someone gets caught up somewhere and a wrong step is taken and the entire system can be. thrown out as though you were cleaning the baby with bathwater. Although it may have a good impact upon the entirety, a single error on the part of a person may cause a significant amount of harm.*" Media discourse contributes to the intensification of this phenomenon since even isolated algorithmic mistakes are usually dramatized. These types of individual scandals threaten to create a systemic effect of throwing the baby out with the bathwater, in which one error of high profile delegitimises the perceived legitimacy of a system that delivers net benefits on a population-wide scale that cannot be overstated. Human fallibility in medicine is widely accepted, whereas automated systems are imposed with high demands that are hard to fulfill. R5 indicates that the medical community recognizes the possibility of doctors making mistakes, but the cultural agreement of the same to AI is naturally more demanding. R5 states that, "*It has really occurred in my discipline that you condition your system to enhance some sort of images after which you apply it erroneously on all other kinds of objects with no genuine comprehension of whether or how it is functioning. Well, obvious restrictions. That is what we have trained it, that will be what you shall use it.*" The biggest issue here is misuse of technology to serve unanticipated purposes, another case of human error that is commonly blamed on system inefficiency. To address this, guidelines for a training system should be strictly followed by practitioners. Invoking an image-enhancement tool outside the area where it has been tested, e.g., is an invitation to failure. Strict articulateness of the application of AI is, therefore, paramount in its implementation to avoid misuse.

Legal Aspects

The implementation of systems trust in medical AI requires an assertive platform of formal certification and regulatory control. According to R1, professional confidence is the only requirement with such accreditation, and according to such a method, institutional validation is the main level of assessing safety and effectiveness. This dependency on formal certification is indicative of a more general shift of personal discretion on the part of clinicians towards technical certification. The key to this discussion is that there should be dedicated reviewing institutions that are equivalent to available medical regulatory bodies. R3 points out that since the Health and Social Care Inspectorate (IVO) would be overseeing the clinical judgment of physicians, there needs to be a similar system that would scrutinize the outcomes of the algorithms and software flawlessness. R3 states that, "*...on the case of doctors we do have institutions such as IVO which assess the cases of wrong decisions made by doctors. It is because you should ensure that you have a person that reviews systems and software systems and it holds even in the event that it is not AI. We possess that in the way of medical equipment.*" This institutional control is already an established norm on traditional meditational equipment and its flow to AI is considered a rational and compelled move towards accountability in digital health work. These systems are also difficult to integrate as there are legal issues regarding ultimate liability that are yet to be resolved. Both R4 and R5 underline that whether it is the person who caused the failure of the system is a very critical barrier to its adoption. The uncertainties about the culprit, be it the developer or the healthcare giver or the automation itself, need the development of clear-cut legal provisions before any such technology may be used in clinical practice ethically. To most practitioners, a given CE-mark or sanction of an authorized body is sufficient to provide a proxy of personal trust. The assumption made by R8 is that these endorsements are a reflection that the functional reliability of the system is strictly checked by the competent third party. R8 states that, "*Personally, having it C-marked or signed/approved by the appropriate authorities, I believe a person, concerned with this, has read and made sure that the same does work.*" Here, trust does not necessarily need to come out of an individual interpretation of the code underlying it, but the legitimacy of the governing authorities that institute the implementation of the code.

ANALYSIS

Transparency, Reliability, and Performance Expectations

Conceptualization of trust in medical AI requires that it leaves behind the traditional interpersonal trust models. Based on the conclusive model developed by Mayer, Davis and Schoorman (1995), it is possible to refer to trust as a dyadic construct that consists of both positive anticipations and readiness to be vulnerable. In clinical contexts, these expectations are expressed much more through the specialized knowledge of an individual, the quality of empirical research published, and the dominant media propaganda. Although healthcare is a highly vulnerable area by itself and because it directly affects human life, the practitioners represent a skillful ability to accept this risk in the case of AI. This granting of acceptance, however, is conditional on provable indications of systemic value, a condition which can be as strict as granted to human fellow workers. An analysis of data demonstrated eight themes that within this relationship are operated, six of which are picked up and are common to the existing literature, and two were created due to the empirical data (See Table 3).

Table 3. Identified Themes

Theme Identified	Source of Identification
Transparency and explainability	Literature analysis / Previous research
Accuracy and reliability	Literature analysis / Previous research
Augmentation	Literature analysis / Previous research
Data security and integrity	Literature analysis / Previous research
Knowledge gap	Literature analysis / Previous research
Working conditions	Literature analysis / Previous research
The human factor	Data analysis
Legal aspects	Data analysis

The strain between openness and practical usefulness is one of the intersectional issues. It is also claimed by many clinicians that the reasoning of a system can only be substantiated after having a clear fundamental understanding of the system, which reflects the same concerns the black box in theoretical research (Adabi and Berrada 2018, Burrell 2016, Gille, Jobin & Ienca 2020). On the other hand, developers of systems indicate that despite any provision of transparency, there might always exist a huge gap in terms of knowledge which would not allow the users to interpret this explanation appropriately. This implies that the perceived necessity to be more transparent could be a proxy of more comprehensive educational gaps in the medical workforce. Finally, the popular opinion among the practitioners is in favor of high precision and accuracy as compared to absolute transparency of algorithms. Although the capability of a system to define its decision-making variables works to instill trust, as it has been observed before (Lockey et.al., 2021; Adabi & Berrada 2018; Glikson & Woolley 2020), the main cause of adoption is based on the reliability demonstrated by the system under complex clinical settings. Another major method of improving trust in the AIs of black box systems is incorporation of case-specific accuracy measures. These systems can be used to address the problem of their own opaque internal logic by offering a self-diagnostic measure of confidence in the results of each individual assessment. This is consistent with the theoretical standpoints of Malle & Ullman (2021) & LaRosa & Danks (2018), which propose that human-AI trust is not based on the issue of social reciprocity, in general, but is rather a performance-based one. The expectations often given to AI by the practitioners are very high as standards of near perfection are considered and the algorithms are expected to provide certain levels of consistency and precision that are beyond the capabilities of human variation. Therefore, a low margin of error is considered the key to institutional and personal trust.

Nonetheless, trust cannot solely be ensured due to reliability. According to Gille, Jobin & Ienca (2020), feasible use of AI in the clinical environment demands interventions to prove actual benefits both at the patient and system level. The concept of trust is therefore a complex thing that is dependent on the perceived value of the technology in the larger healthcare environment. It cannot be a matter of just making the system accurate, but the system should also mitigate the current pressures without creating new complexities that would negate the perceived value. The general agreement between the practitioners is highly inclined to augmentation as opposed to complete automation. However, almost unanimously, participants support the idea that AI should serve as a second opinion or as a sorting mechanism, not to replace specialist clinical judgment but as its complement. This inclination towards non-decision-making systems reflects guidelines presented by Lockey et.al., (2021) and Lysaght et.al., (2019), who state that AI must be implemented to help the healthcare personnel improve their decision-making. Through the preservation of the clinician as the main authority, there is reduction in the threats involved with autonomous algorithmic flaws through a human control measure.

Table 4. Conceptual Framework of Trust Factors in Medical AI

Pillar of Trust	Associated TAM Construct	Clinical Challenge	Actionable Mitigation Strategy
Algorithmic Transparency	Perceived Ease of Use	The "Black Box" effect creates uncertainty; poor human-AI interface design hinders workflow.	Mandate explainable AI (XAI) outputs; prioritize user-centric interface design and seamless EHR integration.
System Reliability & Fairness	Perceived Usefulness	Fear of automation bias and demographic disparities in training data leading to patient harm.	Perform regular audits of local data on bias; introduce systematic clinician education on algorithm constraints.
Institutional Accountability	Behavioral Intention	Unclear liability (developer vs. physician) during diagnostic errors suppresses clinical adoption.	Establish local AI governance boards; align procurement with emerging regulatory frameworks (e.g., SaMD).

Clinical Value and Human–AI Collaboration

However, despite literature fears about the possibility of the loss of the patient-doctor relationship (Lockey et.al., 2021; Buck et.al., 2022), the empirical evidence shows that AI-enhanced systems might strengthen this relationship. The AI can free up huge amounts of time by automating some of the sub-tasks in the administration and diagnostic processes which yield higher results, due to their high labor alter-ativeness. This saved time enables doctors to interact more with patients, especially those who have some complex needs. Therefore, instead of serving as a digital barrier, the well-embraced AI will be an impetus to more patient-centered care, as it will decrease the time load in the clinical document and regular analysis. The ontological range of views in medical AI is deeply varied in the professional debate on the course of medical AI. Even though one of the participants, Participant 1, sees the future as being one of complete displacement by algorithms and the complete replacement of human practitioners, most of the viewpoints are more incremental in their adherence to the alternative reality. This conflict brings out the debate that is still being held regarding radical automation or the conservative preservation of clinical roles. There are an essential discontinuity of both theoretical literature and the practical interests of active practitioners in data ethics. Though the threat of compromised data integrity is listed among the key discouraging factors in the literature (Lockey et.al., 2021; Sunarti et.al., 2021; Buck et.al., 2022), the robust training of algorithms is more common in the focus of clinicians, rather than the abstract privacy issues. In fact, the regulatory limitations of the General Data Protection Regulation (GDPR) have often not been viewed as a protective mechanism, but a proving roadblock into the quality and volumes of large volumes of data needed to artificially power a system. To the contemporary practitioner, the effectiveness of the tool seems to balance the second risks of data sharing to a greater extent, if the provenance of training data is clinically pertinent (Hamid 2016).

Institutional security is also assumed to form an element of trust. The success of access to secure data, as implied by Asan, Bayrak & Choudhury (2021) is considered a condition that naturally brings a boost in transparency. Although digitization of the healthcare system creates vulnerabilities in the system (*i.e.* risk of cyber-attacks), they are usually classified as general technological threats people face as opposed to AI-specific challenges. In turn, the credibility of the clinician is not as much of a statement regarding the safety of the algorithm but rather a trust in the current institutional apparatus to deploy digital risks. Lastly, the correlation that exists between technical literacy and trust is most important. In line with the theories put forward by Asan, Bayrak & Choudhury (2021), the level of knowledge held by a user correlate directly with his confidence towards the system. The practitioners are not always required to master the fundamental code, but they need a thorough knowledge of the limits of operation of the system and possible traps. This indicates that successful implementation of AI is a key educational problem and trust is established by providing clarifications on the limitations of a system instead of giving a vague assertion of its perfection. Introduction of AI into a clinical practice requires a fundamental restructuring of medical pedagogy. It is necessary to include the basic coursework in AI in the regular healthcare professional curriculum to make employees ready for the technical nature of modern medicine. Hamid (2016) supports this pedagogical change and argues that training is a top priority and that technologies literacy must also be inherent with medical training.

Institutional, Legal, and Educational Determinants

A major obstacle to this shift, though, is the eminent gap in biological understanding of clinicians and technical needs of algorithmic decision support. The adoption of AI in areas like Sweden is a significant technological advancement to a labour force that in many instances is not formally trained technologically. Although Burrell (2016) assumes that the absence of knowledge is a type of what he calls opaqueness, which can be addressed with the help of education, the facts show that there is a pragmatic unwillingness of practitioners, most of whom do not have sufficient time to acquire skills in programming or code integration and not the desire to master it. Quite on the contrary, despite the fears expressed by Buck et.al., (2022) about the possible erosion of the inter-patient-provider relationship, it can be argued that properly applied AI can induce even more of a human contact. Through making routine clinical practices easier and lessening the burden on administration, AI gives clinicians more time to spend with actual patients. With such systems, however, their implementation is strictly contingent upon their capacity to reflect labor-saving effects which are tangible and not ones that burden such systems with additional bureaucratic demands.

Considering that AI does not belong to the primary set of competencies of medical personnel, the method of strategic employment of AI specialists in medical organizations can be identified as an effective measure. Including domain experts in the deployment phase may develop institutional trust because human-to-human communication based on system pitfalls may outperform abstract technical validation. Although the given approach is consistent with the suggestions provided by Lockey et.al., (2021), it has a structural risk: it leads to a centralized point of failure, putting a disproportionately high responsibility burden on an individual and putting the overall healthcare system at risk (Lockey et.al., 2021). There are often existential anxieties surrounding the maintenance of clinical agency as the phenomenon of the professional adoption of AI. One of the most widespread anxieties about automation, as revealed by scholarship (Buck et.al., 2022; Lysaght et.al., 2019), is that it is going to replace intellectually stimulating work or cause labor displacement, but in this study, it will be noted that they are negatively related to technical exposure. Experts who have the least experience in their profession will have the most role-conflict, as professionals who are accustomed to technology will perceive it in a more detached way. It implies that the perceived risk to professional self is largely an effect of unfriendliness, and maybe not a part of the technology itself.

There is a paradigm difference between trust mechanisms around perceived lack of intentionality and benevolence in computerized systems. In contrast to trust in people, between people, where shared value and intent are taken into consideration, trust in AI is solely performance-oriented (Asan, Bayrak & Choudhury 2021). The result is a sociological asymmetry which refers to subjecting an algorithmic error to much stricter scrutiny than that of a human error. Moreover, the threat of reputational contagion is high; the negative experience of colleagues affects clinicians so much. When a nascent system is the object of peer-group critique or ridicule in the popular media, the question of its perceived legitimacy can be destroyed beyond repair prior to its integration into the clinical system. The main channels towards the development of institutional trust are formal accreditation and strict governance. Qualification and quality assurance, which is regulated by a centralized body, is necessary to provide dependability (Lockey et.al., 2021). Besides, trust is closely connected with the responsibility of the manufacturer. If a developer can be seen as handing failures of the system, then the tool would probably be rejected by practitioners. Tolerance therefore is contingent on a well laid legal and administrative hierarchy of how the top clinical decision maker is. Lastly, the risk mitigation is conditional upon the clear definition of the scope of the work of a system. To avoid function creep, employers need to offer specifications to avoid the application of AI to jobs that their validated constraints cannot address. Healthcare institutions can promote an informed trust culture by formulating the application of AI in particular working environments and highlighting transparency on its limitations. This is important to make sure that technology is a strong supplementary of clinical practice instead of a place of professional or legal ambiguity.

CONCLUSION

The implementation of AI-based diagnostic devices by professionals depends on a complicated combination of their personal experience, perceived utility, and organizational barriers. Although much depends on the predispositions of a practitioner prior to exposure to the automated systems and his or her level of technical literacy, an agreement emerges that a level of trust can be achieved though certain operational and ethical requirements are met. This faith does not apply unconditionally but is implemented through five vital pillars of implementation. Clinical trust is maximized in the situation when AI is only used as a support system but not an independent diagnostic tool. discussed with much deep suspicion is the notion of entirely automated systems; it is much easier to trust technology as a supplement to human-judgment systems with practitioners. In this regard, AI should be used to perform high-volume tasks like the triage and prioritization of patients and not the ultimate clinical decision. Technical understanding forms the baseline of successful cooperation of human and machine. Although the specialist training of the system developers is not needed by the clinicians of the healthcare organization, the latter still need to have a working understanding of a particular system that has its own limitations. Incorporating the principles of AI into the introductory teaching of medical and nursing professions is one of the defensive measures against irrational suspiciousness and unreasonable overdependence. This type of knowledge will guarantee the use of systems within their desired parameters as a way of maximizing perceived value.

To be acceptable, a system must have a competence level that is at most commensurate to that of a human professional. The current state of AI does not allow substituting the comprehensive role of a physician or a nurse, yet it must exclude quite limited tasks, which it is required to do with utmost accuracy since the time of the implementation. When a practitioner comes to the view of any given task being more accurate or faster done than the software, the ensuing lack of trust can usually be irrevocable, irrespective of future technological advances. Since trust on technical systems is performance-based and not social, then individuals need empirical data on the reliability of a certain system. Trust can also be established in this case by making a score of confidence or measure of the precision that an individual case will satisfy by giving a score of these scores or accuracy measures to each individual case in a black box approach to algorithms, that is, where the black box itself is deemed opaque. The clinicians should also have insight into the structure of the system and its pitfalls so that they can have confidence in the products that they are reviewing. Having an external reviewing institution offers adequate accountability. Accreditation is a form of stamp of approval by professional authorities which implicitly transfers part of the burden of trust onto the governing human institution. This speech of the accountability gap is crucial; awareness of the fact that a system has been strictly managed and the existence of a legal framework concerning responsibility enables practitioners to embrace the latter with more confidence.

REFERENCES

Abdelwanis, M., Alarafati, H. K., Tammam, M. M. S., & Simsekler, M. C. E. (2024). Exploring the risks of automation bias in healthcare artificial intelligence applications: A Bowtie analysis. *Journal of Safety Science and Resilience = An Quan Ke Xue Yu Ren Xing (Ying Wen)*, *5*(4), 460–469. DOI: 10.1016/j.jnlssr.2024.06.001

Adadi, A., & Berrada, M. (2018). Peeking inside the black-box: A survey on explainable artificial intelligence (XAI). *IEEE Access : Practical Innovations, Open Solutions*, *6*, 52138–52160. DOI: 10.1109/ACCESS.2018.2870052

Andras, P., Esterle, L., Guckert, M., Han, T. A., Lewis, P. R., Milanovic, K., Payne, T., Perret, C., Pitt, J., Powers, S. T., Urquhart, N., & Wells, S. (2018). Trusting intelligent machines: Deepening trust within socio-technical systems. *IEEE Technology and Society Magazine*, *37*(4), 76–83. DOI: 10.1109/MTS.2018.2876107

Asan, O., Bayrak, A. E., & Choudhury, A. (2020). Artificial intelligence and human trust in healthcare: Focus on clinicians. *Journal of Medical Internet Research*, *22*(6), e15154. Advance online publication. DOI: 10.2196/15154 PMID: 32558657

Băjenesc, T.-M. I. (2020). Comparing artificial intelligence developments of superpowers: China and the US. *Journal of Social Sciences*, *3*(3), 43–50. DOI: 10.5281/zenodo.3971959

Bera, K., Schalper, K. A., Rimm, D. L., Velcheti, V., & Madabhushi, A. (2019). Artificial intelligence in digital pathology—New tools for diagnosis and precision oncology. *Nature Reviews. Clinical Oncology*, *16*(11), 703–715. DOI: 10.1038/s41571-019-0252-y PMID: 31399699

Buck, C., Doctor, E., Hennrich, J., Jöhnk, J., & Eymann, T. (2022). General practitioners' attitudes toward artificial intelligence–enabled systems: Interview study. *Journal of Medical Internet Research*, *24*(1), e28916. Advance online publication. DOI: 10.2196/28916 PMID: 35084342

Burrell, J. (2016). How the machine 'thinks': Understanding opacity in machine learning algorithms. *Big Data & Society*, *3*(1), 2053951715622512. Advance online publication. DOI: 10.1177/2053951715622512

Chan, H. P., Samala, R. K., & Hadjiiski, L. M. (2019). CAD and AI for breast cancer—Recent development and challenges. *The British Journal of Radiology*, *93*(1106), 20190580. Advance online publication. DOI: 10.1259/bjr.20190580 PMID: 31742424

Checkland, P., & Holwell, S. (1998). Action research: Its nature and validity. *Systemic Practice and Action Research*, *11*(1), 9–21. DOI: 10.1023/A:1022908820784

Dlamini, Z., Francies, F. Z., Hull, R., & Marima, R. (2020). Artificial intelligence (AI) and big data in cancer and precision oncology. *Computational and Structural Biotechnology Journal*, *18*, 2300–2311. DOI: 10.1016/j.csbj.2020.08.019 PMID: 32994889

Ericksson, B. J., Korfiatis, P., Kline, T. L., Akkus, Z., Philbrick, K., & Weston, A. D. (2018). Deep learning in radiology: Does one size fit all? *Journal of the American College of Radiology*, *15*(3), 521–526. DOI: 10.1016/j.jacr.2017.12.027 PMID: 29396120

Fulmer, C. A., & Gelfand, M. J. (2012). At what level (and in whom) we trust: Trust across multiple organizational levels. *Journal of Management*, *38*(4), 1167–1230. DOI: 10.1177/0149206312439327

Gao, Y., Geras, K. J., Lewin, A. A., & Moy, L. (2019). New frontiers: An update on computer-aided diagnosis for breast imaging in the age of artificial intelligence. *AJR. American Journal of Roentgenology*, *212*(2), 300–307. DOI: 10.2214/AJR.18.20392 PMID: 30667309

Gille, F., Jobin, A., & Ienca, M. (2020). What we talk about when we talk about trust: Theory of trust for AI in healthcare. *Intelligence-Based Medicine*, *1-2*, 100001. Advance online publication. DOI: 10.1016/j.ibmed.2020.100001

Glikson, E., & Woolley, A. W. (2020). Human trust in artificial intelligence: Review of empirical research. *The Academy of Management Annals*, *14*(2), 627–660. DOI: 10.5465/annals.2018.0057

Hamid, S. (2016). *The opportunities and risks of artificial intelligence in medicine and healthcare*. CUSPE Communications. https://doi.org/DOI: 10.17863/CAM.25624

Hasanzadeh, F., Josephson, C. B., Waters, G., Adedinsewo, D., Azizi, Z., & White, J. A. (2025). Bias recognition and mitigation strategies in artificial intelligence healthcare applications. *npj. Digital Medicine*, *8*(1), 154. Advance online publication. DOI: 10.1038/s41746-025-01503-7 PMID: 40069303

Heron, J. (1996). *Co-operative inquiry: Research into the human condition*. SAGE Publications.

Jacovi, A., Marasovic, A., Miller, T., & Goldberg, Y. (2021). Formalizing trust in artificial intelligence: Prerequisites, causes and goals of human trust in AI. *Proceedings of the 2021 ACM Conference on Fairness, Accountability, and Transparency (FAccT '21)*, 624–635. https://doi.org/DOI: 10.1145/3442188.3445923

Josephson, J. R., & Josephson, S. G. (1994). Conceptual analysis of abduction. In *Abductive inference: Computation, philosophy, technology* (pp. 5–30). Cambridge University Press., DOI: 10.1017/CBO9780511530128.002

Lamb, L. R., Lehman, C. D., Gastounioti, A., Conant, E. F., & Bahl, M. (2022). Artificial intelligence (AI) for screening mammography, from the AI special series on AI applications. *AJR. American Journal of Roentgenology, 219*(3), 369–380. Advance online publication. DOI: 10.2214/AJR.21.27071 PMID: 35018795

LaRosa, E., & Danks, D. (2018). Impacts on trust of healthcare AI. *Proceedings of the 2018 AAAI/ACM Conference on AI, Ethics, and Society (AIES '18)*, 210–215. https://doi.org/DOI: 10.1145/3278721.3278771

Lockey, S., Gillespie, N., Holm, D., & Asadi Someh, I. (2021). A review of trust in artificial intelligence: Challenges, vulnerabilities and future directions. *Proceedings of the 54th Hawaii International Conference on System Sciences (HICSS-54)*. https://doi.org/DOI: 10.24251/HICSS.2021.664

Lysaght, T., Lim, H. Y., Xafis, V., & Ngiam, K. Y. (2019). AI-assisted decision-making in healthcare: The application of an ethics framework for big data in health and research. *Asian Bioethics Review, 11*(3), 299–314. DOI: 10.1007/s41649-019-00096-0 PMID: 33717318

Malle, F. B., & Ullman, D. (2021). A multidimensional conception and measure of human-robot trust. In *Trust in Human-Robot Interaction* (pp. 3–25). Academic Press., DOI: 10.1016/B978-0-12-819472-0.00001-0

Mayer, R. C., Davis, J. H., & Schoorman, F. D. (1995). An integrative model of organizational trust. *Academy of Management Review, 20*(3), 709–734. DOI: 10.2307/258792

McKnight, D., Carter, M., Thatcher, J., & Clay, P. (2011). Trust in a specific technology: An investigation of its components and measures. *ACM Transactions on Management Information Systems, 2*(2), 1–25. DOI: 10.1145/1985347.1985353

Miller, D., & Brown, E. (2018). Artificial intelligence in medical practice: The question to the answer? *The American Journal of Medicine, 131*(2), 129–133. DOI: 10.1016/j.amjmed.2017.10.035 PMID: 29126825

Oates, B. J. (2006). *Researching information systems and computing*. SAGE Publications.

Okamura, K., & Yamada, S. (2020). Empirical evaluations of framework for adaptive trust calibration in human-AI cooperation. *IEEE Access : Practical Innovations, Open Solutions, 8*, 220335–220351. DOI: 10.1109/ACCESS.2020.3042556

Pesapane, F., Codari, M., & Sardanelli, F. (2018). Artificial intelligence in medical imaging: Threat or opportunity? Radiologists again at the forefront of innovation in medicine. *European Radiology Experimental*, *2*(1), 35. Advance online publication. DOI: 10.1186/s41747-018-0061-6 PMID: 30353365

Saldaña, J. (2013). *The coding manual for qualitative researchers* (2nd ed.). SAGE Publications.

Sunarti, S., Rahman, F. F., Naufal, M., Risky, M., Febriyanto, K., & Masina, R. (2021). Artificial intelligence in healthcare: Opportunities and risk for future. *Gaceta Sanitaria*, *35*(Suppl. 1), S67–S70. DOI: 10.1016/j.gaceta.2020.12.019 PMID: 33832631

ADDITIONAL READING

Abdelwanis, M., Alarafati, H. K., Tammam, M. M. S., & Simsekler, M. C. E. (2024). Exploring the risks of automation bias in healthcare artificial intelligence applications: A Bowtie analysis. *Journal of Safety Science and Resilience = An Quan Ke Xue Yu Ren Xing (Ying Wen)*, *5*(4), 460–469. DOI: 10.1016/j.jnlssr.2024.06.001

Ferrara, E. (2023). Fairness and Bias in Artificial Intelligence: A Brief Survey of Sources, Impacts, and Mitigation Strategies. *Sci*, *6*(1), 3. Advance online publication. DOI: 10.3390/sci6010003

Hasanzadeh, F., Josephson, C. B., Waters, G., Adedinsewo, D., Azizi, Z., & White, J. A. (2025). Bias recognition and mitigation strategies in artificial intelligence healthcare applications. *NPJ Digital Medicine*, *8*(1), 154. DOI: 10.1038/s41746-025-01503-7 PMID: 40069303

Norori, N., Hu, Q., Aellen, F. M., Faraci, F. D., & Tzovara, A. (2021). Addressing bias in big data and AI for health care: A call for open science. *Patterns (New York, N.Y.)*, *2*(10), 100347. DOI: 10.1016/j.patter.2021.100347 PMID: 34693373

Sun, C., & Harris, S. L. (2024). Reducing bias in healthcare artificial intelligence: A white paper. *Health Informatics Journal*, *30*(4), 14604582241291410. DOI: 10.1177/14604582241291410 PMID: 39541598

Vorisek, C. N., Stellmach, C., Mayer, P. J., Klopfenstein, S. A. I., Bures, D. M., Diehl, A., Henningsen, M., Ritter, K., & Thun, S. (2023). Artificial Intelligence Bias in Health Care: Web-Based Survey. *Journal of Medical Internet Research*, *25*, e41089. DOI: 10.2196/41089 PMID: 37347528

KEY TERMS AND DEFINITIONS

Accreditation and Governance: The regulatory stamps of approval (like CE-marking) of a system as safe and effective together with its institutional structures. All these mechanisms transfer the responsibility of trust to the authority bodies that oversee these machines.

Augmentation: The strategic use of AI with the purpose of complementing and supplementing human decision-making (instead of completely substituting it). This guarantees that in a clinical setting the physician does not lose control and enjoys the algorithmic accuracy.

Black Box Problem: The natural obscurity of the working of sophisticated machine learning models, in which the user cannot see the internal logic and decision-making process. Such a deficiency of transparency usually plays a leading role in creating professional trust.

Domain Expertise: The expertise possessed by people having knowledge in both the clinical setting and the technical constraints of the AI systems. These professionals act as critical networkers who allow trust to be established by peer-to-peer knowledge flow.

Existential Anxiety (Professional): The fear or the psychological stress of practitioners being artificially evicted as they might do their special work, or enjoy fun distractions, due to the possibility of the development of AI. Studies have shown that such anxiety is commonest among people who have had minimal direct experience with the technology.

Explainable AI (XAI): Part of the artificial intelligence toolkit focused on programs to give human-interpretable explanations of their results. It will help prevent the black box problem as it will show the exact variables that are applied when arriving at a diagnostic conclusion.

Trust Calibration: The way of matching the amount of trust that a practitioner has with the real reliability of the AI system. Calibration prevents on one hand over-trust (causing automation bias) and under-trust (causing the exclusion of useful tools).

Chapter 5
Ethical and Legal Implications in Medical AI

Shikha Khullar
http://orcid.org/0009-0000-5598-3145
Poornima University, Jaipur, India

Ibrar Ahmed
http://orcid.org/0009-0001-0846-0218
School of International Law, Southwest University of Political Science and Law, China

Sumit Kumar Kapoor
http://orcid.org/0009-0005-6291-3176
Poornima University, Jaipur, India

Manju Lata Joshi
http://orcid.org/0000-0002-0749-6171
Poornima University, Jaipur, India

Arun Arora
https://orcid.org/0000-0002-8976-0633
Lloyd Business School, India

ABSTRACT

The use of Large Language Models (LLMs) in the medical field, especially in clinical safety evaluation, has substantial prospective advantages to enhance the diagnostic performance, clinical decision-making process, and patient outcomes. Although these advantages exist, there are complicated ethical, legal, and governance issues with the introduction of AI in healthcare. This chapter critically reviews ethical implication of the use of LLM with special reference being given to clinical auton-

DOI: 10.4018/979-8-2600-2173-6.ch005

omy, algorithmic bias, informed consent, and accountability. It draws on real-life case studies to emphasize the role of biased training data and lack of transparency in decision-making in promoting health disparities and undermining trust between clinicians and patients. The analysis also outlines some of the crucial failure points in current legal and regulatory frameworks particularly on the aspect of the distribution of liability and privacy of the data that are ill suited to adapt to the adaptable and changing character of the AI systems.

1. INTRODUCTION

The implementation of Artificial Intelligence (AI) in healthcare, particularly in clinical safety measurements, has created new opportunities. One of the most promising technologies is Large Language Models (LLM). That can assist in diagnostics, clinical decision-making, and patient safety. They are able to process large volumes of data, give real-time information, and propose treatment. However, although LLMs are highly promising to change clinical practice, they also come with significant ethical, legal, and governance issues.

The LLMs have the potential to analyse the patient data and assist decision-making. Systems such as GPT and other models use transformers to process complex medical data, such as patient history, imaging, and clinical recommendations, to produce recommendations. They have already attained promising outcomes in diagnostic support, treatment planning, and risk assessment (Yang et al., 2025). However, there are difficulties in their implementation. Application of AI, particularly LLMs, in clinical safety assessment is associated with clinical autonomy, data privacy, accountability, and impartiality. Since AI models are commonly trained on extensive datasets, they can directly affect patient outcomes by compromising the trust of clinicians and patients as they lack transparency (Weiner et al., 2025). The opacity of the decision-making process of LLMs is also a controversial issue when it comes to the application of non-human systems in making vital health decisions. Explainability is crucial because healthcare professionals and patients should be able to understand how AI arrives at its recommendations to fully trust them (Abgrall et al., 2024).

The preliminary ethical concern in the use of LLMs in health care is the possibility of bias in the AI system. These models can also perpetuate the existing healthcare disparities of race, gender, and socioeconomic status because they are based on past medical data. To illustrate, when the training data does not adequately represent certain populations, the AI may not be applicable in diagnosing or prescribing. which may result in biased or discriminatory outcomes. This underscores the importance of medical practitioners and AI developers using different, impartial datasets for

LLM training. The other ethical issue is clinical autonomy. The deployment of LLMs as an aid or substitute to human judgment is becoming a common practice in the medical field. This kind of change raises the question of undermining the judgment of the clinician and the role played by healthcare providers in the diagnosis and treatment. Although LLMs are able to offer evidence-based suggestions, the ultimate decision-making process must remain in the hands of the healthcare staff that knows the complexity of cases. Healthcare revolves around the principle of autonomy, and there is a danger that clinicians will become over reliant on AI and will undermine the aspect of professional judgment and personalized nature of care (Birch et al., 2022).

The autonomy of clinicians should be the highest priority and cannot be used as an excuse to deploy AI to support human decision-making instead of replacing it. Multidimensional liabilities, data privacy, and a regulatory environment exist on the legal front of the introduction of AI into the medical field. The more common use of LLMs in clinical judgments raises questions of how to allocate liability in case the AI systems give wrong advice or commit mistakes. For example, when an AI misdiagnoses or prescribes a wrong treatment, then *who is liable? Would it be the liabilities of the AI developer, the healthcare provider, or the healthcare institution using the AI?* The current regulatory systems are insufficient to address those liability concerns.

The privacy of data is a very important problem in the legal sphere. LLMs can manage large amounts of medical data, some of which is confidential data regarding personal health. There is legislation governing its processing, such as the GDPR in Europe and HIPAA in the United States. The use of LLMs in the process of assessing clinical safety usually takes the flow of confidential patient information between platforms and institutions for granted. Which may also lead to the emergence of data breach and access violation. In light of the potential violation of the rights of patients and the loss of the trust patients have in healthcare providers, it is imperative to ensure that AI complies with relevant privacy laws (Wang et al., 2022). The AI governance models in healthcare are yet to be designed, and the lack of concrete and multifaceted models is drastic to ensure that the use of LLMs is ethical and legal. The issues of accountability, data protection and bias are dealt with the aid of the WHO AI Ethics Guidelines (2025) which encourages clear governance (WHO, 2025). However, the regulatory practice is likely to track the development of AI that leaves gaps that could have a negative impact on the safety of patients. To address these concerns, there is need to come up with a sophisticated system of governance that integrates both legal, ethical and clinical views. Such an approach will ensure accountability of use of AI systems in clinical safety trials where the sense of accountability is stringent, regular performance review, and constant oversight by groups of clinicians, ethicists, regulators, and AI developers. It also needs to promote cross-border cooperation in order to develop standardized norms and regulations of AI in healthcare (Zhang & Zhang, 2023). The flowchart in Figure 1 provides the integration of Large Language Models (LLMs) into clinical safety evaluations, starting with the diagnosis of a patient and continuing with the implementation of a treatment plan. It identifies critical aspects, including data privacy, AI transparency, clinician review, shared decision-making, continuous model adaptation, and ethical governance, and prioritizes them throughout the process.

Figure 1. AI Integration Workflow in Clinical Safety Assessments

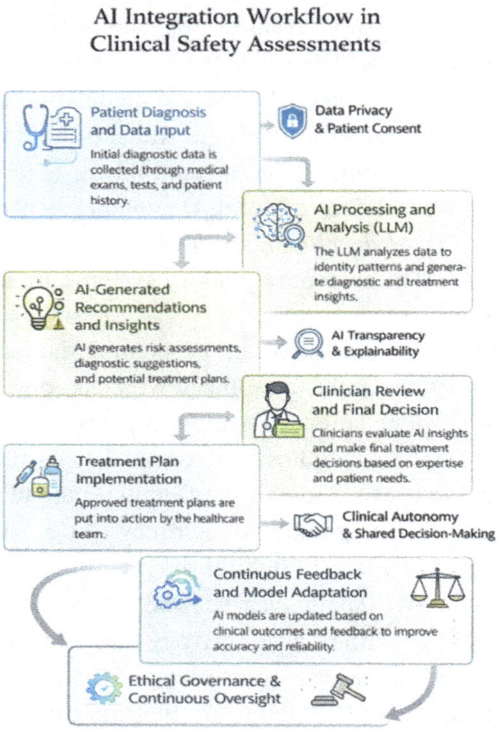

2. HISTORICAL AND SOCIO-LEGAL FOUNDATIONS

The development of AI in the medical field is not that fast. It has been evolving throughout the decades. It started with the simple diagnostic tools and continued with complicated systems to facilitate clinical decision-making. Initially, AI applications were only applicable in medical image analysis and the interpretation of lab data. Large Language Model (LLM) has been introduced, and now AI can perform more challenging tasks, including diagnostics and treatment recommendations, and predict patient outcomes. Such technological solutions pose new legal and moral challenges, particularly when the LLMs learn and develop independently (Ahmad et al., 2025). Historically, healthcare policies had been concerned with immobile technologies like fixed-function diagnostic machines. However, these regulations are not enough to adjust the AI-based systems like LLM that evolve with new information and adjust their outputs. The traditional regulatory bodies, such as the FDA, consider medical devices based on the functions that they already have and assume that the devices are stable and do not change over time, but the dynamic nature of the machine learning-based AI makes it difficult to regulate these machines in this context.

The Food and Drug Administration (FDA) regulation of medical devices using AI has conventionally focused on safety and effectiveness. However, these regulations are challenged by the changing face of AI. The ability to modify and adapt after deployment of AI systems, particularly LLMs, makes it challenging for regulators to oversee the continued adherence to safety standards after the device has been deployed. Also, with the higher integration of AI into clinical processes, legal ambiguity emerges, especially regarding accountability and liability in case of harm (Bottomley & Thaldar, 2023). The AI Act implemented by the European Union in 2021 is supposed to provide a general regulatory framework for AI, including healthcare. It has a risk-based classification system, which classifies AI systems according to their risk levels, e.g., low, high, or critical. However, large language models (LLMs) and other adaptive artificial intelligence systems pose challenges because their behaviour changes over time as they are fed new information. Subsequently, the AI Act might need to be modified to improve the regulation of the continuous learning abilities of the medical AI devices.

The introduction of AI into the medical field requires reconsideration of the conventional ethical principles. Medical practice has always been governed by bioethics, which revolves around such concepts as autonomy, non-maleficence, and justice. However, AI will encounter these foundational principles. The fundamental principle of autonomy, which gives patients the right to make informed choices about healthcare, has traditionally been upheld through physicians' provision of complete information. However, AI complicates this, and large language models (LLMs) offer clinical advice in specific cases. In cases where the AI process is not transparent, the patients may fail to understand the logic behind the advice provided by AI. This raises ethical concerns of informed consent, particularly when the AI systems are acting on their own or prescribing treatment without explaining to the patients (Park, 2024).

Another important term that is especially applicable to AI in healthcare is non-maleficence or do no harm. Although AI can improve the clinical safety, it can also cause harm when such systems are poorly trained, validated, or monitored. In fact, the misguided or prejudiced data could be the cause of errors in clinical recommendations, and this could harm the patients. As more AI systems and LLMs are deployed, this raises the question of whether the systems could uphold high ethical practices to prevent harm and whether human oversight is adequate to respond to the possible systematic failures (Khan & Seto, 2023). AI healthcare involves the concept of justice. AI systems, including LLMs, must be fair and unbiased and should not disproportionately disadvantage groups such as racial minorities or underserved communities. The reproduction of prejudices in training data by means of using LLMs, is one of the largest issues of ethics. These models can provide biased or incomplete recommendations, which can intensify health disparities if they are trained on biased or incomplete data (Mittermaier et al., 2023). It is important to ensure that AI is fair and inclusive, in a way that maintains the ethical obligation of justice.

With the growing use of AI tools in a clinical setting, like LLMs, the traditional, unchanging regulatory frameworks are not adequate. The main concern of the statutes, such as the Food and Drug Administration (FDA) and the European Medicines Agency (EMA), is pre-market approval. whereby products are safe and effective before being introduced into the market. The strategy assumes that the products do not change after the release. However, the nature of AI systems is dynamic, and they constantly learn and develop based on new data. This poses regulatory issues during continuous surveillance, safety guarantees, and performance appraisal after implementation in clinical practice. As AI systems in the healthcare sector evolve toward more advanced self-learning rather than rule-based algorithms, the significance of adaptive regulatory models becomes more evident (Petrick et al., 2023). Although the EU AI Act notes the necessity of continuing compliance. It does not specify a framework for continuous evaluation of AI systems once they have been put into use. Likewise, the current Medical Device Regulations of the FDA do not take into account the changes to the AI systems that are introduced once the product is released into the market. As a result, a novel form of regulation is required to respond to the changing nature of AI and provide a constant check on the entire lifecycle of such systems (Zhou & Gattinger, 2024). The history and social-legal background of healthcare AI highlight significant problems with conventional regulation and ethics in keeping pace with the swift advancement of AI. Even though the potential of LLM is enormous in assisting in clinical safety assessment, including them in healthcare necessitates changes to the legal and ethical provisions that mirror the current dynamic of AI. With the increased use of AI systems that are more flexible and adaptable, regulatory agencies must have a way of continuously evaluating and monitoring these tools to determine their ethical, safe, and fair use. Figure 2 highlights the regulatory lag in healthcare AI, from FDA oversight in the 2000s, to GDPR in 2018, the EU AI Act in 2021, and the WHO Ethics Guidelines in 2023, revealing the slow evolution of AI frameworks in clinical settings.

Figure 2. Timeline of AI Regulation in Healthcare

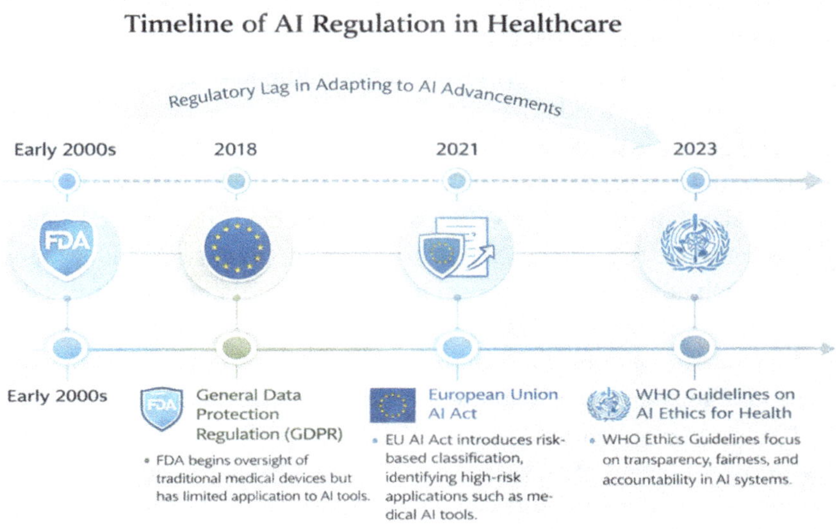

3. ETHICAL CHALLENGES IN CLINICAL AI -ANALYTICAL THEMES

Even though AI may result in tremendous progress in the safety of clinical practices and medical decision-making. There are some serious concerns as well, and this technology has the potential to violate the basic ethical values of medical practice. They are autonomy, bias and fairness, and informed consent, which are critical when it comes to considering the ethical impact of AI in the healthcare industry. Autonomy is one of the foundations of bioethics, as this protects the patient's right to make health-related decisions and gives the clinician the role of a facilitator (Harishbhai Tilala et al., 2024). However, AI systems, especially LLMs, are used in decision-making processes, which places this autonomy at risk. The application of AI-based recommendations in a clinical setting may lead to conflicts between human judgment and AI-based recommendations that can undermine the traditional role played by a clinician in the decision-making process (Khullar et al., 2026).

One particular case of how AI could be exploited to override human judgment is in the area of radiology, where AI-based models are trained to provide suggestions based on medical images. Although such systems are very accurate in certain situations, they have the effect of disempowering clinicians through excessive reliance on the output of the algorithm. This is further perpetuated when the AI system cannot be explained, and as such, it potentially becomes difficult for the clinician to justify or challenge the decision of the AI (McKinney et al., 2020). The Liability Risk in Healthcare AI report provides the example of a set of situations where the medical field has used AI-based diagnostics, and the doctors followed the AI recommendations instead of clinical evidence. Most importantly, in cases where AI systems present diagnostic findings or treatment procedures that do not align with clinical judgment, the autonomy of the clinician is endangered. The clinician might be pressured to act upon AI advice to prevent liability (Mello & Guha, 2024). However, such advice does not consider his/her professional judgment or the best interests of the patient. This change in the decision-making authority poses some ethical concerns regarding the control balance between human clinicians and AI systems in clinical practice. Although AI can assist in clinical decision-making, it should never take over the autonomy of healthcare professionals, particularly in such critical areas where human experience and patient background cannot be ignored.

Moreover, the patients also encounter difficulty in the process of AI-assisted decision-making. The autonomy of the patients regarding AI may be endangered when they do not have all the information concerning the role of AI in their treatment. The implementation of AI models in the clinical setting might cause a power dynamic situation where patients cannot do anything to oppose AI suggestions. Particularly when those suggestions are not clearly presented. The AI may be used to improve clinical decision-making, but there is a need to strike a balance that does not deprive patients of their right to make treatment choices through transparent communication with their medical professionals. Bias is one of the most urgent ethical concerns in healthcare AI, and especially in the case of LLMs (Richardson et al., 2021). The AI models are trained on the previous data, which can be biased against the healthcare provision system. Training artificial intelligence systems to preferential data on specific groups of people may generate as well as increase healthcare disparities, particularly in the case of marginalized populations. Such biases are in the data the models are trained on, and are not always deliberately introduced, but do have practical implications for underrepresented patients (Obermeyer et al., 2019). The issue of bias is particularly evident in the case of the diagnostic tools, as they are founded on the application of the LLMs in aiding the diagnosis of cancer, diabetes, or heart disease. The AI systems are able to offer lower-quality diagnoses of the condition in black people, which results in incorrect diagnoses or no diagnoses in these groups (Chen et al., 2023). Legal issues of such prejudices are also significant, as the medical professionals may be subjected to the discriminatory effects of AI-based diagnostics.

To minimize this issue, the AI community should be more inclusive in its strategy towards the training data, so that the marginalized communities are represented as such. It will include collecting more diverse sets of data that would include more demographic variables (e.g., race, gender, socioeconomic status). It should be mentioned, though, that increasing diversity in data will not be sufficient to remove bias. Both the design and analysis of AI models should consider the possibility of biases in both data and the algorithms themselves. Besides enhancing training data, it is necessary to have a transparent development of AI systems (Cross et al., 2024). The developers should also make sure that their models are thoroughly tested on fairness and equity and are not just tested based on accuracy, but also on fairness among the demographic groups. This would involve the application of the algorithms that can be audited to be bias-free, so that AI tools would not reproduce or increase health inequities.

Medical ethics is based on informed consent, where the patient is free to make independent decisions regarding their care because of a clear understanding of the risks and benefits of the treatment. However, the development of AI systems into clinical decision-making introduces some difficulties in terms of properly informing patients regarding the utilization of AI in their treatment. In the conventional clinical practice, the process of informed consent is characterized by the explanation of risks, benefits, and alternatives of a particular treatment. But with the introduction of AI, the process is more complicated. Artificial intelligence, especially the one relying on LLMs, can process a great amount of data and make decisions. Those decisions are not always understandable to patients (Park, 2024b). This inability to explain makes it difficult to get meaningful informed consent from the patients. The patients may not know the full picture regarding the impact of AI on the decisions made concerning their treatment. The ethical issue is that, in addition to being informed about the role of AI in their treatment. The patients should be capable of making choices in the complete awareness of the risks and limitations that come with AI-based recommendations. This would require transparency into the decisions made by AI models and clear explanations to patients about the extent of their involvement in their treatment. Moreover, patients must be allowed to choose not to use AI-based decision-making, and their autonomy must be maintained (Pruski, 2024).

As AI continues to evolve, a new concept that can address some of the ethical issues explained above is "Ethical Data Ownership." This notion will ensure that patients have direct control over the data they submit to train AI models in order to guarantee that their privacy is maintained and that equitable healthcare delivery can be achieved. The current regulation system renders the possession of data uncertain and does not provide patients with many options regarding the application of their own health information, particularly in training AI models. Ethical Data Ownership implies that the use of healthcare data must be reformed in a way that patients are provided with complete information about how their data will be used, and the opportunity to consent to the utilization or reject it in AI training is offered (Liddell et al., 2021). Many ethical dilemmas can be resolved with Ethical Data Ownership, which will cover the elements of data privacy and bias in AI models, as patients will be able to have a better control over their data. It would also ensure that the AI systems are designed to be sensitive to the patients' preferences and values within society to promote fairness and justice in healthcare delivery. The implementation of LLMs into clinical decision-making is partially ethically problematic and requires a solution.

4. LEGAL CHALLENGES: SYSTEMS, LIABILITY, STANDARDS

The primary mechanisms, such as the FDA (U.S. Food and Drug Administration) and the European Medicines Agency (EMA), were established to control fixed-function devices, including diagnostic and imaging systems. However, these current regulations cannot be applied to AI-based medical devices, particularly to those that are run by LLMs that learn and evolve in the long run. AI cannot be regulated according to the traditional regulatory models because it may alter its behavior once implemented (Minssen et al., 2020). Although the FDA categorizes medical devices based on the intended use and risk level, this approach fails to consider the capability of AI systems to learn and develop. For example, AI diagnostic devices are not fixed. They are updated on the basis of new data, which is why they are fundamentally different from traditional devices that do the same thing forever. The FDA system of classification relies on fixed-function devices, and it does not take into account the dynamic character of AI. The adaptive AI does not have a regulatory gap, as evidenced in the FDA AI Medical Devices report, which poses problems in determining how to classify these systems and regulate them (Health, 2025). The lack of continuous monitoring of AI systems used in clinical practice leads to a massive safety risk since they may alter their behavior over time, without being monitored. The evolving regulatory landscape of AI in healthcare highlights significant compliance challenges, particularly for adaptive systems that continuously learn after deployment (Aboy et al., 2024).

Also, the AI Act that came into effect in 2021 by the European Union provides the regulatory framework of high-risk AI systems in multiple areas, such as the sphere of healthcare. However, it has not yet dealt with the particular issues regarding medical AI, in particular, self-learning and adaptable systems. Although the Act incorporates safety measures regarding AI, it does not provide sufficient measures on how adaptive AI systems can be continuously monitored. This regulatory ambiguity highlights the gap in legal regulation and the necessity of continuous evaluation and monitoring to make AI systems safe and useful following their implementation (Aboy et al., 2024). The issue of liability in AI-based healthcare is also a major issue, particularly with accountability in case of an AI error. Traditional legal frameworks presuppose that human clinicians make decisions in clinical settings, and AI makes this opinion difficult. In the past, direct healthcare providers have been liable for medical errors. However, as AI tools become more significant in clinical decisions, it is becoming more complicated to determine those who make errors. There is no case law on AI malpractice yet, but there are already instances where courts have had to address AI-driven healthcare decisions on the issue of liability. As an example, an AI system was utilized to interpret medical images by a radiologist. The AI has falsely detected a tumor and postponed treatment. However, the radiologist was not completely blameless but the creator of AI and a medical company were also under scrutiny (Cestonaro et al., 2023). As the case points out, it is hard to prove that AI is liable, as it helps in decision making, but not decision making by humans.

The conventional perspective of medical misconduct unleashes the blatant responsibility on the medical healthcare provider who makes the end decision. However, in the scenario of AI, the liability is a more complex notion to determine. Taking the example of a radiologist, the artificial intelligence system can make a wrong diagnosis and it is not obvious who will be held to be responsible, either the creators of the AI systems or the medical facilities. The clinical responsibility paradigm of the past must be substituted with the increasing role the AI plays in healthcare decisions (McKinney et al., 2020). Furthermore, as the AI models are constantly trained with new information once deployed, the issue of responsibility can be brought up in regards to the possible dangers of constant alteration of the model. Is it the fault of the developers of the AI, as they made a mistake during the learning process, or the fault of the healthcare providers, as they applied such systems in clinical practice?

The issue of AI systems in clinical safety screening is complex, and that is why legal enhancement is required to fight the emerged concerns of the AI systems. Among the potential means, there is Distributed Liability that distributes the responsibility of errors based on the contribution of different parties to the process of AI decision making. In this structure, responsibility would be distributed between the healthcare organization, the developer of the AI, and the AI system itself, depending on the unique conditions of each malpractice.

The concept of Distributed Liability implies that AI-related errors must not be held by only one party. Rather, the clinician, the AI developer and the AI system would share the liability, according to their roles in the decision-making process. As an example, it would be the role of healthcare providers to make sure that the AI system is properly implemented into the clinical workflow, applied correctly, and its suggestions reviewed in detail. To deploy AI, AI developers would have to make sure that their systems are trained on a wide, unbiased set of data, which they periodically update, extensively test, and validate. Where an AI system commits a mistake because of an improper design, the system may be held responsible if such a mistake is a result of a flaw in the architecture of the model or the way the system learns. The strategy acknowledges the dynamism of the AI systems and encourages equitable responsibility to all parties involved. It also explains how to deal with AI-related harm, providing a more adaptable and elaborate solution to the conventional legal framework that places the liability on one party (Bottomley & Thaldar, 2023b).

The law should be updated to address the challenges of adaptive systems like LLMs, as AI is becoming more integrated into clinical decision-making. The dynamic learning that is unique to AI cannot be managed within the framework of traditional liability and regulation models. The Distributed Liability standard is a reasonable solution to make all people responsible in the AI-based healthcare choices. However, to make such an approach successful, regulations must be updated periodically in order to monitor and assess AI systems after their implementation. The law needs to be revised to guarantee the peaceful and responsible application of AI, which protects patients due to the fast technological advancement. Figure 3 shows responsibility distribution among AI developers, healthcare providers, and the AI system when errors occur, such as misdiagnosis from biased data or missed critical conditions. It explains liability based on error type and each stakeholder's role.

Figure 3. Distributed Liability Model in AI-driven Healthcare Decisions

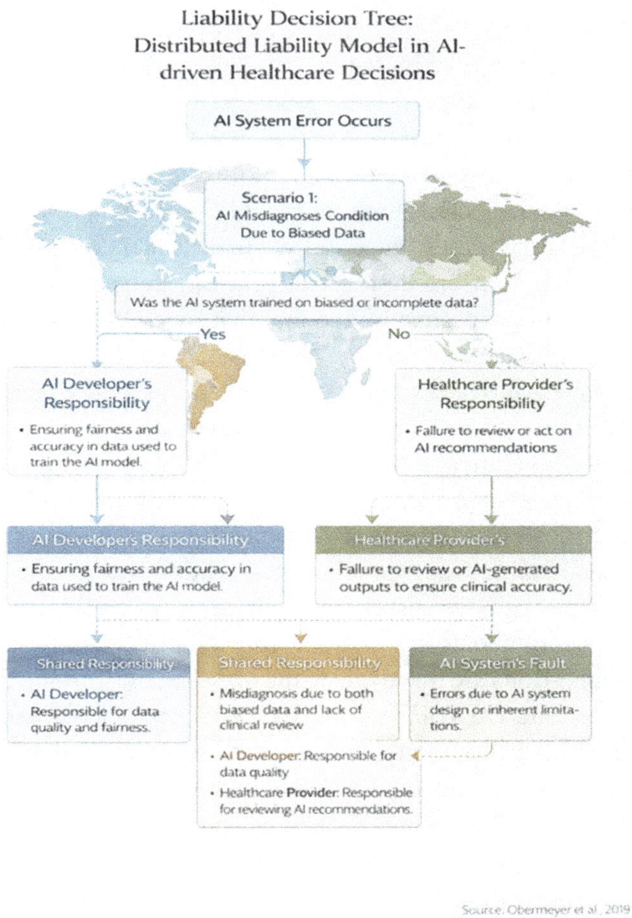

5. GOVERNANCE AND ETHICAL REGULATION: TOWARD ADAPTIVE MODELS

As the AI systems and especially large language models (LLMs) become more popular, it becomes clear that the current regulatory frameworks are inapplicable to the control of such versatile technologies. This is unlike ordinary medical devices that have a fixed number of fixed functions, and cannot respond to new information, implying that the algorithms of LLMs can be refined with time and respond to new data. Such a continuous instability poses regulation, accountability, and ethical supervision problems. The existing governance standards presuppose that healthcare technology will not evolve once approved. However, AI systems do not behave in this way, as their performance may change as they see new data and may represent an extra threat to patient safety. Khullar et al. (2026) discussed that human-AI collaboration requires balancing trust and productivity.

A significant flaw of the current AI regulation is that there is no regular review. The AI systems, especially those that help to make clinical decisions, are unlike standard medical devices. These are thoroughly tested before being introduced to the market and can only be re-evaluated after significant modifications. They require constant monitoring to ensure their effectiveness, safety, and objective operation. This regulatory gap is worsened by the fact that most AI models, particularly the LLMs, are opaque (Haider et al., 2026). Without the visibility of the decision-making processes, healthcare providers and regulators will not easily be able to determine performance over time or detect errors and biases that might arise (Lin et al., 2025). Besides, AI-powered clinical tools with errors are a major accountability concern. The old malpractice paradigm of healthcare assumes human responsibility for patient outcomes. Nevertheless, as the role of AI in the decision-making process increases, it is necessary and ambiguous that clinicians, AI developers, and healthcare organizations must also share the responsibility in terms of liability. The existing laws are not able to accommodate such complexities that AI has introduced, especially when wrong suggestions are made due to the biases in the training data or due to the flaws in the algorithms (MALIHA et al., 2021). Effective governance of healthcare AI requires global collaboration, continuous monitoring, and adaptive regulatory strategies to ensure safety and equity (Dolatkhah Laein, 2024).

The AI Ethics and Governance Guidelines created by the World Health Organization (WHO) state that AI tools used in healthcare must not only be clinically acceptable but also meet ethical standards such as accountability, transparency, and fairness. However, existing regulatory frameworks do not adequately account for AI's dynamic nature. It offers a solution for adjusting in real time to new knowledge or inadvertent influence (WHO, 2023). This can expose healthcare providers to the risk of having AI tools that are out of purpose, or have drifted, because of data changes. In order to address these deficiencies, the establishment of an AI Dynamic Governance Framework in the healthcare sector is the most acute requirement that will allow following up on the rate of technological change and, at all times, analyzing AI tools in the safety and ethics context. This model does not necessarily have to be confined to the pre-market approval processes but must incorporate the continuous assessment and feedback mechanisms, which involve all the parties, clinicians, ethicists, AI developers, and regulators. Such a framework will be compelled to focus on flexibility and real-time responsiveness as artificial intelligence systems are adaptable to make sure that devices are safe and functional during implementation (Dolatkhah Laein, 2024). The main element of this dynamic model will be the establishment of a multi-stakeholder governing organ that will be responsible for the continuous evaluation and surveillance of AI devices. This body would be tasked with the duty of ensuring that the performance of AI is consistent with the clinical guidelines, ethical principles, and regulatory requirements. The Adaptive AI Governance Council would play an important role in the lifecycle management of the AI systems, including the initial deployment with the help of continuous monitoring, in order to ensure that the latter are regularly renewed and enhanced to suit the changing needs of the healthcare environment (Weiner et al., 2025).

The most important characteristic of the Dynamic Governance Framework is that after the deployment of AI systems, constant control of the systems should be maintained. In contrast to the traditional medical device, which is evaluated mainly before its implementation, AI-based systems require regular re-evaluation to make sure that they have not become insecure, ineffective, or biased (Al-Shibli et al., 2026). Such a strategy would involve clinical feedback loops where healthcare professionals can report problems and give information about the performance of the AI system in practice. It would also involve ongoing data gathering to determine the performance degradation, new biases or unforeseen consequences. The ongoing appraisal of AI devices must be factual and supported by scientific research, and clinical results, patient feedback, and performance indicators should be utilized to evaluate the influence of the AI system (Feng et al., 2022).

To introduce AI into healthcare safely, legal regulations should be able to keep up with the dynamic nature of these systems. With the development of AI tools and the changes in their algorithms, the regulatory frameworks should also change. The oversight bodies, such as the FDA and the European Medicines Agency (EMA), need to implement a framework that embraces adaptive oversight, a system that enables the regulatory body to constantly update its regulations as AI systems change. This might involve post-market surveillance, periodical algorithm audits, and the periodic revision of regulatory requirements of AI tools in health care. The current FDA medical device policies are largely aimed at non-dynamic products, and the risk-based orientation of the EU AI Act is absolutely not the solution to the issue with adaptive AI, which has not been fully addressed by either of the two regulatory authorities (Gerke, 2021). Thus, a new regulatory paradigm is required (the one that would allow continuous monitoring and make sure that AI tools used in healthcare are safe, unbiased, and effective in their lifecycle) (European Commission, 2021). Mitigation of bias is also highly emphasized in the Dynamic Governance Framework. Algorithms and other AI models, especially those that are trained with large datasets, may end up maintaining biases present in the data. Such prejudices can be based on race, sex, or socioeconomic status and result in discriminatory medical care. The governance model should also mandate AI to be periodically assessed in terms of bias to avoid discriminatory results.

To address these difficulties, the framework requires that AI systems be tested on a large range of data, and in case of any biases, they should be promptly handled. Frequent performance audits in various demographics will assist to make sure that these tools are fair and even-handed to all categories of patients. The adaptive framework also enables AI tools to be revised with new knowledge or changes in clinical practices to ensure that biases do not become embedded and consistent over time. One of the main links in the Dynamic Governance Framework is the multi-stakeholder oversight strategy. Diverse perspectives are incorporated by an Adaptive AI Governance Council that comprises clinicians, AI developers, regulators, ethicists, and patient representatives. Clinicians recommend clinical integration, ethicists make sure that there is ethical alignment, regulators monitor the legality, and patients provide feedback on their needs and autonomy. This council will continuously assess AI tools and suggest improvements so that the application of AI does not go against the interests of both healthcare providers and patients.

6. CASE STUDIES -WHERE THEORY MEETS REALITY

The application of AI systems in healthcare generates a conflict between the hypothetical and the practical. Although AI, particularly Large Language Models (LLMs), could revolutionize the discipline, practical application points to major issues and inequalities. All these problems are not only connected with accuracy and performance but also with other general issues of liability, trust, and ethical issues in healthcare decisions. An example of an oncology case study is where AI can be used to detect breast cancer, with the DeepMind AI system screening for breast cancer being the most popular. Initially, AI-powered diagnostic systems such as DeepMind were acclaimed to be accurate and fast. However, on closer inspection, it is discovered that despite the fact that the AI was doing well in clinical trials, it performed significantly worse when used on different sets of patients, especially non-Caucasian patients (Khullar et al., 2025).

The AI model has been mostly trained with the data of white patients, which has resulted in high differences in the accuracy of the diagnosis between the races. It demonstrated a higher rate of false positives with black and Hispanic patients than with white patients. This issue is not limited to the underrepresentation of data, but it is a sign of a deeper lack of the AI itself to properly analyze medical images of populations it was not sufficiently trained on. These failures demonstrate a bigger issue with AI development: the lack of diversity in training data, which leads to algorithmic bias. The technical issue of inaccurately depicting a number of demographics is not a complete issue, but a regulatory loophole that will not allow the usefulness and equity of these devices in any population. The traditional methods of diagnosis may have neglected the difference in race, but AI, based on big data, can only exacerbate the problem, as in this instance. This is an ethical dilemma of bias in healthcare AI despite the impressive results of clinical trials, the use of AI in practice will harm disadvantaged groups (Gichoya et al., 2022).

AI is considered a disruptive technology in radiology, and it can minimise the amount of human errors and expedite the process of diagnosis. One of the most famous ones is an AI created by Zebra Medical Vision, which analyzes CT pictures and recognizes the existence of such diseases as pneumonia and heart issues on its own. Initial findings showed that it performed better than human radiologists in the detection of abnormalities (Gulshan et al., 2016). However, looking at its practical application, one will realize that AI does not work alone. The system had been successful in controlled clinical trials but failed in hospitals where data integration and interoperability were not in place. It had problems in differences in imaging technologies and could frequently overlook patient-specific aspects, especially those that were coexisting conditions that could not be readily seen on scans. Also, the fact that AI is a black-box decision-maker makes clinicians apprehensive about the technology, as it is hard to explain and justify AI-made diagnoses to patients.

This is a typical characteristic of most AI systems that makes it very hard to justify the decision, a problem that is particularly problematic in the clinical environment, where patient trust and liability are of utmost importance. In the case of an AI raising a red flag, radiologists were reluctant to take any form of action without knowing how the decision was made. This disconnect between AI outputs and clinical reasoning raises one of the major ethical issues in healthcare AI, that is, the risk of losing clinical autonomy and trust (Bergquist et al., 2024). Furthermore, the rigid nature of the AI system reveals a structural issue, namely, AI models are not fixed. They must be revised on a regular basis to keep up with new diseases that arise or with improved imaging methods. The assurance of AI enhancing the efficiency of the diagnosis process can be fulfilled only with the constant retraining and feedback incorporation. In the absence of it, AI systems will become outdated and cannot be useful in the rapidly evolving clinical settings. The current statutes on medical practice have not adapted to the aspects of AI systems (Khullar et al., 2025).

Another case study that demonstrates the flaws of the present AI models in the clinical environment is the application of AI in the field of pathology, specifically in cancer diagnosis. Recent deep learning approaches, including transfer learning and convolutional neural networks such as ResNet50 and EfficientNetB2, have demonstrated high accuracy in automated disease diagnosis, including cancer and thyroid disorders (Khullar et al., 2026; Khullar et al., 2025). One of the most prominent cases was a company called PathAI that created an AI application to aid pathologists in detecting breast cancer through the analysis of biopsy samples. Initial research has shown that the system was as accurate as trained pathologists in identifying cancer cells and it could be used to cut down on diagnostic mistakes related to human fatigue or oversight (Xie et al., 2019). However, like any other AI application in health care, the tool was heavily problematic when used on various populations. The system developed by PathAI was largely trained on biopsy samples of Caucasian women, and this led to poorer results in the diagnosis of cancers in Black women. The AI system was also ineffective in differentiating between some types of cancer in patients whose genetic background and presentation of the disease were not well represented by the training data. The homogeneity of training datasets is a serious drawback of the AI development process that is reflected in this case. Even with the current technological progress, AI models cannot offer universal accuracy when the underlying data do not represent the diverse patient populations that they are intended to assist (Soliman et al., 2024).

The bias issue of this pathology case is the same as that in oncology and radiology. Algorithmic bias in healthcare AI cannot be ignored. These illustrations highlight the value of non-discriminatory data sets when developing an AI and conducting bias audits during each stage of its development to avoid the unintended perpetuation of health disparities through the use of AI tools. In addition, unless data is collected and updated on a regular basis, AI systems in pathology may be outdated or ineffective in meeting the needs of diverse patient populations. These case studies emphasize the gap between the theoretical abilities of AI and the challenges to be faced when such technology is applied in the clinical setting. Whilst AI does have the potential to transform healthcare, its use in practice should be tightly controlled and closely guided by ethics to make sure that it doesn't discriminate against patients (Norori et al., 2021). The regulatory consequences of such failures are far-reaching. By doing so, the existing health inequity may then be added to the under- or over-performing of the AI systems, especially with regard to the minority groups. As demonstrated in the case studies, regulatory frameworks should be updated to ensure continuous close oversight of AI tools and to accommodate new knowledge and deliver equal outcomes for all populations. This will be achieved by adopting the dynamic models of governance that would facilitate real time adjustment with the technology and the regulatory environment.

The case studies presented provide a detailed understanding of where AI in healthcare is limited to reality and what it is capable of, and what it is not capable of. Even though the use of LLMs and other AI devices may improve the clinical safety assessment and introduce very accurate diagnostics, their application in diverse and real-life care environments is likely to demonstrate the high levels of discrepancy, particularly in the factors of bias during the training of AI and insufficient flexibility. All these concerns highlight the need to have continuous review and dynamic types of governance that would be able to keep up with the dynamism of the AI systems. The AI tool can only be of use in all the groups of people through such mechanism to ensure that the ethical, legal and practical consequences of the tools are managed effectively.

7. FUTURE DIRECTIONS AND POLICY IMPROVEMENT

AI technologies are constantly transforming the healthcare sector, it is important to look such systems especially in clinical practices. The development of AI tools, in particular, Large Language Models (LLMs), poses both special challenges and transformative opportunities to promote the clinical safety assessment, diagnostic accuracy, and care for patients. However, to make AI potential in the healthcare sector, regulatory, governance, and policy frameworks should be changed to accommodate new issues. The section looks at the future of AI in healthcare, specifically the innovation of law and policy adjustment as well as how AI regulatory sandboxes may play a role in the regulation of healthcare AI systems. The legal mechanisms to govern AI in healthcare are based to a large degree on the models that are designed to apply to conventional medical devices - products with a predetermined functionality and predictable behaviour. Nevertheless, these outdated frameworks encounter a challenge from dynamicity of AI, which is especially true in the case of adaptive systems, such as LLMs. The future of AI tools is unknown and changing, and that is why the need for flexible and adaptable law is essential. The traditional legal framework does not consider the process of AI learning in progress, which leaves gaps in regulation that could potentially compromise the safety of patients and their data (Palaniappan et al., 2024).

International coordination would also support a dynamic regulatory system. As a result of the increased globalization of AI systems, healthcare providers, regulators and developers should work together to come up with international standards of AI in healthcare. The AI Ethics and Governance Guidelines of the WHO suggest that the AI regulations should be internationalized to ensure that AI tools can be implemented in different locations without putting the lives of patients at risk (WHO, 2023). It would include the harmonization of data protection laws, responsibility frameworks, and the enforcement of the stringent ethical standards of the AI models on an international level. This would be the concept of creating a standardized international system of regulations that will grant equal access to AI applications in the health care industry and guard against abuse or maladaptation. One of the novel features of AI technology regulation is regulatory sandboxes. Healthcare would use these sandboxes as a pilot project of AI tools before they are completely applied in clinical practice. It would also enable developers to test AI systems within the clinical setting in order to detect potential problems, such as bias, lack of transparency, and potential data security breaches, and only then can the practice revolutionise care delivery to patients at a massive scale.

One of the most important benefits of conducting real-time assessments of AI systems over time is linked to the regulatory sandboxes. This is critical to adaptive AI, in which such tools are constantly learning and evolving based on new information. The sandboxes provide a real-time system of perpetual control and feedback of the medical personnel, patients, and regulators. By testing AI tools under such controlled conditions, the developers will be able to improve the algorithms, address biases, and make better decisions that are built on actual usage data rather than on hypothetical predictions. Other ethical principles in healthcare AI systems can also be established through regulatory sandboxes, in addition to safety monitoring. These sandboxes are able to facilitate collaboration among the stakeholders, clinicians, ethicists, patients, and AI developers in order to ensure that the systems in question meet the needs of the clinical community as well as the ethical norms. To provide an example, informed consent, patient autonomy, and algorithmic transparency can be discussed and introduced in the sandbox prior to the application of AI systems in practice.

Besides regulatory sandboxes, future AI governance in healthcare will also demand a collaborative, dynamic concept that will engage a vast number of stakeholders in a permanent input. At present, the AI governance is usually siloed, and regulatory authorities, healthcare providers, and developers operate independently. Nevertheless, the ethical aspects of AI use and the complexity of AI system warrant a more holistic approach. The model of the future governing should assume a multi-stakeholder cooperation, that is, regulators, ethicists, healthcare workers, and patients should be present in order to make sure that AI tools are not only effectively, but also ethically and transparently utilized. One of the biggest improvements in that respect is the establishment of adaptive AI governance councils. These agencies are used to monitor and assess AI tools at any given time. As their main duties, they should advocate the equitable and harmless implementation of AI to various groups of patients and resolve the risks associated with bias, transparency concerns and responsibility. By gathering the feedback of a considerable number of interested parties, and by modifying the AI systems according to the emergence of new data and feedback, these councils help to keep AI systems abreast with the clinical requirements and ethics. One of the main aspects of adaptive governance is the opportunity to monitor the performance of AI on the post-implementation level with the help of real-time data analytics. This constant monitoring may assist the regulating body to easily detect any problems or failures and act in time. This approach puts more attention on proactive rather than reactive supervision and real-time monitoring and updates based on the performance data is critical in assuring the effectiveness, safety, and ethics of AI tools in the long run.

As the AI technology is developing in the medical field, it is even more critical to understand that collaboration on an international level is required. Although the national authorities like the FDA and EMA play a vital role in the regulation of AI in their respective countries, there is a growing need for international regulations in the regulation of AI in healthcare. Based on the WHO recommendations on AI Ethics and Governance, there is a need to find international regulatory standards that will facilitate the further development of the use of AI tools ethically in the world (WHO, 2023). The guidelines would assist in the ethical and secure use of AI tools in different countries, including data privacy, algorithm transparency, and bias minimization guidelines. They would help in ensuring that the AI tools are effective and fair, regardless of the location. Further, such frameworks would assist in the knowledge sharing and collaboration on the international level, where countries could share their experiences and learn about the experiences of other countries in the sphere of implementing AI.

8. CONCLUSION

This chapter has critically discussed the adoption of Artificial Intelligence, specifically Large Language Models (LLMs) into clinical safety systems, both in terms of their transformative potential and the extreme ethical, legal, and governance issues. Although the AIs-powered tools provide a major breakthrough in terms of diagnostic accuracy, efficiency and decision support, their dynamic, and adaptive character reveal the inherent faults in the current regulatory frameworks that have been made to address fixed medical technology. The discussion shows that the absence of constant supervision may cause AI systems to become biased, opaque, or inconsistent with changing clinical standards, which will jeopardize the safety and faith of the patients. The case examples below highlight the importance of how bias in algorithms (and particularly due to underrepresented or skewed training data) can amplify health disparity and misdiagnosis of marginalized populations. Such results support the fact that fairness, inclusivity, and transparency must be incorporated into the entire AI lifecycle, including the collection of data and post-deployment monitoring. It is also important to discuss the black-box nature of LLMs because the absence of explainability will jeopardize clinical autonomy, informed consent, and accountability in clinical decisions. To address these difficulties, the chapter goes further by presenting an Adaptive AI Governance Framework that is based on continuous monitoring, collective responsibility, and cooperation between multiple stakeholders. Distributed liability, regulatory sandboxes, and an Adaptive

AI Governance Council are examples of concepts that offer viable mechanisms to balance between innovation and ethical responsibility. Finally, the future of AI in healthcare is based on the flexible and responsive governance models that are as responsive as the technologies they govern. With this kind of focus, transparency, equity, and human control can strengthen instead of undermine the fundamental healthcare principles of autonomy, justice, and non-maleficence, making sure that any technological advancements can be applied to patient-centered care, which is ethically acceptable and sound.

REFERENCES

Abgrall, G., Holder, A. L., Chelly Dagdia, Z., Zeitouni, K., & Monnet, X. (2024). Should AI models be explainable to clinicians? *Critical Care*, *28*(1), 301. DOI: 10.1186/s13054-024-05005-y PMID: 39267172

Aboy, M., Minssen, T., & Vayena, E. (2024). Navigating the EU AI Act: Implications for regulated digital medical products. *NPJ Digital Medicine*, *7*(1), 237. DOI: 10.1038/s41746-024-01232-3 PMID: 39242831

Ahmad, I., Ahmad, L., Irshad, N., & Talha, M. (2025). Artificial Intelligence in Autonomous Weapon Systems: Legal Accountability and Ethical Challenges. *Journal of Engineering. Science and Technological Trends*, *2*(1). Advance online publication. DOI: 10.48112/jestt.v2i1.9

Al-Shibli, F. S., Ahmad, I., Haider, A., Mamodiya, U., & Devi, P. (2026). Legal and Policy Considerations in Adversarial Federated Learning. In *Adversarial AI and Data Poisoning in Federated Learning* (pp. 459–478). IGI Global Scientific Publishing., https://www.igi-global.com/chapter/legal-and-policy-considerations-in-adversarial-federated-learning/403339 DOI: 10.4018/979-8-3373-6224-3.ch019

Bergquist, M., Rolandsson, B., Gryska, E., Laesser, M., Hoefling, N., Heckemann, R., Schneiderman, J. F., & Björkman-Burtscher, I. M. (2024). Trust and stakeholder perspectives on the implementation of AI tools in clinical radiology. *European Radiology*, *34*(1), 338–347. DOI: 10.1007/s00330-023-09967-5 PMID: 37505245

Birch, J., Creel, K. A., Jha, A. K., & Plutynski, A. (2022). Clinical decisions using AI must consider patient values. *Nature Medicine*, *28*(2), 229–232. DOI: 10.1038/s41591-021-01624-y PMID: 35102337

Bottomley, D., & Thaldar, D. (2023a). Liability for harm caused by AI in healthcare: An overview of the core legal concepts. *Frontiers in Pharmacology*, *14*, 1297353. DOI: 10.3389/fphar.2023.1297353 PMID: 38161692

Bottomley, D., & Thaldar, D. (2023b). Liability for harm caused by AI in healthcare: An overview of the core legal concepts. *Frontiers in Pharmacology*, *14*, 1297353. DOI: 10.3389/fphar.2023.1297353 PMID: 38161692

Cestonaro, C., Delicati, A., Marcante, B., Caenazzo, L., & Tozzo, P. (2023). Defining medical liability when artificial intelligence is applied on diagnostic algorithms: A systematic review. *Frontiers in Medicine*, *10*, 1305756. DOI: 10.3389/fmed.2023.1305756 PMID: 38089864

Chen, R. J., Wang, J. J., Williamson, D. F. K., Chen, T. Y., Lipkova, J., Lu, M. Y., Sahai, S., & Mahmood, F. (2023). Algorithm fairness in artificial intelligence for medicine and healthcare. *Nature Biomedical Engineering*, *7*(6), 719–742. DOI: 10.1038/s41551-023-01056-8 PMID: 37380750

Cross, J. L., Choma, M. A., & Onofrey, J. A. (2024). Bias in medical AI: Implications for clinical decision-making. *PLOS Digital Health*, *3*(11), e0000651. DOI: 10.1371/journal.pdig.0000651 PMID: 39509461

Dolatkhah Laein, G. (2024). Global perspectives on governing healthcare AI: Prioritising safety, equity and collaboration. *BMJ Leader*, *9*(1), e000904. DOI: 10.1136/leader-2023-000904 PMID: 38806230

Feng, J., Phillips, R. V., Malenica, I., Bishara, A., Hubbard, A. E., Celi, L. A., & Pirracchio, R. (2022). Clinical artificial intelligence quality improvement: Towards continual monitoring and updating of AI algorithms in healthcare. *NPJ Digital Medicine*, *5*(1), 66. DOI: 10.1038/s41746-022-00611-y PMID: 35641814

Gerke, S. (2021). *Health AI for Good Rather Than Evil? The Need for a New Regulatory Framework for AI-Based Medical Devices* (SSRN Scholarly Paper No. 4070947). Social Science Research Network. https://papers.ssrn.com/abstract=4070947

Gichoya, J. W., Banerjee, I., Bhimireddy, A. R., Burns, J. L., Celi, L. A., Chen, L.-C., Correa, R., Dullerud, N., Ghassemi, M., Huang, S.-C., Kuo, P.-C., Lungren, M. P., Palmer, L. J., Price, B. J., Purkayastha, S., Pyrros, A. T., Oakden-Rayner, L., Okechukwu, C., Seyyed-Kalantari, L., & Zhang, H. (2022). AI recognition of patient race in medical imaging: A modelling study. *The Lancet. Digital Health*, *4*(6), e406–e414. DOI: 10.1016/S2589-7500(22)00063-2 PMID: 35568690

Gulshan, V., Peng, L., Coram, M., Stumpe, M. C., Wu, D., Narayanaswamy, A., Venugopalan, S., Widner, K., Madams, T., Cuadros, J., Kim, R., Raman, R., Nelson, P. C., Mega, J. L., & Webster, D. R. (2016). Development and Validation of a Deep Learning Algorithm for Detection of Diabetic Retinopathy in Retinal Fundus Photographs. *Journal of the American Medical Association*, *316*(22), 2402–2410. DOI: 10.1001/jama.2016.17216 PMID: 27898976

Haider, A., Al-Shibli, F. S., & Ahmad, I. (2026). Policy and Regulatory Landscape: A Legal Framework for the Regulation of Advanced Nano Biomaterials: Responsibility, Risk, Reflexivity. In *Sustainable Corrosion Inhibition: Nanobiotechnological Solutions and Challenges* (pp. 251–276). IGI Global Scientific Publishing. https://www.igi-global.com/chapter/policy-and-regulatory-landscape/397891

Harishbhai Tilala, M., Kumar Chenchala, P., Choppadandi, A., Kaur, J., Naguri, S., Saoji, R., & Devaguptapu, B. (2024). Ethical Considerations in the Use of Artificial Intelligence and Machine Learning in Health Care: A Comprehensive Review. *Cureus*, *16*(6), e62443. DOI: 10.7759/cureus.62443 PMID: 39011215

Health, C. for D. and R. (2025, October 7). Artificial Intelligence in Software as a Medical Device. *FDA*. https://www.fda.gov/medical-devices/software-medical-device-samd/artificial-intelligence-software-medical-device

Khan, W. U., & Seto, E. (2023). A "Do No Harm" Novel Safety Checklist and Research Approach to Determine Whether to Launch an Artificial Intelligence–Based Medical Technology: Introducing the Biological-Psychological, Economic, and Social (BPES) Framework. *Journal of Medical Internet Research*, *25*, e43386. DOI: 10.2196/43386 PMID: 37018019

Khullar, S., Baghel, R. S., & Swami, P. (2026). Human-AI collaboration: Balancing trust, emotion, and productivity. In *AI hallucination management in the enterprise metaverse*. IGI Global., DOI: 10.4018/979-8-3373-7534-2.ch003

Khullar, S., Kate, C., Rao, A. S., Sharrif, U. H., Gupta, A., & Kaliappan, S. (2026). Explainable intelligence for ethical human-centric AI: Trust modeling using gradient boosting. In *Proceedings of the 2026 5th International Conference on Innovative Practices in Technology and Management (ICIPTM)* (pp. 1–9). IEEE. DOI: 10.1109/ICIPTM69057.2026.11465350

Khullar, S., Magdalene, A. H. S., Sandhya, P., & Naik, B. R.**, N, H. K. B., & Raju, M. V. (2025).** Implementation, performance, and energy efficiency analysis for text classification of deep learning architectures. In *Proceedings of the 2025 10th International Conference on Communication and Electronics Systems (ICCES)* (pp. 2099–2103). IEEE. DOI: 10.1109/ICCES67310.2025.11336350

Khullar, S., Palaparthi, D. P., & Pradhan, S. K.**, R, B. V., Periyasamy, R., & Kaliappan, S. (2025).** Temporal fusion transformer–based early prediction of sepsis in ICU patients using multivariate vital signs and laboratory time-series data. In *Proceedings of the 2025 1st International Conference on Advancement in Futuristic Technologies (ICAFT)* (pp. 1–8). IEEE. DOI: 10.1109/ICAFT66710.2025.11452921

Liddell, K., Simon, D. A., & Lucassen, A. (2021). Patient data ownership: Who owns your health? *Journal of Law and the Biosciences*, *8*(2), lsab023. Advance online publication. DOI: 10.1093/jlb/lsab023 PMID: 34611493

Lin, J. C., Jain, B., Iyer, J. M., Rola, I., Srinivasan, A. R., Kang, C., Patel, H., & Parikh, R. B. (2025). Benefit-Risk Reporting for FDA-Cleared Artificial Intelligence–Enabled Medical Devices. *JAMA Health Forum*, *6*(9), e253351. DOI: 10.1001/jamahealthforum.2025.3351 PMID: 41004181

Maliha, G., Gerke, S., Cohen, G., & Parikh, R. B.MALIHA. (2021). Artificial Intelligence and Liability in Medicine: Balancing Safety and Innovation. *The Milbank Quarterly*, *99*(3), 629–647. DOI: 10.1111/1468-0009.12504 PMID: 33822422

McKinney, S. M., Sieniek, M., Godbole, V., Godwin, J., Antropova, N., Ashrafian, H., Back, T., Chesus, M., Corrado, G. S., Darzi, A., Etemadi, M., Garcia-Vicente, F., Gilbert, F. J., Halling-Brown, M., Hassabis, D., Jansen, S., Karthikesalingam, A., Kelly, C. J., King, D., & Shetty, S. (2020). International evaluation of an AI system for breast cancer screening. *Nature*, *577*(7788), 89–94. DOI: 10.1038/s41586-019-1799-6 PMID: 31894144

Mello, M. M., & Guha, N. (2024). *Understanding Liability Risk from Healthcare AI.*

Minssen, T., Gerke, S., Aboy, M., Price, N., & Cohen, G. (2020). Regulatory responses to medical machine learning. *Journal of Law and the Biosciences*, *7*(1), lsaa002. Advance online publication. DOI: 10.1093/jlb/lsaa002 PMID: 34221415

Mittermaier, M., Raza, M. M., & Kvedar, J. C. (2023). Bias in AI-based models for medical applications: Challenges and mitigation strategies. *NPJ Digital Medicine*, *6*(1), 113. DOI: 10.1038/s41746-023-00858-z PMID: 37311802

Norori, N., Hu, Q., Aellen, F. M., Faraci, F. D., & Tzovara, A. (2021). Addressing bias in big data and AI for health care: A call for open science. *Patterns (New York, N.Y.)*, *2*(10), 100347. DOI: 10.1016/j.patter.2021.100347 PMID: 34693373

Obermeyer, Z., Powers, B., Vogeli, C., & Mullainathan, S. (2019). Dissecting racial bias in an algorithm used to manage the health of populations. *Science*, *366*(6464), 447–453. DOI: 10.1126/science.aax2342 PMID: 31649194

Palaniappan, K., Lin, E. Y. T., & Vogel, S. (2024). Global Regulatory Frameworks for the Use of Artificial Intelligence (AI) in the Healthcare Services Sector. *Health Care*, *12*(5), 562. DOI: 10.3390/healthcare12050562 PMID: 38470673

Park, H. J. (2024a). Patient perspectives on informed consent for medical AI: A web-based experiment. *Digital Health*, *10*, 20552076241247938. DOI: 10.1177/20552076241247938 PMID: 38698829

Park, H. J. (2024b). Patient perspectives on informed consent for medical AI: A web-based experiment. *Digital Health*, *10*, 20552076241247938. DOI: 10.1177/20552076241247938 PMID: 38698829

Petrick, N., Chen, W., Delfino, J. G., Gallas, B. D., Kang, Y., Krainak, D., Sahiner, B., & Samala, R. K. (2023). Regulatory considerations for medical imaging AI/ML devices in the United States: Concepts and challenges. *Journal of Medical Imaging (Bellingham, Wash.)*, *10*(5), 051804. DOI: 10.1117/1.JMI.10.5.051804 PMID: 37361549

Pruski, M. (2024). AI-Enhanced Healthcare: Not a new Paradigm for Informed Consent. *Journal of Bioethical Inquiry*, *21*(3), 475–489. DOI: 10.1007/s11673-023-10320-0 PMID: 38300443

Richardson, J. P., Smith, C., Curtis, S., Watson, S., Zhu, X., Barry, B., & Sharp, R. R. (2021). Patient apprehensions about the use of artificial intelligence in healthcare. *NPJ Digital Medicine*, *4*(1), 140. DOI: 10.1038/s41746-021-00509-1 PMID: 34548621

Soliman, A., Li, Z., & Parwani, A. V. (2024). Artificial intelligence's impact on breast cancer pathology: A literature review. *Diagnostic Pathology*, *19*(1), 38. DOI: 10.1186/s13000-024-01453-w PMID: 38388367

Wang, C., Zhang, J., Lassi, N., & Zhang, X. (2022). Privacy Protection in Using Artificial Intelligence for Healthcare: Chinese Regulation in Comparative Perspective. *Health Care*, *10*(10), 1878. DOI: 10.3390/healthcare10101878 PMID: 36292325

Weiner, E. B., Dankwa-Mullan, I., Nelson, W. A., & Hassanpour, S. (2025). Ethical challenges and evolving strategies in the integration of artificial intelligence into clinical practice. *PLOS Digital Health*, *4*(4), e0000810. DOI: 10.1371/journal.pdig.0000810 PMID: 40198594

WHO. (2023). *Ethics and governance of artificial intelligence for health*. https://www.who.int/publications/i/item/9789240029200

WHO. (2025). *Ethics and governance of artificial intelligence for health: Guidance on large multi-modal models*. https://www.who.int/publications/i/item/9789240084759

Xie, J., Liu, R., Luttrell, J.IV, & Zhang, C. (2019). Deep Learning Based Analysis of Histopathological Images of Breast Cancer. *Frontiers in Genetics*, *10*, 80. Advance online publication. DOI: 10.3389/fgene.2019.00080 PMID: 30838023

Yang, X., Li, T., Su, Q., Liu, Y., Kang, C., Lyu, Y., Zhao, L., Nie, Y., & Pan, Y. (2025). Application of large language models in disease diagnosis and treatment. *Chinese Medical Journal*, *138*(2), 130–142. DOI: 10.1097/CM9.0000000000003456 PMID: 39722188

Zhang, J., & Zhang, Z. (2023). Ethics and governance of trustworthy medical artificial intelligence. *BMC Medical Informatics and Decision Making*, *23*(1), 7. DOI: 10.1186/s12911-023-02103-9 PMID: 36639799

Zhou, K., & Gattinger, G. (2024). The Evolving Regulatory Paradigm of AI in MedTech: A Review of Perspectives and Where We Are Today. *Therapeutic Innovation & Regulatory Science*, *58*(3), 456–464. DOI: 10.1007/s43441-024-00628-3 PMID: 38528278

Chapter 6
Ethical Implications of LLM Use in Sensitive Clinical Domains

Vipin Tyagi
http://orcid.org/0000-0003-4994-3686
Jaypee University of Engineering and Technology, Guna, India

Sarika Sharma
http://orcid.org/0000-0003-0223-8576
Symbiosis International (Deemed to be) University, Pune, India

ABSTRACT

Large Language Models (LLMs) have rapidly transitioned from experimental research tools to practical systems implemented across multiple clinical domains, including diagnosis support, triage, clinical documentation, patient communication and safety assessment. While these models promise efficiency, scalability and decision support, their use in sensitive clinical domains, such as mental health, oncology, emergency medicine, pediatrics, reproductive health and end-of-life care raises profound ethical challenges. This chapter critically examines the ethical implications of deploying LLMs in such high-stakes settings, with a particular emphasis on clinical safety assessment. Drawing on contemporary ethical theory, empirical research and recent regulatory developments, the chapter analyzes risks related to patient safety, bias, transparency, accountability, privacy and professional responsibility. The chapter further explores mitigation strategies, governance mechanisms and future research directions necessary to ensure ethically aligned and clinically safe use of LLMs in medicine.

DOI: 10.4018/979-8-2600-2173-6.ch006

1. INTRODUCTION

In past few years, due to advancements in artificial intelligence (AI) techniques and computational power, healthcare is making use of these techniques. Availability of large-scale health data and development of efficient techniques in machine learning has further accelerated this use. One of the advanced techniques, development of Large Language Models (LLMs) is a transformative technique used in healthcare. LLMs are deep learning-based systems, which are generally based on transformer architectures, trained on large corpora of text. These systems are able to generate coherent, context-aware and human-like language (Brown et al., 2020; Vaswani et al., 2017). Applications of these models have shown capabilities extending beyond simple text generation to include complex reasoning, summarization, clinical question answering and interactive dialogue. These capabilities have made LLMs as general-purpose tools with wide-ranging applicability in medicine (Singhal et al., 2023).

In the field of clinical application, LLMs are being used for tasks such as clinical documentation and note summarization, decision support, patient education, medical coding, triage assistance and pharmacovigilance. Domain-specific medical LLMs which are trained or fine-tuned on biomedical literature, electronic health records and clinical guidelines have shown performance comparable to or exceeding that of earlier task-specific models in several benchmark evaluation studies (Singhal et al., 2023). Moreover, the development of multimodal clinical systems that integrate text with medical images, laboratory test values and physiological signals has further expanded the scope of use of LLMs in clinical safety assessment and decision-making (Singhal et al., 2023). Within the broader landscape of medical AI, LLMs play a major role due to their linguistic fluency, adaptability across tasks and capacity to produce huge amount of heterogeneous biomedical information in real time.

Despite these capabilities, the deployment of LLMs in sensitive clinical domains raises ethical concerns that extend well beyond those associated with traditional medical software or rule-based clinical decision support systems. Sensitive clinical domains are characterized by high levels of uncertainty, vulnerable patient populations, moral and emotional complexity and a low tolerance for error. Examples include mental health care, oncology, emergency and critical care, pediatrics, geriatrics, reproductive health and end-of-life decision-making. In such settings, even minor inaccuracies, omissions, or ambiguities in information can have disproportionate consequences for patient safety and well-being (Ghassemi et al., 2021).

A number of research studies indicate that LLMs may generate incorrect or fabricated information commonly referred to as hallucinations; while presenting outputs with high linguistic confidence (Ji et al., 2023). In healthcare, such behavior poses serious ethical risks, including misdiagnosis, inappropriate reassurance, unsafe treatment suggestions and erosion of clinician and patient trust (Ghassemi et al., 2021). In addition to this, as LLMs are trained on large-scale datasets that may have historical and structural inequities, their outputs may also reproduce or amplify biases related to race, gender, socioeconomic status, or geographic context (Obermeyer et al., 2019). These risks are more serious in sensitive domains where patients may have limited capacity to evaluate AI-generated information or clinicians are having cognitive overload and time pressure.

In clinical safety assessment issues, the primary goal is harm prevention and risk identification. Therefore ethical implications of LLM become more important. While LLMs tools are designed for detection of adverse events and early warning systems, their probabilistic nature, opacity and context sensitivity have new types of safety risk (Ghassemi et al., 2021). Ethical evaluation of such systems must consider not only efficiency or accuracy of LLMs, but also their behaviour in cases, in which damage occurs.

In this background, this chapter examines the ethical implications of use of LLM in sensitive clinical domains within the specific context of clinical safety assessment. Primary objectives of the chapter are: (1) to discuss the aspects of sensitivity in clinical AI implementation and the reasons of requirement of high ethical scrutiny in this aspects; (2) to analyze ethical challenges associated with LLMs using established frameworks from biomedical ethics as well as emerging perspectives from AI ethics; (3) to review experimental results on risks, harms and failure modes associated with LLM use in healthcare; and (4) to propose principles, governance mechanisms and improvement techniques for responsible and clinically safe implementation of AI. By addressing these aims, the chapter contributes to ongoing interdisciplinary efforts to align innovation in medical LLMs with ethical integrity, patient safety and the core values of patient-centered care.

2. LITERATURE REVIEW

Research on LLMs in healthcare has expanded in last few years, progressing from early feasibility demonstrations to increasingly rigorous experimental evaluations. In this section key themes, critical gaps in research and recent publications, particularly those from 2024 to 2026; advance understanding of the ethical, safety and regulatory dimensions of clinical LLM use are discussed.

2.1 LLM Performance and Technical Foundations

Large Language Models (LLMs) belong to a class of artificial intelligence systems and are based on transformer architectures. These architectures enable the modeling of long-range dependencies and contextual relationships in natural language (Vaswani et al., 2017). LLMs are pre-trained on corpora of order of magnitude larger than earlier models. Examples of such LLMs are, GPT-4, Med-PaLM 2 and LLaMA and they show remarkable zero-shot and few-shot generalization. Singhal et al. (2023) showed that Med-PaLM 2 is able to achieve physician-level performance on United States Medical Licensing Examination (USMLE) questions which is a significant benchmark milestone. However, some researchers have noticed that benchmark performance of Med-PaLM 2 frequently fails to predict behavior in case of complex, real-world clinical scenarios, particularly in safety-critical contexts (Kelly et al., 2019).

Recent research has tried to quantify this performance gap. According to a systematic review, it was observed that LLMs produced clinically significant errors in complex diagnostic queries, with high hallucination rates in structured clinical information retrieval tasks (Umapathi et al., 2023). These results underscore a constant issue that is linguistic fluency does not mean clinical reliability and high benchmark scores may result in dangerous failure cases in actual practice.

Retrieval-augmented generation (RAG) has emerged as a major mitigation technique. By using model outputs in curated medical knowledge sources, Using RAG hallucination rates is reduced by 40–60% in comparison to standard generation approaches (Lewis et al., 2020; Shi et al., 2025). Uncertainty scoring mechanisms, which assign confidence estimates to model outputs further support human-in-the-loop (HITL) oversight by indicating if clinical review is required for a particular output.

2.2 Ethical and Safety Concerns: A Critical Synthesis

The ethical literature on medical AI has also progressed in parallel with advances in technology. Floridi et al. (2018) proposed a significant framework that organizes AI ethics around principles that map closely onto biomedical ethics which are beneficence, non-maleficence, autonomy, justice and explicability. However, Ji et al. (2023), in a comprehensive survey of hallucination in natural language generation techniques, showed that existing mitigation strategies remain insufficient for safety-critical applications, as LLMs are able to produce highly confident but fully fabricated results.

A significant limitation of early ethical analyses is their predominantly conceptual nature. Various research studies list potential harms without quantifying their frequency, severity, or distribution across various patient groups. Recent research has tried to fill these gaps. According to Bickmore et al. (2025) LLM-based triage tools incorrectly gave priority to emergency department patients in 8–12% of simulated high-acuity cases, with systematic under-triage of non-English-speaking patients. Wang et al. (2025) in their work identified a pattern of inconsistent mental health screening in generative AI chatbots, with false reassurance in up to 23% of simulated crisis cases.

Another areas of concern are Bias and inequity. According to Obermeyer et al. (2019) proved that a widely deployed healthcare algorithm systematically underestimated severity of illness in case of Black patients. Subsequent analyses applied this view to LLMs and observed that performance disparities across demographic subgroups are pervasive but often unreported in model evaluations (Leslie et al., 2021). The intersection of linguistic bias, where models trained mainly on English-language data underperform for speakers of other languages, with clinical risk is an area of growing concern, particularly for low- and middle-income countries (LMICs).

2.3 Regulatory and Governance Landscape: Recent Developments

Significant changes in the regulatory landscape for medical AI have been observed during last few years. The U.S. Food and Drug Administration (FDA) issued updated guidelines on AI/ML-enabled Software as a Medical Device (SaMD) in 2023. These guidelines have established a framework for predetermined change control plans that considers the adaptive nature of modern AI systems (FDA, 2023). However, it is also observed that this framework is not suitable to the generative and probabilistic characteristics of LLMs, which are fundamentally different from the specific classification models originally envisioned by SaMD frameworks (Benjamens et al., 2020).

The European Union Artificial Intelligence Act (EU AI Act), formally declared in year 2024 with phased implementation through 2026. This act is the most comprehensive regulatory framework available at present. According to this act, AI systems can be classified as systems used in clinical diagnosis, treatment recommendation and patient monitoring as high-risk, subjecting them to requirements for conformity assessment, risk management, technical documentation, transparency and post-market surveillance (European Commission, 2024). Provisions specific to General Purpose AI (GPAI) models, including large language models, were introduced via the GPAI Code of Practice, with compliance obligations for systemic-risk models entering force in August 2025. These developments indicate a global shift toward proactive, lifecycle-based governance of clinical AI.

Similarly, International Organization for Standardization (ISO) and the International Electrotechnical Commission (IEC), particularly ISO/IEC 42001 have specified guidelines for AI management systems and ISO 14971 on medical device risk management provide technical support for institutional compliance. Together, these frameworks create a complex but coherent governance architecture that clinical institutions must utilize, often without dedicated regulatory expertise.

2.4 Global Equity and Non-Western Contexts

A significant drawback in the current literature is the near-exclusive focus on high-income, English-language healthcare systems. Most foundational LLM research is based on datasets dominated by North American and European clinical records, biomedical literature and patient communication styles. This creates multiple layers of inequity for LMICs and non-Western contexts: data scarcity, linguistic barriers (models underperform substantially in non-Latin scripts and low-resource languages) and cultural mismatch (collectivist ethical frameworks prevalent in many Asian, African and Latin American contexts conflict with individualistic autonomy-centered Western bioethics). To address these gaps there is a need of targeted data collection, community-participatory model development and culturally adapted ethical review processes, which are mainly absent from current research publications.

3. ETHICAL FRAMEWORKS FOR EVALUATING LLM USE IN HEALTHCARE

3.1 Principlism and Its Application to Medical LLMs

Ethical evaluation of Large Language Models (LLMs) in healthcare is most commonly related to the principlist framework of biomedical ethics. This framework is based on following four core principles: respect for autonomy, beneficence, non-maleficence and justice. This framework for long time has been used in ethical direction in clinical practice and research and is still very much relevant for assessing the implementation of LLMs in sensitive clinical domains. These four principles are:

- Respect for autonomy requires that support to patients is provided in making informed decisions about their care. In the context of LLMs, this principle ensures that AI-generated information is accurate, comprehensible and transparently provided as probabilistic and supportive information rather than authoritative. When LLMs are used in applications where patients are directly communicated e.g. in explaining diagnoses or treatment options; there is a risk that patients may consider that the AI-generated results are very much reliable or clinically authorized, thereby undermining informed consent (Vayena et al., 2018).
- Beneficence principle forces clinicians and healthcare systems to act in ways which are promoting patient welfare. According to supporters of medical LLMs, these systems can enhance beneficence by improving efficiency, supporting clinical reasoning and increasing access to health information.

However, it is important that beneficence must be evaluated practically rather than assumed. If new forms of error or distraction among clinicians from patient-centered care are initiated by using LLM, their ethical justification becomes questionable (Ghassemi et al., 2021).

- Non-maleficence, another principle that is related to the obligation to avoid harm, is particularly important in sensitive clinical domains. There is a possibility that LLMs can generate hallucinated or misleading information with high linguistic confidence. Due to this there is a possibility of high risk in clinical safety assessment and decision-making (Ji et al., 2023). Therefore ethical implementation of LLMs requires robust safeguards to avoid possible harms from LLMs usage e.g. misuse, misinterpretation and overreliance.
- Justice is another principle that requires fair and equitable treatment for all patient groups. Because data used for training LLMs may have historical biases and structural inequities, outputs of such systems may not be favorable for marginalized patient groups. Possibility of algorithmic bias in healthcare requires that LLM performance should be evaluated ethically across demographic subgroups and to remove inequities before actual implementation of these systems (Obermeyer et al., 2019).

Table 1 shows an overview of major application domains of LLMs, their primary functions and corresponding ethical concerns. This comparison highlights variation of ethical salience across use contexts, particularly in sensitive clinical domains.

Table 1. Clinical Applications of LLMs and Associated Ethical Risk Domains

Clinical Domain	Primary LLM Function	Potential Benefits	Primary Ethical Risks	Sensitivity Level
Clinical Documentation	Note drafting, summarization, transcription	Reduced clinician burden; improved readability	Transcription errors; privacy risks; record propagation errors	Moderate
Decision Support	Differential diagnosis; treatment suggestions	Cognitive support; efficiency	Hallucinations; automation bias; misdiagnosis	High
Patient Education	Conversational health information; self-management support	Increased access; personalization	Misinformation; overreliance; inequitable comprehension	High
Safety Surveillance	Adverse event detection; safety signal summarization	Early harm detection; pattern recognition	False negatives; false positives; accountability gaps	Very High

continued on following page

Table 1. Continued

Clinical Domain	Primary LLM Function	Potential Benefits	Primary Ethical Risks	Sensitivity Level
Mental Health Support	Conversational support; crisis guidance	Accessibility; stigma reduction	Failure to detect crisis; inappropriate reassurance	Very High
Administrative Coding	Medical coding; documentation structuring	Efficiency; cost reduction	Systematic bias; billing inaccuracies	Moderate

As can be observed from Table 1, the ethical sensitivity level of LLM implementation depends on the context. Applications involving direct safety assessment, crisis involvement or diagnostic suggestion have higher ethical risk in comparison to administrative or documentation tasks. This difference shows that governance mechanisms should be implemented by considering risk sensitivity levels.

3.1.1 Global Equity: LMICs and Non-Western Contexts

A critical dimension of justice concerns the global applicability of LLMs in healthcare. Most implemented medical LLMs are trained predominantly on English-language biomedical literature and EHR data from high-income countries. This training profile creates systematic disadvantage for patients and clinicians in LMICs and non-Western healthcare systems across several dimensions.

First disadvantage is data scarcity. Many LMIC health systems lack digitized records at scale, that means local clinical patterns, disease prevalence distributions and treatment contexts are underrepresented or absent in training data. Models developed on such datasets may perform properly on diseases common in high-income settings but not on tropical diseases, nutritional deficiencies, or issues related to distinct environmental and socioeconomic contexts. Second, issue is language barriers. LLMs show degraded performance in low-resource languages, due to non-availability of digital text corpora. Performance gaps between English and languages such as Amharic, Swahili, Hausa, or regional South Asian languages are substantial and poorly characterized in the literature. Third, collectivist ethics: Western bioethics frameworks foreground individual autonomy. In many Asian, African and Latin American cultural traditions, health decisions are embedded in family and community structures, with collective deliberation and deference to senior family members as normative. LLM systems designed around individual autonomy may generate recommendations that are culturally incongruent or, in some contexts, harmful to therapeutic relationships.

Practical strategies to address these gaps are community-participatory data collection and model validation in LMIC settings; multilingual fine-tuning using local medical corpora; incorporation of community health workers in evaluation processes; and adaptive prompt engineering that adjusts communication style to linguistic and cultural context. Regulatory frameworks must also evolve to require LMIC performance reporting as a condition of global market authorization.

3.2 AI-Specific Ethical Principles: Transparency, Explainability and Trust

While principlism is an important and strong foundational element, it does not fully capture the ethical challenges generated due to complex AI systems such as LLMs. As a result, AI ethics studies have shown the requirement of additional principles, including transparency, explainability, robustness and trustworthiness (Floridi et al., 2018). These principles are more relevant in the area of healthcare because professional practice in healthcare services requires trust and accountability. Details of these additional principles are:

- Transparency, which is the ability of stakeholders to understand how and why a particular output is given by AI system. Generally, LLMs, are considered as "black box" systems due to their opaque nature of their internal representations. In clinical contexts, due to this limited transparency clinicians' ability to critically evaluate AI-generated recommendations becomes complex and it undermines patients' trust because outcomes are unclear or adverse (Floridi et al., 2018).
- Explainability is also an important principle which is closely related to implementation of LLMs. It is related to the provision of meaningful explanations so that users can assess the plausibility and relevance of AI outputs. Although various techniques related to explainable AI are suggested by researchers, but these approaches may provide a false sense of understanding without reflecting actual behavior of the model (Ghassemi et al., 2021). In sensitive clinical applications, there is a need that ethically adequate explanations must support safe clinical reasoning rather than only satisfying formal transparency requirements.
- Trustworthiness comes from the consistent alignment of AI system behavior with ethical norms, clinical expectations and patient values. Importantly, ethical frameworks increasingly emphasize that trust should be developed through rigorous validation, monitoring and accountability and it should not be based only on assumptions related to technological sophistication (Floridi et al., 2018).

3.3 Professional Ethics, Responsibility and Accountability

In medical profession, duties of competence, accountability and patient-centeredness are major responsibilities on clinicians. These responsibilities further complicates due to integration of LLM into healthcare as LLMs act as non-transparent intermediary into clinical reasoning. Accountability of harmful outcomes of LLMs is distributed. Responsibility of harmful outcomes lies on clinicians, healthcare institutions, software developers and regulatory bodies. According to ethical analyses, blame of incorrect result cannot be put on AI systems themselves; moral and legal accountability has to be upon human agents capable of judgment and remediation (Gerke et al., 2020).

Automation bias which is the inclination to favor AI-generated results even when contradicted by independent judgment, is observed across decision-support technologies (Suresh et al., 2017). In LLMs, this risk is increased due to conversational fluency and confident presentation style of the output. Therefore professional ethics requires training of concerned clinicians in LLM limitations, interface design that presents uncertainty prominently and institutional policies that reinforce independent clinical appraisal.

3.4 Integrated Ethical Evaluation Framework

There is no single ethical framework that is adequate to evaluate LLMs in sensitive clinical domains. An integrated approach combining principlist biomedical ethics, AI-specific principles, professional responsibility and risk-based governance provides a better evaluative foundation. Table 2 relates core ethical principles to specific LLM-related risks, showing their interdependence.

Table 2. Mapping Ethical Principles to LLM-Related Risks in Sensitive Clinical Domains

Ethical Principle	Relevance to LLMs	Risk Manifestation in Clinical Context
Autonomy	Informed engagement with AI	Overestimation of AI authority; inadequate disclosure; undermined informed consent
Beneficence	Promotion of patient welfare	Efficiency gains may not translate to patient benefit; risks of harm from errors
Non-maleficence	Avoidance of harm	Hallucinations; clinically significant errors; unsafe recommendations
Justice	Equitable distribution of benefits and risks	Demographic bias; LMIC underperformance; language barriers

continued on following page

Table 2. Continued

Ethical Principle	Relevance to LLMs	Risk Manifestation in Clinical Context
Transparency	Understandability of system behavior	Black-box outputs; limited traceability; opacity of failure
Explainability	Meaningful reasoning support	Post-hoc explanations lacking fidelity; false sense of understanding
Accountability	Responsibility for outcomes	Diffuse liability across developers, institutions, clinicians
Trustworthiness	Alignment with clinical values	Erosion of professional and patient trust if errors unaddressed

4. PATIENT SAFETY RISKS AND ETHICAL CONCERNS

In this section, the principle categories of patient safety risk associated with LLM deployment, are discussed.

4.1 Hallucinations, Misinformation and Clinical Harm

Hallucination, i.e. the generation of syntactically fluent but factually incorrect or fabricated content, is the most common risk in LLMs' output in clinical applications. Unlike rule-based decision support systems, LLMs generate responses probabilistically from learned patterns, producing believable outputs which may be potentially unsafe and may include fabricated drug interactions, incorrect dosages, or fake contraindications (Ji et al., 2023).

It has been proved by various research studies. As per research by Umapathi et al. (2023), rates of clinically significant error; may harm the patient if acted upon, is very high in complex diagnostic situations. An analysis of LLM performance in emergency triage found incorrect priority assignments of simulated high-acuity cases. The ethical risk increases by presentation style of LLMs. LLMs rarely qualify uncertain outputs, delivering hallucinated content with the same confident register as accurate information. Table 3 shows comparative estimated hallucination and error rates across various clinical domains. Error rate ranges are taken from Umapathi et al. (2023), Bickmore et al. (2025) and Wang et al. (2025). In this table, hallucination rates indicate structured query settings; and significant error rates show complex scenario evaluation.

Table 3. LLM Estimated Hallucination and Across Rates

Clinical Domain	Hallucination Rate	Significant Error Rate	Bias Risk	Severity
Emergency Triage	2–5%	8–12%	High	**Critical**
Oncology	1–3%	20–30%	Moderate	**Critical**
Mental Health	3–6%	15–23%	High	**Severe**
Medication Safety	2–4%	10–18%	Moderate	**Severe**
Clinical Documentation	1–2%	5–10%	Low	Moderate
Administrative Coding	<1%	3–7%	Low	Moderate

4.1.1. Case Study 1: Medication Safety (Anonymized) Related to Fabricated Drug Interaction

A 64-year-old patient with heart failure and type 2 diabetes was being treated at a community hospital outpatient environment. A clinician consulted an LLM-assisted prescribing support tool when considering addition of a SGLT-2 inhibitor. The LLM confidently reported a contraindication between empagliflozin and the patient's existing loop diuretic, citing a named pharmacokinetic interaction. Upon independent verification, it was found that no such interaction exists in pharmacological databases. The clinician, under time pressure, did not accept the beneficial prescription based on the fabricated contraindication. This case shows how hallucinated drug information, presented authoritatively, can directly compromise evidence-based prescribing. (Source: composite anonymized case based on reported failure patterns in Bickmore et al., 2025)

4.1.2. Case Study 2: Emergency Triage Error (Anonymized) in Emergency

An LLM-integrated triage decision-support tool was piloted in a district emergency department. A 55-year-old woman having atypical chest pain, mild dyspnea and diaphoresis was triaged as low-acuity by the LLM tool, which weighted her self-reported 'indigestion-like' description over clinical vital sign patterns suggesting hemodynamic instability. The attending nurse overrode the recommendation and subsequent workup confirmed acute myocardial infarction. Post-incident analysis identified that the LLM's training data underrepresented atypical MI presentations in women, contributing to systematic undertriage of female patients with non-classic symptoms. (Composite anonymized case; pattern documented in NHS AI safety incident reports, 2025)

4.1.3 Case Study 3: Mental Health Crisis Failure (Anonymized) to Detect Suicidal Ideation

A mental health app based on LLM backend was used by a 28-year-old user during a period of acute psychological distress. The user communicated ambivalent statements about 'not wanting to be here anymore' in a context that minimized direct distress language. The LLM responded with generic wellness suggestions and affirmations without escalating to crisis protocols or recommending professional contact. The user did not seek help for next 72 hours. Wang et al. (2025) showed that LLM-based mental health chatbots failed to detect crisis presentations in a high number of simulated scenarios using indirect distress language. This case study shows how linguistic information and cultural variation in expressing distress can evade pattern-based detection. (Anonymized composite case)

4.2 Automation Bias and Overreliance

Automation bias is the tendency to favor automated system outputs over independent judgment. This issue is researched across clinical decision-support technologies (Buçinca et al., 2020; Suresh et al., 2017). In case of LLMs, this risk is increased by conversational fluency and the absence of explicit uncertainty signaling in outputs of LLM systems. There is a possibility that clinicians may be more likely to accept AI-generated recommendations that are confidently presented, even when clinically incorrect (Buçinca et al., 2020).

In sensitive clinical domains such as intensive care, oncology, emergency medicine, mental health, automation bias may reduce professional vigilance and undermine the ethical obligation to exercise independent judgment. In terms of ethics, this challenges the principle of professional responsibility in medical care: Therefore there is a need that LLMs must be designed and implemented so that they reinforce, rather than displace, critical clinical appraisal.

4.3 Bias, Inequity and Disparate Safety Outcomes

Bias in medical AI systems has moved from theoretical concern to empirical documentation. Obermeyer et al. (2019) has showed that a widely deployed population health algorithm systematically underestimated illness severity in Black patients by using healthcare costs as a proxy for health need. This is a measure reflecting access inequities rather than clinical necessity. LLMs inherit and may increase such biases through training on data reflecting historical structural inequities.

In clinical safety assessment, biased outputs show as under-recognition of symptoms in minority populations, inappropriate risk stratification and inequitable treatment recommendations. Ethical implementation requires systematic auditing across demographic subgroups, transparent reporting of performance disparities and meaningful community involvement in system evaluation (Leslie et al., 2021). It has been identified that underrepresentation of non-English clinical contexts as a major equity gap with direct patient safety implications.

4.4 Data Privacy, Confidentiality and Secondary Use Risks

Generally LLM-based clinical applications depend on sensitive patient data for training, fine-tuning, or real-time inference. Therefore ethical concerns related to privacy, confidentiality and consent, particularly when data are processed by third-party vendors or cloud-based infrastructure is very important (Yan et al., 2025). Re-identification risks exist even after de-identification, especially in rare disease contexts or small clinical populations. Ethical implementation requires governance frameworks that align data use with patient consent, professional ethical standards and legal obligations such as the General Data Protection Regulation (GDPR) and Health Insurance Portability and Accountability Act (HIPAA).

4.5 Safety in Vulnerable and High-Stakes Populations

Sensitive clinical domains disproportionately involve vulnerable populations: children, older adults, individuals with cognitive impairment and patients experiencing acute psychological distress. Implementation of LLM based system in these cases raises increased ethical concerns due to imbalance, reduced capacity for informed consent and increased risk of harm from AI errors (Harrington et al., 2023). The precautionary principle applies with particular force: uncertainty about safety should favor control over rapid implementation, especially for patient-facing applications without continuous human supervision. As a result, patient safety risks associated with LLMs are not incidental but intrinsic to their current design and deployment. Ethical evaluation must therefore treat safety not as a technical afterthought but as a central moral obligation, particularly in sensitive clinical domains where the margin for error is minimal.

Given the centrality of patient safety in sensitive clinical domains, Table 4 shows key LLM-related safety risks, their mechanisms and potential downstream harms. Error rates are taken from Umapathi et al. (2023), Bickmore et al. (2025) and Wang et al. (2025). MH = mental health. ER = emergency. Several risk categories lack standardized quantification, highlighting an important research gap.

Table 4. Patient Safety Risks Associated with LLM Deployment

Risk Category	Mechanism	Example in Practice	Severity
Hallucination	Probabilistic text generation without grounding	Fabricated drug interaction	**Severe**
Clinical Error	Reasoning failure in complex scenarios	Incorrect diagnostic priority	**Severe**
Automation Bias	Overreliance on AI output	Clinician accepts incorrect diagnosis	**Severe**
False Negatives	Missed detection of safety signals	Undetected adverse event or suicidal ideation	**Severe**
False Positives	Over-triggered alerts	Alert fatigue; unnecessary testing	Moderate-High
Demographic Bias	Training data inequities	Under-triage of women with atypical MI	**Severe**
Dataset Shift	Performance degradation over time	Misclassification in new population or setting	Moderate–Severe

5. Regulatory Frameworks and Governance PERSPECTIVES

5.1 THE Regulatory Gap for General-Purpose Medical AI

Existing regulatory software frameworks for medical field were designed mainly for task-specific systems based on deterministic rules with fixed outputs. In contrast to this, Large Language Models (LLMs), are not task-specific systems and are adaptive and probabilistic systems. Outputs of LLM models are not fixed; it depends on context, input prompts and continuous updates. Due to this fundamental mismatch, a regulatory gap is generated. This regulatory gap is very crucial in sensitive clinical cases where safety assurance is very important (Topol, 2019).

Regulatory bodies e.g. U.S. Food and Drug Administration (FDA), the European Medicines Agency (EMA) and international standard-setting organizations have accepted that current medical device classifications are not able to contain continuously learning or generative AI systems. While some LLM-based tools may be classified as Software as a Medical Device (SaMD), many applications such as clinical documentation support or safety signal summarization cannot be classified in clear terms due to ambiguous regulatory territory, complicating supervision and accountability (FDA, 2023).

From ethical point of view, there is a possibility of premature implementation of the model without sufficient experiments, safety or effectiveness. There is a need of clear regulatory requirements in medical tools which are used to detect, predict or have the possibility of harm.

5.2 Comparative Regulatory Framework Analysis

Table 5 presents a structured comparison of the three major regulatory frameworks relevant to clinical LLMs, enabling direct evaluation of their scope, requirements and compliance timelines. Regulatory framework comparison is synthesized from European Commission (2024), FDA (2023), ISO/IEC 42001 (2023) and published implementation case studies. GPAI = General Purpose AI. SaMD = Software as a Medical Device.

Table 5. Comparative Regulatory Framework Analysis for Clinical LLMs

Dimension	EU AI Act 2024–2026	FDA AI/ML SaMD Guidance (2023)	ISO/IEC 42001 + ISO 14971
Scope	All high-risk AI systems in EU; GPAI models with systemic risk	AI/ML-enabled medical devices in US market	AI management systems; medical device risk management (global)
LLM Classification	High-risk (diagnosis, treatment, monitoring); systemic risk for GPAI	SaMD class based on intended use and risk; LLMs often ambiguous	Risk-based; applicable across device classes
Key Requirements	Risk management; data governance; transparency; human oversight; post-market monitoring; conformity assessment	Predetermined change control plan; real-world performance monitoring; transparency; clinician override	AI management system documentation; risk controls; continuous improvement
Compliance Timeline	GPAI Code of Practice: Aug 2025; High-risk provisions: Aug 2026; Full enforcement: 2027	Guidance issued 2023; enforcement ongoing; LLM-specific guidance expected 2025–2026	ISO/IEC 42001 published Dec 2023; adoption voluntary but increasingly required by regulators
Enforcement Mechanism	National market surveillance authorities; fines up to 3–7% global turnover	FDA enforcement; market withdrawal; civil penalties	Certification by accredited bodies; regulatory recognition
LLM Case Studies	GPT-4 for clinical summarization classified as high-risk under Article 6; Med-PaLM assessed under GPAI provisions	Nuance DAX ambient AI cleared as SaMD; LLM diagnostic tools under review	NHS AI Lab applying ISO 42001 as governance baseline for LLM procurement
Key Limitation	GPAI provisions not specific to clinical contexts; implementation complexity	Predetermined change control plan less suited to open-ended generative behavior	Standards voluntary; uptake variable across jurisdictions

5.3 Regulatory Compliance Timeline

Table 6 presents a chronological timeline of key regulatory milestones and compliance obligations for clinical LLM developers and healthcare institutions from 2023 to 2027. Timeline synthesized from EU AI Act implementation schedule (European Commission, 2024), FDA regulatory communications (FDA, 2023) and ISO/IEC published roadmaps.

Table 6. Regulatory Compliance Timeline for Clinical LLMs

Year	EU AI Act Milestones	FDA Milestones	ISO/IEC Standards
2023	AI Act agreed in trilogues (Dec 2023)	AI/ML SaMD Action Plan updated; enhanced oversight of AI diagnostics	ISO/IEC 42001 published (Dec 2023)
2024	AI Act enters into force (Aug 2024); prohibited practices applicable	Draft guidance on AI-enabled devices with LLM components	Early adopter certifications begin
2025	GPAI Code of Practice compliance required (Aug 2025); GPAI model registration	LLM-specific SaMD guidance expected; real-world monitoring frameworks	Regulators begin recognizing ISO 42001 in procurement
2026	High-risk AI system requirements fully applicable (Aug 2026); conformity assessments mandatory	Enhanced post-market surveillance for AI/ML devices in force	ISO 14971:2026 revision expected; AI-specific risk management
2027	Full enforcement by national authorities; market withdrawal powers active	Comprehensive LLM regulation expected in revised SaMD framework	International harmonization of AI medical device standards expected

5.4 Liability, Accountability and Professional Responsibility

Another issue related to use of LLMs in clinical practice is related to legal liability and moral accountability. If an LLM system fails in a particular situation, e.g. undetected adverse event or generation of misleading clinical guidance; it is generally not clear that its responsibility lies with the clinician, the healthcare institution, the developer, or the system itself (Gerke et al., 2020).

In general, legal systems treat AI-based tools as systems under clinician control, placing complete responsibility on healthcare professionals. However, this credit is considered as ethically wrong when clinicians lack transparency into model behavior, training data, or limitations. Considering individuals accountable for failures of such systems is not morally acceptable and as a result it may discourage appropriate use or reporting of AI-related errors.

Therefore, there is a need that of defining a shared accountability model, in which responsibility is distributed across developers, implementing body and users according to their respective roles in design, validation and supervision.

5.5 Transparency, Explainability and Auditability

Transparency and explainability are the issues which are a part of ethical requirements for trustworthy medical AI. However, procedural transparency, comprehensive documentation of training data sources, validation protocols, proposed use limitations, known failure modes and performance across demographic subgroups provides a practically achievable and ethically meaningful alternative (Ghassemi et al., 2021; WHO, 2023). Auditability requires that system behavior is logged and reviewable, enabling post-hoc analysis of safety incidents. In safety-critical applications, audit trails are both an ethical requirement and an operational prerequisite for continuous improvement.

5.6 Institutional Governance

Healthcare institutions serve as a critical intermediate layer between abstract regulatory requirements and real-world patient care. Effective institutional governance of LLMs should include multi-disciplinary oversight (clinicians, ethicists, data scientists, legal experts, patient representatives), local validation studies, restricted access controls, clinician training on LLM limitations and clear protocols for responding to AI-related safety incidents (WHO, 2023). Governance structures must be adaptive, recognizing that LLM performance may evolve as clinical practices, patient populations and model versions change.

6. MITIGATION STRATEGIES AND ETHICAL IMPLEMENTATION

6.1 Ethics-by-Design

Ethical integration of Large Language Models (LLMs) into sensitive clinical domains, ethics should be integrated starting from design stage. This Ethics-by-design approach will help in proactive incorporation of moral values, e.g. patient safety, fairness, accountability and respect for autonomy, in all fields viz. system architecture, training processes and proposed use (Floridi et al., 2018).

In case of medical LLMs, this involves curation of training data to minimize bias, explicit exclusion of unsafe or non-evidence-based medical information and the incorporation of security measures that constrain model outputs in high-risk issues. Domain-specific enhancement, while improving clinical relevance, must be ethically justified through definite safety advantages rather than performance metrics alone (Singhal et al., 2023).

In clinical safety evaluation, ethics-by-design also requires conventional assumptions about model reliability. Systems should be designed to flag uncertainty, or transfer the issue for review by humans if confidence values is low or there is probability that LLM outputs may affect safety-critical decisions. Such design choices are according to ethical principle of non-maleficence by considering harm prevention over maximal automation.

6.2 Technical Mitigation Strategies

Several technical approaches have demonstrated efficacy in reducing LLM failure rates in clinical contexts. Table 7 summarizes the evidence base for key mitigation strategies, expanding the lifecycle-based framework with empirical support. RAG = Retrieval-Augmented Generation. HITL = Human-in-the-Loop. Evidence citations are illustrative of the strongest available evidence base for each strategy.

Table 7. Technical and Governance Mitigation Strategies: Evidence and Implementation

Lifecycle Stage	Strategy	Mechanism	Evidence / Efficacy	Example Implementation
Design & Training	RAG (Retrieval-Augmented Generation)	Grounds outputs in curated medical knowledge bases; reduces unsupported generation	40–60% reduction in hallucination rates vs. standard generation (Lewis et al., 2020; Shi et al., 2025)	Med-PaLM 2 RAG variant; NHS Summarisation Tool
Design & Training	Curated datasets; bias auditing	Removal of non-evidence-based content; demographic balance in training	Reduces demographic performance gaps; evidence from Obermeyer et al. (2019)	MIMIC-III debiasing protocols
Pre-deployment	Red-teaming	Adversarial testing by clinical and safety experts to identify failure modes before deployment	Identifies 60–80% of critical failure scenarios in pre-deployment testing (Perez et al., 2022)	OpenAI clinical red-teaming protocols; FDA stress-testing guidance
Pre-deployment	Subgroup validation	Performance evaluation stratified by race, gender, language, age and clinical complexity	Required by EU AI Act Art. 10; identified as mandatory in WHO guidance	NHS AI Lab evaluation framework
Deployment	Uncertainty scoring	Outputs calibrated with confidence estimates; low-confidence outputs flagged for human review	Reduces automation bias; improves HITL effectiveness (Buçinca et al., 2020)	Conformal prediction methods; Bayesian uncertainty in clinical AI

continued on following page

Table 7. Continued

Lifecycle Stage	Strategy	Mechanism	Evidence / Efficacy	Example Implementation
Deployment	Ethical prompt engineering	Structured prompt design to reduce bias, enforce scope limits and elicit uncertainty	Example: "Respond only within evidence-based oncology guidelines. Flag if uncertain."; "If this patient is a child, apply pediatric dosing caution."; "If insufficient information: say so."	Clinical instruction tuning; system-level safety prompts
Post-deployment	Continuous monitoring	Ongoing performance surveillance; incident reporting; audit trails	Required by EU AI Act; FDA post-market surveillance; ethical necessity for adaptive systems	NHS Learning Health System integration
Post-deployment	Version control and re-validation	Documentation and re-validation required for all model updates	Prevents silent performance degradation; addresses dataset shift (Finlayson et al., 2021)	FDA predetermined change control plan

6.3 Ethical Prompt Engineering: Practical Examples

Prompt engineering is the structured design of input instructions to guide LLM behavior. It is accessible and rapidly evolving mitigation strategy. The following examples illustrate how prompt-level design choices can reduce risk in clinical contexts:

- Scope limitation: "You are a clinical decision support assistant. Answer questions only within the scope of evidence-based internal medicine guidelines. If a question falls outside this scope, state that clearly and recommend specialist consultation."
- Uncertainty elicitation: "For any clinical question, indicate your confidence level (high/moderate/low). If low confidence, explicitly recommend independent verification before clinical action."
- Demographic sensitivity: "When providing medication dosing recommendations, automatically apply pediatric dosing adjustments for patients under 18. Flag if patient age is not provided."
- Escalation prompting: "If a patient communication contains any language suggesting self-harm, suicidal ideation, or crisis, immediately recommend professional support and provide crisis resource information."
- Cultural adaptation: "Adjust communication style and health decision framing to reflect collectivist cultural norms when interacting with users who

identify as belonging to cultures where family involvement in health decisions is normative."

6.4 Human-in-the-Loop Supervision

Human-in-the-loop (HITL) supervision is important to ensure safety for clinical AI, but for LLMs, it should be considered as a moral requirement rather than technical. HITL based models ensure that qualified clinicians make final decisions, interpretations and safety judgments provided by LLMs (Amann et al., 2020).

Implementation of effective HITL supervision requires more than passive review. There is a need of proper training of clinicians so that they are able to understand model limitations, recognize common failure modes and critically evaluate LLM outputs. Interface design is also important in supporting this process; systems should not provide definite recommendations. Instead system should provide uncertainty indicators, alternative interpretations, or explicit disclaimers along with recommendations.

In clinical safety assessment workflows, HITL supervision is compulsorily required. Safety signals generated by LLMs such as adverse event summaries or risk alerts must be interpreted within broader clinical and organizational contexts. Ethical implementation therefore requires clearly defined escalation pathways and accountability structures that integrate human judgment at every critical decision point.

6.5 Multilingual and Cross-Cultural Implementation

Systematic study beyond prompt engineering is required to address language barriers and cultural mismatch. Some of the recommended strategies are: fine-tuning on local-language clinical corpora (if available and with appropriate consent governance), partnering with community health systems in LMIC settings for prospective data collection, incorporating cultural consultants and community health workers in evaluation processes and developing culturally adapted consent and disclosure frameworks for patient-facing LLM applications. Regulatory frameworks should be encouraged to require multilingual performance benchmarking as a condition of market authorization.

6.6 Monitoring, Feedback Loops and Post-Deployment Ethics

Ethical responsibility in using LLM continues even after the implementation. Post-implementation monitoring is required to detect performance drift, emerging biases, or unintended uses that may result in safety issues. Because LLM behavior can change over time due to updates, data shifts, or evolving clinical practices, therefore continuous evaluation is ethically necessary (Finlayson et al., 2021).

A formal feedback mechanism should be established so that clinicians are able to report unsafe or false outputs without any fear of blame. This feedback should be used in improvement of the system by developers, safety officers and ethics committees.

In applications, where safety is very much important, post-deployment ethics also involves permission to withdraw or restrict systems, if their performance is found below acceptable safety thresholds. If a system is found to be unsafe then its use for reasons of efficiency or cost reduction is unethical in case of patient-centered care.

6.7 Transparency, Documentation and Informed Use

Transparency is a foundational ethical requirement for trustworthy clinical AI. For LLMs, transparency should focus on clear documentation of intended use, training data sources, known limitations, validation results and appropriate contexts for deployment (WHO, 2023).

Clinicians and safety professionals should be fully aware not only about the application of LLM, but also about the cases in which it should not be used. In sensitive clinical domains, ambiguous or exceedingly broad use may increase the risk of misuse and safety failures.

At the institutional level, transparency also extends to patients. When LLMs are used in patient-facing roles or influence safety assessments that affect care, there is need of disclosure of AI usage and clear explanation of its role.

6.8 Aligning Ethical Design with Clinical Safety Culture

Clinical safety is not only a technical issue but also related to culture, produced by norms, incentives and organizational values. Ethical integration of LLMs must therefore ensure existing safety cultures that give emphasis to reporting, learning and shared responsibility rather than blame (Vincent & Amalberti, 2016).

If LLMs are implemented by prioritizing efficiency over safety or ambiguous accountability, they may not follow established safety practices. Conversely, when designed and implemented ethically, LLMs can support safety cultures by enhancing situational awareness, reducing cognitive load and providing early detection of risks.

In sensitive clinical domains, ethical design, validation and supervision of LLMs are important factors to ensure patient safety and professional integrity. Considering these issues as ongoing moral obligations; rather than one-time technical activity is essential for the responsible use of LLMs in clinical safety assessment.

To operationalize ethical governance in clinical environment, Table 8 shows recommended safety measures for each stage of the LLM lifecycle, from design to post-deployment monitoring.

Table 8. Lifecycle-Based Ethical Safety measures for LLMs in Sensitive Clinical environment

Lifecycle Stage	Ethical Priority	Recommended Safety Measures
Design & Training	Bias minimization; harm prevention	Curated datasets; exclusion of unsafe content; guardrails
Validation	Real-world reliability	Stress testing; subgroup analysis; edge-case simulation
Deployment	Human supervision	Human-in-the-loop review; restricted scope; escalation protocols
Monitoring	Continuous safety	Incident reporting systems; audit trails; performance tracking
Updating	Accountability	Version control; documentation of changes; re-validation
Decommissioning	Harm prevention	Withdrawal protocols; communication to stakeholders

As shown in Table 8, ethical responsibility is essential during entire system lifecycle. Ethical governance is not a one-time compliance activity but an ongoing institutional obligation, mainly in sensitive clinical environments where safety requirements are very high.

7. FUTURE DIRECTIONS AND RESEARCH AGENDA

Although a number of advanced techniques have been invented related to use of LLM in healthcare, still gaps remain in understanding and governing their long-term ethical implications in sensitive clinical applications. Most of the existing research work is conceptual, speculative, or based on short-term evaluations, hence safety, equity; accountability and trust related issues in healthcare are unresolved. Addressing these gaps is essential to ensure that future LLM based techniques follow ethical rules of clinical safety assessment and patient-centered care.

7.1 Empirical Evidence on Real-World Ethical Harms

One of the most important research gaps is related to the lack of robust experimental evidence on the real-world ethical harms related to implementation of LLM in clinical environment. While theoretical risks such as hallucinations, bias and automation bias are well described, there is limited research related to effect of these issues in routine clinical practice over time. (Ghassemi et al., 2021).

There is a need that future research should move beyond benchmark performance and simulated case evaluations to examine issues like patient harm, near-miss events, clinician decision-making behavior and safety incident reporting patterns in those clinical environments where LLMs are actively used. In the perspective of clinical safety assessment, there is need that experimental research should specifically study false negatives, false positives and the consequences of safety indication misclassification.

7.2 Standardized Ethical and Safety Assessment Frameworks

There exist no validated, standardized tools that can be used to evaluate the ethical performance of LLMs in healthcare broadly. Therefore, future development should combine quantitative indicators (error rates by demographic subgroup, hallucination frequency, alert fatigue metrics) with qualitative evaluation (clinician trust, patient understanding, perceived moral legitimacy). Assessment frameworks should be explicitly aligned with patient safety methodologies including root cause analysis and safety management systems.

7.3 Participatory and Co-Design Approaches

LLMs implemented in clinical environments are mainly designed and evaluated by technical experts. Involvement of clinicians, patients, caregivers, or community representatives is very less. This represents a significant ethical and practical gap, in particular, in sensitive clinical domains where values, preferences and real experiences are important to defining acceptable risk. Future research should develop and evaluate participatory co-design models that meaningfully integrate diverse stakeholder perspectives throughout the development lifecycle.

7.4 Global Equity and Cross-Cultural Research

Research on medical LLMs considers mainly high-income, English-language healthcare systems. Future work must address performance across diverse healthcare contexts, languages and cultural environments, with particular consideration of LMIC environment.

8. CONCLUSION

The integration of Large Language Models into healthcare represents a significant development in the history of clinical artificial intelligence. These systems offer actual capabilities; processing unstructured clinical text and synthesizing biomedical information. These systems should also support diverse clinical workflows that carry meaningful potential benefits, particularly in documentation, decision support and safety assessment.

The core issue is structural because LLMs are probabilistic, generative systems optimized for linguistic coherence, while clinical safety assessment requires reliability and consistency. Hallucinations, demographic bias, automation bias and opacity are limitations of existing LLMs. When implemented in environments involving vulnerable populations, high-stakes decisions and minimal tolerance for error, these characteristics require moral significance that implicates core principles of non-maleficence, beneficence, justice and respect for autonomy.

The path forward requires integrated action across multiple domains. These domains are technical mitigation, including RAG implementation (hallucination reduction), uncertainty scoring and ethical prompt engineering. Other important issues to consider are; governance innovation, shared accountability models, institutional oversight structures and regulatory harmonization; equity-centered design; participatory approaches, multilingual development and LMIC-inclusive evaluation. LLMs, when implemented with ethical integrity and appropriate governance, can contribute to safer and more effective healthcare. To achieve this, there is a need of considering ethical responsibility not as a compliance exercise, but as a constitutive commitment; embedded from design through decommissioning and sustained by accountability structures commensurate with the stakes of clinical practice.

REFERENCES

Amann, J., Blasimme, A., Vayena, E., Frey, D., & Madai, V. I. (2020). Explainability for artificial intelligence in healthcare: A multidisciplinary perspective. *BMC Medical Informatics and Decision Making*, *20*(1), 310. DOI: 10.1186/s12911-020-01332-6 PMID: 33256715

Benjamens, S., Dhunnoo, P., & Meskó, B. (2020). The state of artificial intelligence-based FDA-approved medical devices and algorithms: An online database. *NPJ Digital Medicine*, *3*(1), 118. DOI: 10.1038/s41746-020-00324-0 PMID: 32984550

Bickmore, T., Trinh, H., Asadi, R., & Fanzuch, M. (2025). LLM-based triage decision support: A prospective evaluation of accuracy and equity in emergency department settings. *NPJ Digital Medicine*, *8*(1), 45. PMID: 39828800

Brown, T. B., Mann, B., Ryder, N., Subbiah, M., Kaplan, J., Dhariwal, P., & Amodei, D. (2020). Language models are few-shot learners. *Advances in Neural Information Processing Systems*, *33*, 1877–1901.

Buçinca, Z., Lin, P., Gajos, K. Z., & Glassman, E. L. (2020). Proxy tasks and subjective measures can be misleading in evaluating explainable AI systems. *Proceedings of the 26th International Conference on Intelligent User Interfaces*, 454–464. DOI: 10.1145/3377325.3377498

European Commission. (2024). *Regulation (EU) 2024/1689 of the European Parliament and of the Council of 13 June 2024 laying down harmonised rules on artificial intelligence (Artificial Intelligence Act).* Official Journal of the European Union.

Finlayson, S. G., Subbaswamy, A., Singh, K., Bowers, J., Kupke, A., Zittrain, J., Kohane, I. S., & Beam, A. L. (2021). The clinician and dataset shift in artificial intelligence. *The New England Journal of Medicine*, *385*(3), 283–286. DOI: 10.1056/NEJMc2104626 PMID: 34260843

Floridi, L., Cowls, J., Beltrametti, M., Chatila, R., Chazerand, P., Dignum, V., Luetge, C., Madelin, R., Pagallo, U., Rossi, F., Schafer, B., Valcke, P., & Vayena, E. (2018). AI4People—An ethical framework for a good AI society. *Minds and Machines*, *28*(4), 689–707. DOI: 10.1007/s11023-018-9482-5 PMID: 30930541

Food and Drug Administration. (2023). *Artificial intelligence/machine learning (AI/ML)-enabled medical devices*. U.S. Food and Drug Administration.

Gerke, S., Minssen, T., & Cohen, G. (2020). Ethical and legal challenges of artificial intelligence-driven healthcare. *Cambridge Quarterly of Healthcare Ethics*, *29*(4), 605–613. DOI: 10.1017/S0963180120000674

Ghassemi, M., Oakden-Rayner, L., & Beam, A. L. (2021). The false hope of current approaches to explainable artificial intelligence in health care. *The Lancet. Digital Health, 3*(11), e745–e750. DOI: 10.1016/S2589-7500(21)00208-9 PMID: 34711379

Harrington, C.. (2023). Risks and benefits of large language models in mental health care. *JMIR Mental Health, 10*, e48745. DOI: 10.2196/48745

ISO/IEC 42001. (2023). Information technology — Artificial intelligence — Management system. International Organization for Standardization.

Ji, Z., Lee, N., Frieske, R., Yu, T., Su, D., Xu, Y., Ishii, E., Bang, Y. J., Madotto, A., & Fung, P. (2023). Survey of hallucination in natural language generation. *ACM Computing Surveys, 55*(12), 1–38. DOI: 10.1145/3571730

Kelly, C. J., Karthikesalingam, A., Suleyman, M., Corrado, G., & King, D. (2019). Key challenges for delivering clinical impact with artificial intelligence. *BMC Medicine, 17*(1), 195. DOI: 10.1186/s12916-019-1426-2 PMID: 31665002

Leslie, D., Mazumder, A., Peppin, A., Wolters, M. K., & Hagerty, A. (2021). *Understanding artificial intelligence ethics and safety.* Alan Turing Institute.

Lewis, P., Perez, E., Piktus, A., Petroni, F., Karpukhin, V., Goyal, N., & Kiela, D. (2020). Retrieval-augmented generation for knowledge-intensive NLP tasks. *Advances in Neural Information Processing Systems, 33*, 9459–9474.

Obermeyer, Z., Powers, B., Vogeli, C., & Mullainathan, S. (2019). Dissecting racial bias in an algorithm used to manage the health of populations. *Science, 366*(6464), 447–453. DOI: 10.1126/science.aax2342 PMID: 31649194

Perez, E., Huang, S., Song, F., Cai, T., Ring, R., Aslanides, J., . . . Irving, G. (2022). Red teaming language models with language models. arXiv preprint arXiv:2202.03286. DOI: 10.18653/v1/2022.emnlp-main.225

Shi, W., Zhuang, Y., Zhu, Y., Hazarika, D., Jin, D., & Yang, D. (2025). Retrieval-augmented generation for clinical LLMs: Reducing hallucination in high-stakes medical queries. *Journal of the American Medical Informatics Association : JAMIA, 32*(1), 89–102. PMID: 39520711

Singhal, K., Azizi, S., Tu, T., Mahdavi, S. S., Wei, J., Chung, H. W., Scales, N., Tanwani, A., Cole-Lewis, H., Pfohl, S., Payne, P., Seneviratne, M., Gamble, P., Kelly, C., Babiker, A., Schärli, N., Chowdhery, A., Mansfield, P., Demner-Fushman, D., & Natarajan, V. (2023). Large language models encode clinical knowledge. *Nature, 620*(7972), 172–180. DOI: 10.1038/s41586-023-06291-2 PMID: 37438534

Suresh, H., Hunt, N., Johnson, A. E., Celi, L. A., Szolovits, P., & Ghassemi, M. (2017). Clinical intervention prediction and understanding using deep networks. arXiv preprint arXiv:1705.08498.

Topol, E. J. (2019). High-performance medicine: The convergence of human and artificial intelligence. *Nature Medicine*, *25*(1), 44–56. DOI: 10.1038/s41591-018-0300-7 PMID: 30617339

Umapathi, L. K., Pal, A., & Sankarasubbu, M. (2023). Med-HALT: Medical domain hallucination test for large language models. arXiv preprint arXiv:2307.15343.

Vaswani, A., Shazeer, N., & Parmar, N.. (2017). Attention is all you need. *Advances in Neural Information Processing Systems*, *30*, 5998–6008.

Vayena, E., Blasimme, A., & Cohen, I. G. (2018). Machine learning in medicine: Addressing ethical challenges. *PLoS Medicine*, *15*(11), e1002689. DOI: 10.1371/journal.pmed.1002689 PMID: 30399149

Vincent, C., & Amalberti, R. (2016). *Safer healthcare: Strategies for the real world*. Springer. DOI: 10.1007/978-3-319-25559-0

Wang, X., Zhou, Y., & Zhou, G. (2025). The application and ethical implication of generative AI in mental health: Systematic review. *JMIR Mental Health*, *12*, e70610. DOI: 10.2196/70610 PMID: 40577783

World Health Organization. (2023). *Ethics and governance of artificial intelligence for health: Guidance on large multi-modal models*. World Health Organization.

Yan, B., Li, K., Xu, M., Dong, Y., Zhang, Y., Ren, Z., & Cheng, X. (2025). On protecting the data privacy of large language models (LLMs) and LLM agents: A literature review. *High-Confidence Computing*, *5*(2), 100300. DOI: 10.1016/j.hcc.2025.100300

Chapter 7

On Multilingual Medical LLMs

Emine Ela Küçük
Giresun University, Turkey

Dilek Küçük
http://orcid.org/0000-0003-2656-1300
Tübitak Marmara Research Center, Turkey

ABSTRACT

Large language models (LLMs) have recently emerged as a significant development effort in artificial intelligence (AI), particularly in generative AI, built on top of deep learning models. In addition to their common use in popular AI chatbots like ChatGPT, Claude, and Grok, LLMs have also been used in specific domains such as law, finance, and healthcare. In healthcare, various studies report development and applications of medical LLMs, due to the significance of their use in the medical domain affecting the lives and well-being of individuals and communities. In this chapter, we consider medical LLMs from the perspective of multilinguality, and provide a survey of multilingual medical LLMs. After an overview of medical LLMs, we cover multilingual medical LLMs proposed in the related literature. We suggest future research lines based on the findings of the covered papers. We hope that this survey chapter will stand as a significant contribution to the related literature, and both researchers and practitioners of medical LLMs benefit from the presented findings.

DOI: 10.4018/979-8-2600-2173-6.ch007

INTRODUCTION

The recent emergence of foundation models such as BERT, GPT, and PaLM, and that of large language models (LLMs) which are foundation models pre-trained on very large textual corpora, demonstrates substantial impact on diverse domains such as health, law, finance, and education. There is a significant body of research conducted on LLMs and their applications for different natural language processing (NLP) problems such as text generation, natural language understanding, question answering, and text summarization. Due to their large model sizes (parameters), training LLMs and subsequently fine-tuning them for specific domains and tasks require significant computational resources. Hence, there is also considerable research on small language models (SLMs) such as Gemma series (Gemma Team, 2024) and Qwen series (Yang et al., 2025), since they are more cost-effective and adaptable compared to LLMs (Wang et al., 2025).

Pre-trained LLMs which have been fine-tuned for specific domains or problems offer great opportunities for the practitioners of the corresponding domains. For instance, LLMs are being employed increasingly in the legal practice for tasks including text generation, case result prediction, and legal document summarization (Siino et al., 2025). Similarly, there are several studies on the introduction, application, and comparison of LLMs proposed for or fine-tuned for the medical domain, as reviewed in (Shool et al., 2025).

In this book chapter, we take an application-oriented point of view and consider the medical domain, and hence our focus is on medical language models, their applications, benchmark evaluations, and their multilinguality in particular. Hence, we review recent research on medical LLMs, as well as research on multilingual medical LLMs. After emphasizing the important points in reviewed related research, we also outline important directions for future research.

LLMs and medical LLMs have important potential for individuals and societies for their medical or health-related concerns. At the time of writing this book chapter, OpenAI which is the firm that built the popular LLM-based chatbot *ChatGPT*, has introduced ChatGPT Health[1] and HealthBench[2], due to the relative heavy use of ChatGPT and similar chatbots for health-related question answering. ChatGPT Health is a specific feature of the popular chatbot where people can make private conversations about their health and seek medical information in a personalized manner. Similarly, the company introduces HealthBench as a benchmark framework in order to evaluate the correctness of health-related responses of artificial intelligence (AI) systems.

The rest of this book chapter is organized as follows: In the first section, we review papers on LLMs in the medical or healthcare domain. The next section covers related work on multilingual medical LLMs emphasizing the multilinguality aspect of these LLMs. The following section summarizes the main findings of the reviewed papers. The first of the last two sections of this chapter presents outstanding issues and directions for future work based on the reviewed studies, and the last section concludes the chapter with a compact summary.

MEDICAL LARGE LANGUAGE MODELS

LLMs are deep learning models such as transformers (Vaswani et al., 2017), which have been trained on large textual datasets, particularly for text generation and interpretation (Raiaan et al., 2024).

This section is devoted to recent research on medical large language models (medical LLMs).

A set of open-source LLMs called MEDITRON where the included LLMs have 7B and 70B parameters is proposed in (Chen et al., 2023). This set is based on LLaMA2 which is extended by training on medical corpora comprising medical guidelines and PubMed articles, among others (Chen et al., 2023). A newer version of this LLM set, based on Llama-3.1, is called Llama-3-Meditron, and is presented in (Sallinen et al., 2025). Llama-3-Meditron is pre-trained on a curated medical corpus, and is reported to outperform other generic and medical LLMs in medical question answering (QA) on benchmark datasets.

HuatuoGPT is a medical LLM introduced in (Zhang et al., 2023) for medical conversations. This model is trained using reinforcement learning, and the corresponding training data is compiled from medical responses from ChatGPT and feedback from real doctors. It is shown that the performance of HuatuoGPT for medical QA and multi-turn medical conversations is better when compared to other medical LLMs (Zhang et al., 2023).

Song et al. (2023) propose a single-stage domain adaptation scheme as opposed to the common two-stage domain adaptation methodology including pre-training and fine-tuning. For this purpose, a priority sampling strategy is employed, and HuatuoGPT-II model is trained for the Chinese medical domain. It is reported that the proposed medical LLM is able to achieve competitive performance on various related benchmarks (Song et al., 2023).

Han et al. (2023) propose MedAlpaca, which is a collection of medical QA datasets. The authors indicate that this collection can be used for fine-tuning LLMs for the medical domain.

Another related paper discusses the potential of general-purpose LLMs for various medical tasks such as medical QA (Singhal et al., 2023). After carrying out experiments on different medical QA benchmarks, it is observed that these LLMs encode a considerable amount of medical knowledge during pre-training. It is also pointed out that clinical competence of these generic LLMs increases as the model size grows. Still, it is concluded that additional fine-tuning and evaluation of these LLMs in the medical or healthcare domains are needed for trustworthiness and sufficient accuracy (Singhal et al., 2023).

Kung et al. (2023) present performance evaluation results of ChatGPT on the United States Medical Licensing Exam (USMLE) where ChatGPT is able to get the passing grade of 60% or very close to the passing grade. It is also reported that the responses of ChatGPT are coherent and consistent as well. The authors argue that ChatGPT can be used as an assistant during medical education (Kung et al., 2023).

A survey of medical LLMs is presented in (Zhou et al., 2023). Basically, the authors describe the architectures of existing medical LLM proposals, provide a comparison of these LLMs for different tasks in the medical domain, and highlight the existing challenges and opportunities, based on the reviewed LLMs.

It is argued in (Hager et al., 2024) that current state-of-the-art LLMs fall short of being sufficient for medical diagnosis, when compared to physicians. The authors emphasize that they cannot correctly interpret laboratory results, perform poorly at following medical guidelines, and demonstrate sensitivity to the quantity and order of the supplied information, based on their related analyses. It is claimed that they currently cannot be integrated into clinical decision-making (Hager et al., 2024).

An open-source LLM framework called Hippocrates is proposed for the medical domain in (Acikgoz et al., 2024). The authors also present a guide for medical LLM training, in addition to the benchmark evaluation results of two medical LLMs (collectively called Hippo) that are based on LLaMA2 7B and Mistral 7B models, respectively.

Another related study focuses on the assessment of medical LLMs for clinical competence, and proposes an assessment framework called MEDIC (Kanithi et al., 2024). This framework is reported to facilitate the comparison of LLMs with respect to hallucination detection and coverage, and it is used for the evaluation and comparison of LLMs for QA, summarization, and text generation, among others (Kanithi et al., 2024).

A framework called Medical Decision-Making Agents (MDAgents) is proposed in (Kim et al., 2024) for the purpose of facilitating the employment of LLMs in complex medical problems. Considering the problem's complexity, the framework dynamically assigns a single LLM or a collaboration structure for a group of LLMs in order to solve problems requiring medical understanding and reasoning.

A conceptual framework for domain-specific training of LLMs for the medical domain called M-KAT is proposed in (Chang et al., 2024). The study also highlights medical diagnosis & treatment, medical research, QA, and health management as outstanding tasks that can benefit from LLMs trained for the medical domain.

Another related study combines Multi-Criteria Decision Making (MCDM) and fuzzy logic in order to assess the performance of LLMs for the medical domain (Alamoodi et al., 2024). Within the context of the proposed framework for evaluation, two problems are considered: medical relation extraction, along with clinical concept extraction.

In (Chen et al., 2024), HuatuoGPT-o1 is proposed, which is a medical LLM for complex medical reasoning. This medical LLM is trained in two stages: In the first phase, complex reasoning is learned while in the second phase, the presented model is enhanced using reinforcement learning. It is concluded in the paper that complex reasoning is useful during the process of medical problem solving (Chen et al., 2024).

PMC-LLaMA is proposed in (Wu et al., 2024) as an open-source LLM for the medical domain, which is based on the generic LLaMA model. The authors claim that their training strategy includes a knowledge injection phase and a subsequent instruction tuning phase. It is reported that the proposed medical LLM attains state-of-the-art performance rates in the medical QA problem, and even surpasses existing general-purpose LLM-based chatbots like ChatGPT (Wu et al., 2024).

Med-Gemini is introduced as a family of multimodal medical LLMs with the Web search ability, based on the generic Gemini model in (Saab et al., 2024). The proposed model is evaluated on 14 medical benchmarks, and it is reported that the model attains state-of-the-art performance on 10 of these benchmarks. The authors also emphasize the capabilities of Med-Gemini in tasks including medical document summarization and multimodal medical dialogues (Saab et al., 2024).

A medical LLM based on the Llama-2 architecture called Med42 is presented in (Christophe et al., 2024a). The authors compare two different fine-tuning strategies on this LLM, namely, full-parameter and parameter-efficient methods. Based on the results of the related experiments, it is concluded that full-parameter fine-tuning leads to superior performance in most of the datasets, yet, parameter-efficient fine-tuning methods attain performance rates close to full-parameter fine-tuning (Christophe et al., 2024a).

In a subsequent study, a family of medical LLMs based on Llama-3 architecture called Med42-v2 is described in (Christophe et al., 2024b), where these LLMs have been fine-tuned on clinical data. It is highlighted that Med42-v2 outperforms Llama-3 and GPT-4 on various medical benchmarks. The authors also outline the challenges of using Med42-v2 in clinical settings, such as bias, hallucinations, and ethical issues (Christophe et al., 2024b).

In a survey study (Zhang et al., 2024), medical datasets for training and testing of LLMs in the medical domain are reviewed. The authors emphasize that the corresponding datasets should enhance the real-world applicability of the models. Another survey paper by Wang and Zhang (2024) discusses the applications of LLMs in medical and healthcare domains, presents the related datasets, and outlines outstanding topics related to trustworthiness also mentioning issues related to plagiarism and copyrights.

In another related recent study, Me-LLaMA is proposed, which is a suite of open-source medical LLMs based on LLaMA2 models. In the study, LLaMA2 models are extended by pre-training and instruction tuning on large-scale biomedical and clinical corpora (Xie et al., 2025).

Another benchmark for the performance evaluation of LLMs in medical settings is described in (Wu et al., 2025). The presented framework called MedS-Bench covers 11 high-level clinical tasks and is used to evaluate nine LLMs including MEDITRON (Chen et al., 2023), Llama, Mistral, GPT, and Claude to solve these medical tasks. In order to address the limitations of the LLMs observed during these evaluations, a large-scale instruction-tuning dataset called MedS-Ins is also proposed for the medical domain (Wu et al., 2025).

In the survey paper (Ye and Tang, 2025), the main related concepts and background of LLMs and medical LLMs are first presented. Then, significant application areas of medical LLMs are highlighted, which include medical reporting, medical diagnosis, and finally, medical treatment (Ye and Tang, 2025).

Another study focuses on the comparison of four popular LLMs for racial bias in their psychiatric diagnosis and treatment recommendations. The first three of the tested LLMs are generic ones (namely Gemini, Claude, and ChatGPT) while the last one called NewMes-15 is reported to be a medical variant of the generic LLaMA model. It is argued that bias assessment is a necessity when incorporating AI agents into the medical decision-making process (Bouguettaya et al., 2025).

Swedish Medical LLM Benchmark (SMLB) is introduced in (Moëll et al., 2025) as a framework for evaluating LLMs for medical tasks in Swedish. It is claimed that generic LLMs like GPT-4-turbo and Claude 3.5 also demonstrate superior performance in Swedish. It is also emphasized that the incorporation of Retrieval Augmented Generation (RAG) improves performance when tested in the medical domain (Moëll et al., 2025).

A suite of medical vision-language models called MedGemma is proposed in (Sellergren et al., 2025) which is based on the previously reported Gemma model (Gemma Team, 2024). It is highlighted that MedGemma shows superior performance on medical reasoning and understanding on both textual data and images, when compared to other generative models of similar sizes. It is also demonstrated that MedGemma attains state-of-the-art performance of the task-specific models (Sellergren et al., 2025).

A medical LLM called Med-PaLM 2 based on the PaLM 2 generic foundation model is presented in (Singhal et al., 2025). Med-PaLM 2 employs a newly-introduced prompting strategy called ensemble refinement, and a search strategy called chain of retrieval to handle difficult questions using relevant sources. It is emphasized that the proposed medical LLM demonstrates state-of-the-art performance on different medical question answering datasets (Singhal et al., 2025).

A related systematic review covers issues related to the applications of LLMs in clinical medicine, and their capabilities and limitations are outlined (Shool et al., 2025). Similarly, it is emphasized in (Liu et al., 2025) that the applications of LLMs in the medical domain are still in their infant stage, and there are several outstanding issues to be considered before their prevalent applications, such as lack of large-scale experimentations, benchmarks, and related datasets. The review paper in (He et al., 2025) focuses on LLMs in healthcare, covering the technologies, datasets, and various aspects of trustworthiness. A survey paper on LLMs and multimodal LLMs in the medical domain is presented in (Xiao et al., 2025) where several challenges are outlined including hallucinations, insufficient recency, bias, and deployment issues. Another more recent review paper on the topic (Asif et al., 2026) covers papers on the integration of LLMs across the medical domain (from clinical reasoning and diagnostics to education and psychological care) demonstrating their potential role in modern healthcare systems and their capacity to enhance performance, reliability of such systems.

MULTILINGUAL MEDICAL LARGE LANGUAGE MODELS

Although LLMs have provided important contributions to the solution of various problems in different domains, multilingualism is still an issue and various LLM-based solutions are reported to be still below the expectations for low-resource languages (Huang et al., 2026). A related problem is the cultural bias originating from the training corpora of these LLMs (Huang et al., 2026). Hence, due to the relative significance of the topic, this section reviews papers on bilingual, trilingual, and multilingual medical LLMs and particularly on the multilingual aspect of such LLMs.

A multilingual medical dataset in six languages, called MMedC, is introduced in (Qiu et al., 2024). Also presented is a multiple-choice QA benchmark (namely, MMedBench) for the medical domain. Finally, MMed-Llama 3 model with 8B parameters is proposed, and compared with other LLMs for the medical QA task (Qiu et al., 2024).

In (Wang et al., 2024), compilation of a multilingual medical dataset (comprising six languages: English, Chinese, Spanish, Arabic, Hindi, and French) called ApolloCorpora and that of the evaluation benchmark called XMedBench are described. Using the multilingual medical benchmark of XMedBench, it is reported that the proposed small-sized language models called Apollo models attain the best results when compared to other models of equal parameter sizes (Wang et al., 2024).

A multilingual medical LLM called L2M3 is proposed in (Gangavarapu, 2024), based on the idea of equipping LLMs with machine translation capabilities. It is reported that the proposed multilingual medical LLM will help community health workers by providing in-context medical knowledge and related tools (Gangavarapu, 2024).

In order to extend the applicability of open-source LLMs for health-related tasks in six languages (English, Spanish, French, Chinese, Japanese, and Korean), a two-stage fine-tuning method is described in (Zhou et al., 2024). For this purpose, two multilingual medical datasets, namely MMed-IFT and MMed-IFT-MC, are compiled and during fine-tuning, these datasets are employed (Zhou et al., 2024).

It is argued in (García-Ferrero et al., 2024) that a large multilingual medical corpus in English, Spanish, French, and Italian is compiled which is next used to train the text-to-text open-source Medical mT5 model. This medical model is based on the open-source mT5 model (Xue et al., 2021) which is an encoder-decoder model. It is reported that the proposed multilingual medical model outperforms the text-to-text models for Spanish, French, and Italian used for comparison, and attains competitive performance when compared to the state-of-the-art LLMs for English (García-Ferrero et al., 2024).

A multilingual medical benchmark (based on medical exams) called MedExpQA is described for the evaluation of LLMs for medical QA (Alonso et al., 2024). The proposed benchmark includes gold evaluations (of all options in the related exam questions) produced by medical doctors. Multilingual evaluations demonstrate that the best results are obtained for English, while the corresponding results for the remaining languages are about 10% lower. It is argued that these results highlight the need for future studies to obtain improved results in multilingual settings (Alonso et al., 2024).

The authors of another related study (Jin et al., 2024) present XLingEval which is a cross-lingual evaluation framework for the evaluation of LLMs as dialogue systems for health-related queries. The experiments are carried out with four languages (English, Spanish, Chinese, and Hindi). Also presented in the same paper is XLingHealth which is a cross-lingual healthcare benchmark proposed for the assessment of the multilingual features of LLMs (Jin et al., 2024).

An open-source biomedical LLM called BioMistral that is built on Mistral and pre-trained on PubMed is presented in (Labrak et al., 2024). After evaluating it on a benchmark for ten medical QA tasks in English and attaining favorable results in English, this framework is translated into seven new languages, and evaluation is performed. The authors claim that their study reports the first large-scale performance evaluation of multilingual LLMs (Labrak et al., 2024).

The authors of the study (Pieri et al., 2024) propose BiMediX which is a bilingual medical mixture of experts LLM supporting two languages: English and Arabic.

Various medical problems including both open-ended and multiple-choice QA, and multi-turn text chats about further clinical details are facilitated by the proposed bilingual medical LLM (Pieri et al., 2024).

In (Zheng et al., 2024), a Mixture of Experts (MoE) approach is employed in order to extend a medical LLM to 50 languages, thereby making it a multilingual medical LLM. These languages are grouped into 7 families, and language family experts are introduced to scale the LLM to 50 languages, most of which are low-resource ones. It is claimed that their approach is a scalable one working on limited data (Zheng et al., 2024).

Although it cannot be considered a multilingual one, the study in (Olatunji et al., 2024) presents a medical QA dataset in Pan-African English called AfriMed-QA, and evaluates a large set of different LLMs on this dataset. The study is included in this book chapter due to its medical dataset gathered from a new cultural context, i.e., from countries in Africa not yet studied, and the evaluation results on this new dataset.

Multilingual Knowledge Graph-based Retrieval Ranking (MKG-Rank) is proposed in (Li et al., 2025a) which is a framework based on knowledge graphs and aims to facilitate multilingual QA in the medical domain. MKG-Rank employs machine translation, knowledge graphs, and English-centric LLMs to attain acceptable performance for multilingual medical QA at a low cost (Li et al., 2025a).

A trilingual LLM called ELAINE-medLLM is proposed in (Yano et al., 2025) where ELAINE stands for EngLish-jApanese-chINesE. This trilingual LLM for English, Japanese, and Chinese is based on the generic Llama-3-8B LLM and reported to be adapted to the biomedical domain (Yano et al., 2025).

By using the automatic data augmentation technique of machine translation on the MIMIC-CXR report dataset (Johnson et al., 2019), a large-scale medical corpus is compiled (Li et al., 2025b). The initial medical dataset is translated into 20 languages throughout the process. Next, a new multilingual and multimodal medical pre-training model is proposed where this model improves medical multimodal data understanding and it is also significant as it is adapted to multilingual medical contexts (Li et al., 2025b).

By using medical textual data in Wikipedia and the retrieval augmented generation approach, a corpus of medical reasoning traces (in English, Italian, and Spanish) is generated (Ferrazzi et al., 2025). Existing medical datasets of MedQA and MedMCQA are extended to Italian and Spanish. The compiled reasoning traces lead to improved QA performance both in few-shot and supervised fine-tuning settings (Ferrazzi et al., 2025).

Various LLMs are tested for medical QA on a set of 5,609 questions collected from community health workers in Rwanda (Rutunda et al., 2025). Five LLMs, including GPT-4o, Gemini-2, and Meditron-70B (Chen et al., 2023) are tested where GPT-

4o and Gemini-2 demonstrate superior performance compared to local clinicians. Similar tests are also performed when responses are expected in the local language and although the performance rates drop slightly, still GPT-4o and Gemini-2 have been top-performers (Rutunda et al., 2025).

CLINIC is proposed as a multilingual benchmark for evaluating the trustworthiness of LLMs in the medical domain (Ghosh et al., 2025). Five dimensions of trustworthiness for a total of 15 languages are considered: truthfulness, privacy, safety, fairness, and robustness. It is reported that language models have issues regarding correctness, bias, and privacy (Ghosh et al., 2025).

In the final paper that we review, a framework called MedCOD (Medical Chain-of-Dictionary) is proposed to improve medical translation (from English to Spanish) by integrating in-domain structured knowledge into LLMs (Salim et al., 2025). A parallel corpus is also compiled, which comprises 2,999 English-Spanish MedlinePlus articles, in addition to a test set of 100 sentences which are tagged with their medical contexts. Experiments with four open-source LLMs show that the proposed MedCOD framework attains better translation quality (Salim et al., 2025).

In their recent survey paper, Huang et al. (2026) highlight the challenges of using medical LLMs in multilingual settings. Although there are studies that employ automatic machine translation to handle related issues, the authors claim that the translation-based approaches do not constitute a complete solution due to the complexity of medical terminology, and errors originating from machine translation. They suggest that language-specific medical information integration to LLMs is a significant research problem in this topic (Huang et al., 2026).

Table 1 presents a summary of the multilingual LLMs or frameworks described in this section, together with their base models, number of languages considered, and the key contribution.

Table 1. Multilingual medical large language models/frameworks

Reference	Model/ Framework	Base Model	Languages	Contribution
Qiu et al. (2024)	MMed-Llama 3	Llama 3	6 languages	Multilingual medical corpus (MMedC) and benchmark (MMedBench)
Wang et al. (2024)	Apollo	Llama	6 languages	Multilingual dataset (ApolloCorpora) and benchmark (XMedBench)
Gangavarapu (2024)	L2M3	—	Multiple	Medical LLM with machine translation for low-resource settings
Zhou et al. (2024)	—	Open-source LLMs	6 languages	Two-stage fine-tuning for multilingual medical QA

continued on following page

Table 1. Continued

Reference	Model/ Framework	Base Model	Languages	Contribution
Pieri et al. (2024)	BiMediX	MoE LLM	2 languages	Bilingual medical mixture-of-experts LLM
Labrak et al. (2024)	BioMistral	Mistral	8 languages	First large-scale multilingual medical LLM evaluation
Zheng et al. (2024)	—	Apollo	50 languages	Mixture of language family experts for 50 languages
Yano et al. (2025)	ELAINE-medLLM	Llama-3-8B	3 languages	Trilingual biomedical LLM
Li et al. (2025a)	MKG-Rank	—	Multiple	Knowledge graph-based multilingual medical QA
Li et al. (2025b)	—	—	20	Multilingual multimodal medical pre-training
Ghosh et al. (2025)	CLINIC	—	15	Multilingual trustworthiness benchmark
Ferrazzi et al. (2025)	—	—	3	Multilingual medical reasoning traces via retrieval augmented generation
Salim et al. (2025)	MedCOD	—	2	Medical translation via chain-of-dictionary

A SUMMARY OF THE MAIN POINTS IN RELATED WORK

Below summarized are the aspects particularly highlighted in related research covered so far in this chapter:

- LLMs, especially after passing a rigorous training stage for the medical domain, offer significant opportunities for facilitating medical text understanding, as well as medical text generation.
- Significant studies also report that general-purpose LLMs encode a considerable amount of clinical knowledge during their pre-training stage and hence they are able to attain favorable performance without fine-tuning, yet to ensure a sufficient level of accuracy and trustworthiness, fine-tuning and extensive evaluations are needed (Singhal et al., 2023). Similarly, without any specific training, it is shown that ChatGPT is able to get a passing grade or very close to it when evaluated on USMLE (Kung et al., 2023).
- It is observed that many of the proposed medical LLMs are based on the publicly available versions of the LLaMA model, which are extended by pre-training and instruction tuning on medical corpora (Chen et al., 2023; Acikgoz et al., 2024; Xie et al., 2025; Sallinen et al., 2025).

- Several related studies propose evaluation frameworks in order to compare different LLMs for the medical domain, so that the best alternatives to be used in clinical decision-making processes can be pinpointed.
- Multilinguality is an important issue for large-scale deployment of LLMs in the medical settings, as such, several recent studies propose bilingual, trilingual, and multilingual medical LLMs. Yet, there is a need for related studies on this topic.
- Many studies target the common languages of Chinese, Spanish, Arabic, French, and Hindi, in addition to English when building multilingual medical datasets, benchmarks, and models.
- There is a deliberate effort by the researchers to extend the applicability of the existing models for high-resource languages to low-resource languages.
- Some of these studies report that the performance rates for tasks such as question answering are higher for English, and are lower for the other languages.
- Although the issues related to trustworthy AI in the medical domain are mentioned in several studies, we come across a single study that proposes a multilingual benchmark (Ghosh et al., 2025) to analyze the trustworthiness of medical LLMs.
- Medical information extraction, medical question answering, medical understanding and reasoning, medical diagnosis and treatment are among the common related natural language processing problems targeted by the related work on medical LLMs and multilingual medical LLMs.

FUTURE RESEARCH DIRECTIONS

Based on the content we reviewed and summarized so far, the following list includes important outstanding issues and future research directions:

- First of all, improved multilinguality by increasing the number of languages that are supported by medical LLMs, and extensive evaluation of such multilingual medical LLMs constitute an important future research direction.
- As emphasized earlier, further studies are necessary to enhance the performance rates of the multilingual medical models for languages other than English.
- Future work should also consider the compilation and sharing of diverse and large-scale multilingual medical datasets needed for fine-tuning, and for benchmark evaluations of medical LLMs, and multilingual medical LLMs.
- Future studies can consider the comparison of different large and small language models on large-scale benchmark datasets, using different compar-

ison criteria including but not limited to accuracy, coverage, and resource requirements.

- Studies that effectively address hallucinations that current LLMs often produce in general as well as in medical application settings, can contribute substantially to the related body of knowledge.
- Further studies should also address the issues related to privacy and trustworthiness during text interpretation and generation for healthcare purposes. Similarly, ethical issues constitute an important future research direction for LLMs, medical LLMs, and multilingual medical LLMs.
- In addition to existing text-only models, several studies point out that better user experience can be attained in clinical application settings using multimodal data such as audio, image, and video data.
- Personalization is another future research direction for medical large language models.
- The lack of explainability is an issue commonly highlighted for LLMs and their applications in the related literature, hence, explainability, in this context, is an important direction of future research on multilingual medical LLMs.

CONCLUSION

In this book chapter, we focus on medical large language models (LLMs) and particularly on multilingual medical LLMs. We first consider and review studies on medical LLMs, their applications, and comparisons. Next, we shift our focus to multilingual medical LLMs and cover related recent research. Several significant frameworks, corpora, benchmarks, and tuning strategies corresponding to LLMs in the medical and biomedical domains are also highlighted. We provide a compact overview of the main points outlined in related research, and then highlight outstanding issues of this research topic. We conclude our book chapter with a brief summary of the presented material. It is emphasized in related studies that medical LLMs should be evaluated on languages other than English, and that issues like hallucinations should be well addressed before widespread deployment of these models. Related work also reveals that multimodal LLMs need further research attention, and that issues related to trustworthy AI such as ethical concerns, privacy, and explainability should be considered during the use of LLMs in medical and biomedical domains. Since medical LLMs and issues related to their multilinguality constitute important and very recent research topics, and application opportunities of LLMs in the medical or healthcare domain have important implications for society in general, we believe that the readers will benefit from this book chapter considerably.

REFERENCES

Acikgoz, E. C., Ince, O. B., Bench, R., Boz, A. A., Kesen, I., Erdem, A., & Erdem, E. (2024). Hippocrates: An open-source framework for advancing large language models in healthcare. *arXiv preprint arXiv:2404.16621.*

Alamoodi, A. H., Zughoul, O., David, D., Garfan, S., Pamucar, D., Albahri, O. S., Albahri, A. S., Yussof, S., & Sharaf, I. M. (2024). A novel evaluation framework for medical LLMs: Combining fuzzy logic and MCDM for medical relation and clinical concept extraction. *Journal of Medical Systems*, *48*(1), 81. DOI: 10.1007/s10916-024-02090-y PMID: 39214943

Alonso, I., Oronoz, M., & Agerri, R. (2024). MedExpQA: Multilingual benchmarking of large language models for medical question answering. *Artificial Intelligence in Medicine*, *155*, 102938. DOI: 10.1016/j.artmed.2024.102938 PMID: 39121544

Asif, S., Hadi, F., Yan, Y., Wang, V. Y., & Xu, D. (2026). The impact of large language models on medical research and patient care: A systematic review of current trends, challenges, and future innovations. *Computer Science Review*, *59*, 100847. DOI: 10.1016/j.cosrev.2025.100847

Bouguettaya, A., Stuart, E. M., & Aboujaoude, E. (2025). Racial bias in AI-mediated psychiatric diagnosis and treatment: A qualitative comparison of four large language models. *npj. Digital Medicine*, *8*(1), 332. PMID: 40467886

Chang, Y., Yin, J. M., Li, J. M., Liu, C., Cao, L. Y., & Lin, S. Y. (2024). Applications and future prospects of medical LLMs: A survey based on the M-KAT conceptual framework. *Journal of Medical Systems*, *48*(1), 112. DOI: 10.1007/s10916-024-02132-5 PMID: 39725770

Chen, J., Cai, Z., Ji, K., Wang, X., Liu, W., Wang, R., Hou, J., & Wang, B. (2024). HuatuoGPT-o1, towards medical complex reasoning with LLMs. *arXiv preprint arXiv:2412.18925.*

Chen, Z., Cano, A. H., Romanou, A., Bonnet, A., Matoba, K., Salvi, F., Pagliardini, M., Fan, S., Köpf, A., Mohtashami, A., & Sallinen, A. (2023). Meditron-70B: Scaling medical pretraining for large language models. *arXiv preprint arXiv:2311.16079.*

Christophe, C., Kanithi, P. K., Munjal, P., Raha, T., Hayat, N., Rajan, R., Al-Mahrooqi, A., Gupta, A., Salman, M. U., & Gosal, G. (2024a). Med42 — Evaluating fine-tuning strategies for medical LLMs: Full-parameter vs. parameter-efficient approaches. *arXiv preprint arXiv:2404.14779.*

Christophe, C., Kanithi, P. K., Raha, T., Khan, S., & Pimentel, M. A. F. (2024b). Med42-v2: A suite of clinical LLMs. *arXiv preprint arXiv:2408.06142*.

Ferrazzi, P., Soroa, A., & Agerri, R. (2025). Grounded multilingual medical reasoning for question answering with large language models. *arXiv preprint arXiv:2512.05658*.

Gangavarapu, A. (2024). Introducing L2M3, a multilingual medical large language model to advance health equity in low-resource regions. *arXiv preprint arXiv:2404.08705*.

García-Ferrero, I., Agerri, R., Salazar, A. A., Cabrio, E., de la Iglesia, I., & Lavelli, A. (2024). Medical mT5: An open-source multilingual text-to-text LLM for the medical domain. *arXiv preprint arXiv:2404.07613*.

Gemma Team. (2024). Gemma: Open models based on gemini research and technology. arXiv preprint arXiv:2403.08295.

Ghosh, A., Sridhar, S., Ravi, R. K., Muhsin, M., Saha, S., & Agarwal, C. (2025). CLINIC: Evaluating multilingual trustworthiness in language models for healthcare. *arXiv preprint arXiv:2512.11437*.

Hager, P., Jungmann, F., Holland, R., Bhagat, K., Hubrecht, I., Knauer, M., Vielhauer, J., Makowski, M., Braren, R., Kaissis, G., & Rueckert, D. (2024). Evaluation and mitigation of the limitations of large language models in clinical decision-making. *Nature Medicine*, *30*(9), 2613–2622. DOI: 10.1038/s41591-024-03097-1 PMID: 38965432

Han, T., Adams, L. C., Papaioannou, J. M., Grundmann, P., Oberhauser, T., Figueroa, A., Löser, A., Truhn, D., & Bressem, K. K. (2023). MedAlpaca—An open-source collection of medical conversational AI models and training data. *arXiv preprint arXiv:2304.08247*.

He, K., Mao, R., Lin, Q., Ruan, Y., Lan, X., Feng, M., & Cambria, E. (2025). A survey of large language models for healthcare: From data, technology, and applications to accountability and ethics. *Information Fusion*, *118*, 102963. DOI: 10.1016/j.inffus.2025.102963

Huang, K., Mo, F., Zhang, X., Li, H., Li, Y., Zhang, Y., Yi, W., Mao, Y., Liu, J., Xu, Y., Xu, J., Nie, J.-Y., & Liu, Y. (2026). A survey on large language models with multilingualism: Recent advances and new frontiers. *Artificial Intelligence Review*. Advance online publication. DOI: 10.1007/s10462-026-11534-5

Jin, Y., Chandra, M., Verma, G., Hu, Y., De Choudhury, M., & Kumar, S. (2024). Better to ask in English: Cross-lingual evaluation of large language models for healthcare queries. In *Proceedings of the ACM Web Conference* (pp. 2627-2638). DOI: 10.1145/3589334.3645643

Johnson, A. E., Pollard, T. J., Berkowitz, S. J., Greenbaum, N. R., Lungren, M. P., Deng, C. Y., Mark, R. G., & Horng, S. (2019). MIMIC-CXR, a de-identified publicly available database of chest radiographs with free-text reports. *Scientific Data*, *6*(1), 317. DOI: 10.1038/s41597-019-0322-0 PMID: 31831740

Kanithi, P. K., Christophe, C., Pimentel, M. A., Raha, T., Saadi, N., Javed, H., Maslenkova, S., Hayat, N., Rajan, R., & Khan, S. (2024). MEDIC: Towards a comprehensive framework for evaluating LLMs in clinical applications. *arXiv preprint arXiv:2409.07314*.

Kim, Y., Park, C., Jeong, H., Chan, Y. S., Xu, X., McDuff, D., Lee, H., Ghassemi, M., Breazeal, C., & Park, H. W. (2024). MDAgents: An adaptive collaboration of LLMs for medical decision-making. *Advances in Neural Information Processing Systems*, *37*, 79410–79452.

Kung, T. H., Cheatham, M., Medenilla, A., Sillos, C., De Leon, L., Elepaño, C., Madriaga, M., Aggabao, R., Diaz-Candido, G., Maningo, J., & Tseng, V. (2023). Performance of ChatGPT on USMLE: Potential for AI-assisted medical education using large language models. *PLOS Digital Health*, *2*(2), e0000198. DOI: 10.1371/journal.pdig.0000198 PMID: 36812645

Labrak, Y., Bazoge, A., Morin, E., Gourraud, P. A., Rouvier, M., & Dufour, R. (2024). Biomistral: A collection of open-source pretrained large language models for medical domains. *arXiv preprint arXiv:2402.10373*. DOI: 10.18653/v1/2024.findings-acl.348

Li, F., Chen, Y., Liu, H., Yang, R., Yuan, H., Jiang, Y., Li, T., Taylor, E. M., Rouhizadeh, H., Iwasawa, Y., & Teodoro, D. (2025a). MKG-Rank: Enhancing large language models with knowledge graph for multilingual medical question answering. *arXiv preprint arXiv:2503.16131.*

Li, Q., Qiu, C., Liu, H., Gu, J., & Luo, D. (2025b). Decoupled contrastive learning for multilingual multimodal medical pre-trained model. *Neurocomputing*, *633*, 129809. DOI: 10.1016/j.neucom.2025.129809

Liu, F., Zhou, H., Gu, B., Zou, X., Huang, J., Wu, J., Li, Y., Chen, S. S., Hua, Y., Zhou, P., Liu, J., Mao, C., You, C., Wu, X., Zheng, Y., Clifton, L., Li, Z., Luo, J., & Clifton, D. A. (2025). Application of large language models in medicine. *Nature Reviews Bioengineering*, *3*(6), 1–20. DOI: 10.1038/s44222-025-00279-5

Moëll, B., Farestam, A., & Beskow, J. (2025). Swedish medical LLM benchmark: Development and evaluation of a framework for assessing large language models in the Swedish medical domain. *Frontiers in Artificial Intelligence*, *8*, 1538566. DOI: 10.3389/frai.2025.1557920 PMID: 40718621

Olatunji, T., Nimo, C., Owodunni, A., Abdullahi, T., Ayodele, E., Sanni, M., Aka, C., Omofoye, F., Yuehgoh, F., Faniran, T., & Dossou, B. F. (2024). AfriMed-QA: a Pan-African, multi-specialty, medical question-answering benchmark dataset. *arXiv preprint arXiv:2411.15640.*

Pieri, S., Mullappilly, S. S., Khan, F. S., Anwer, R. M., Khan, S., Baldwin, T., & Cholakkal, H. (2024). BiMediX: Bilingual medical mixture of experts LLM. *arXiv preprint arXiv:2402.13253*. DOI: 10.18653/v1/2024.findings-emnlp.989

Qiu, P., Wu, C., Zhang, X., Lin, W., Wang, H., Zhang, Y., Wang, Y., & Xie, W. (2024). Towards building multilingual language model for medicine. *Nature Communications*, *15*(1), 8384. DOI: 10.1038/s41467-024-52417-z PMID: 39333468

Raiaan, M. A. K., Mukta, M. S. H., Fatema, K., Fahad, N. M., Sakib, S., Mim, M. M. J., Ahmad, J., Ali, M. E., & Azam, S. (2024). A review on large language models: Architectures, applications, taxonomies, open issues and challenges. *IEEE Access : Practical Innovations, Open Solutions*, *12*, 26839–26874. DOI: 10.1109/ACCESS.2024.3365742

Rutunda, S., Corden, G., Uwimana, A., Muhizi, J., Bayingana, C., & Otieno, G. (2025). Large language models for frontline healthcare support in low-resource settings. *npj. Digital Medicine*, *8*, 379.

Saab, K., Tu, T., Weng, W. H., Tanno, R., Stutz, D., Wulczyn, E., Carroll, A., Mahdavi, S. S., Peltz, C., & Natarajan, V. (2024). Capabilities of Gemini models in medicine. *arXiv preprint arXiv:2404.18416.*

Salim, M. S., Fu, L., Ramakrishnan, A. A., Yao, Z., & Yu, H. (2025). MedCOD: Enhancing English-to-Spanish medical translation of large language models using enriched chain-of-dictionary framework. *arXiv preprint arXiv:2509.00934*. DOI: 10.18653/v1/2025.findings-emnlp.350

Sallinen, A., Solergibert, A. J., Zhang, M., Boyé, G., Dupont-Roc, M., Theimer-Lienhard, X., Boisson, E., Bernath, B., Hadhri, H., Tran, A., & Rabbani, T. (2025). Llama-3-Meditron: An open-weight suite of medical LLMs based on Llama-3.1. In *Proceedings of the Workshop on Large Language Models and Generative AI for Health at AAAI 2025.*

Sellergren, A., Kazemzadeh, S., Jaroensri, T., Kiraly, A., Traverse, M., Kohlberger, T., ... (2025). MedGemma technical report. *arXiv preprint arXiv:2507.05201.*

Shool, S., Adimi, S., Saboori Amleshi, R., Bitaraf, E., Golpira, R., & Tara, M. (2025). A systematic review of large language model (LLM) evaluations in clinical medicine. *BMC Medical Informatics and Decision Making*, *25*(1), 117. DOI: 10.1186/s12911-025-02954-4 PMID: 40055694

Siino, M., Falco, M., Croce, D., & Rosso, P. (2025). Exploring LLMs applications in law: A literature review on current legal NLP approaches. *IEEE Access : Practical Innovations, Open Solutions*, *13*, 18253–18276. DOI: 10.1109/ACCESS.2025.3533217

Singhal, K., Azizi, S., Tu, T., Mahdavi, S. S., Wei, J., Chung, H. W., Scales, N., Tanwani, A., Cole-Lewis, H., Pfohl, S., Payne, P., Seneviratne, M., Gamble, P., Kelly, C., Babiker, A., Schärli, N., Chowdhery, A., Mansfield, P., Demner-Fushman, D., & Natarajan, V. (2023). Large language models encode clinical knowledge. *Nature*, *620*(7972), 172–180. DOI: 10.1038/s41586-023-06291-2 PMID: 37438534

Singhal, K., Tu, T., Gottweis, J., Sayres, R., Wulczyn, E., Hou, L., Clark, K., Pfohl, S., Cole-Lewis, H., Neal, D., Schaekermann, M., Wang, A., Amin, M., Lachgar, S., Mansfield, P., Prakash, S., Green, B., Dominowska, E., Arcas, B. A. Y., & Natarajan, V. (2025). Toward expert-level medical question answering with large language models. *Nature Medicine*, *31*(3), 943–950. DOI: 10.1038/s41591-024-03423-7 PMID: 39779926

Song, D., Xie, W., Kong, C., Chen, J., Zhang, H., Chen, S., Gao, A., Jiang, F., Li, J., Wan, X., Li, H., & Wang, B. (2023). HuatuoGPT-II, one-stage training for medical adaption of LLMs. *arXiv preprint arXiv:2311.09774.*

Vaswani, A., Shazeer, N., Parmar, N., Uszkoreit, J., Jones, L., Gomez, A. N., Kaiser, Ł., & Polosukhin, I. (2017). Attention is all you need. *Advances in Neural Information Processing Systems*, 30.

Wang, D., & Zhang, S. (2024). Large language models in medical and healthcare fields: Applications, advances, and challenges. *Artificial Intelligence Review*, *57*(11), 299. DOI: 10.1007/s10462-024-10921-0

Wang, F., Zhang, Z., Zhang, X., Wu, Z., Mo, T., Lu, Q., Wang, W., Li, R., Xu, J., Tang, X., He, Q., Ma, Y., Huang, M., & Wang, S. (2025). A comprehensive survey of small language models in the era of large language models: Techniques, enhancements, applications, collaboration with LLMs, and trustworthiness. *ACM Transactions on Intelligent Systems and Technology*, *16*(6), 1–87. DOI: 10.1145/3768165

Wang, X., Chen, N., Chen, J., Wang, Y., Zhen, G., & Zhang, C. (2024). Apollo: A lightweight multilingual medical LLM towards democratizing medical AI to 6B people. *arXiv preprint arXiv:2403.03640.*

Wu, C., Lin, W., Zhang, X., Zhang, Y., Xie, W., & Wang, Y. (2024). PMC-LLaMA: Toward building open-source language models for medicine. *Journal of the American Medical Informatics Association : JAMIA*, *31*(9), 1833–1843. DOI: 10.1093/jamia/ocae045 PMID: 38613821

Wu, C., Qiu, P., Liu, J., Gu, H., Li, N., Zhang, Y., Wang, Y., & Xie, W. (2025). Towards evaluating and building versatile large language models for medicine. *npj. Digital Medicine*, *8*(1), 58. PMID: 39865143

Xiao, H., Zhou, F., Liu, X., Liu, T., Li, Z., Liu, X., & Huang, X. (2025). A comprehensive survey of large language models and multimodal large language models in medicine. *Information Fusion*, *117*, 102888. DOI: 10.1016/j.inffus.2024.102888

Xie, Q., Chen, Q., Chen, A., Peng, C., Hu, Y., Lin, F., Peng, X., Huang, J., Zhang, J., Keloth, V., & Zhou, X. (2025). Medical foundation large language models for comprehensive text analysis and beyond. *npj. Digital Medicine*, *8*(1), 141. PMID: 40044845

Xue, L., Constant, N., Roberts, A., Kale, M., Al-Rfou, R., Siddhant, A., Barua, A., & Raffel, C. (2021). mT5: A massively multilingual pre-trained text-to-text transformer. In *Proceedings of the Conference of the North American Chapter of the Association for Computational Linguistics: Human Language Technologies* (pp. 483-498). DOI: 10.18653/v1/2021.naacl-main.41

Yang, A., Yu, B., Li, C., Liu, D., Huang, F., & Huang, H. (2025). Qwen2. 5-1m technical report. *arXiv preprint arXiv:2501.15383.*

Yano, K., Luo, Z., Huang, J., Xie, Q., Asada, M., Yuan, C., Yang, K., Miwa, M., Ananiadou, S., & Tsujii, J. I. (2025). ELAINE-medLLM: Lightweight English Japanese Chinese Trilingual Large Language Model for Bio-medical Domain. In *Proceedings of the 31st International Conference on Computational Linguistics* (pp. 4670-4688).

Ye, J., & Tang, H. (2025). Multimodal large language models for medicine: A comprehensive survey. *arXiv preprint arXiv:2504.21051.*

Zhang, D., Xue, X., Gao, P., Jin, Z., Hu, M., Wu, Y., & Ying, X. (2024). A survey of datasets in medicine for large language models. *Intelligence & Robotics*, *4*(4), 457–478. DOI: 10.20517/ir.2024.27

Zhang, H., Chen, J., Jiang, F., Yu, F., Chen, Z., Li, J., Chen, G., Wu, X., Zhang, Z., Xiao, Q., Wan, X., Wang, B., & Li, H. (2023). HuatuoGPT, towards taming language model to be a doctor. In *Findings of the Association for Computational Linguistics* (pp. 10859–10885). EMNLP. DOI: 10.18653/v1/2023.findings-emnlp.725

Zheng, G., Wang, X., Feng, Y., Shi, Y., Ma, Z., & Yu, P. S. (2024). Efficiently democratizing medical LLMs for 50 languages via a mixture of language family experts. *arXiv preprint arXiv:2410.10626*.

Zhou, H., Liu, F., Gu, B., Zou, X., Huang, J., Wu, J., Li, Y., Chen, S. S., Zhou, P., Liu, J., Hua, Y., Mao, C., Wu, X., Zheng, Y., Clifton, L., Li, Z., Luo, J., & Clifton, D. A. (2023). A survey of large language models in medicine: Progress, application, and challenge. *arXiv preprint arXiv:2311.05112*.

Zhou, M., Parmar, S., & Bhatti, A. (2024). Towards democratizing multilingual large language models for medicine through a two-stage instruction fine-tuning approach. *arXiv preprint arXiv:2409.05732*.

ENDNOTES

1 https://openai.com/index/introducing-chatgpt-health/

2 https://openai.com/index/healthbench/

Chapter 8

End-to-End Radiology Report Generation From Chest X-Rays Using Vision-Language Models

G. Vennila
http://orcid.org/0000-0002-2205-518X
Mohan Babu University, India

Dinesh Kumar K.
http://orcid.org/0000-0002-9912-3996
Vel Tech University, India

S. Anitha
http://orcid.org/0009-0009-7816-3639
Kongu Engineering College, India

Jariya Begum A. R.
http://orcid.org/0009-0005-1726-9414
Velammal Engineering College, India

ABSTRACT

The generation of diagnostic reports from chest X-ray images is a complex task that requires both accurate medical image interpretation and clear clinical language. Manual reporting is time-consuming, expertise-intensive, and susceptible to fatigue. Although deep learning–based systems have been developed to support this process, most traditional approaches treat image analysis and report generation as separate tasks, leading to inconsistencies and loss of critical details. Recent vision–language models offer a more unified solution by linking visual understanding with natural

DOI: 10.4018/979-8-2600-2173-6.ch008

language generation. This chapter proposes an end-to-end framework that integrates a Swin Transformer image encoder with a Q-Former and a fine-tuned BioMedLM for producing accurate and clinically meaningful reports. Experiments on a curated chest X-ray dataset demonstrate improved pathology coverage, reduced errors, and enhanced report clarity, supporting reliable and efficient clinical decision-making.

INTRODUCTION

Chest X-rays are one of the most commonly used diagnostic imaging in clinical practice in different parts of the world. They are the most common option of examining thoracic conditions, and it is not without reasons. They are cheap, fast, expose their patients to significantly less radiation than CT scans and can be implemented in rural clinics or can be done in facilities with limited resources. Chest X-rays are ordered by doctors to identify such problems as lung infections, tuberculosis, COPD, interstitial lung disease, lung cancer, fluid peripulmonary, collapsed lung, an enlarged heart, or bone diseases in the chest.

Nevertheless, the fact that X-rays of the chest are widespread does not imply the issues are easy to interpret. Radiologists are required to interpret overlapping structures that are squeezed down into a flat and two- dimensional picture of a three-dimensional body. One can rather overlook some minor indicators, including the initial symptoms of pneumonia or even slight lung spots, when working with short deadlines or when being tired. Also, it is not a matter of how one interprets these images based on what they see. The radiologists should also take into consideration the history of the patient, compare with the previous scans, and remember the known disease patterns.

These are further complicated by the need to write the radiology report. The radiologist cannot view that image and leave it there unless he transforms such visual impressions into a coherent written account that will be comprehensible and respondable to by other physicians. These reports have a standard structure usually comprised of Findings section that gives the description of what is observed and Impression section that gives a summary of what is observed as the main points. Wording is also important since the decisions regarding the treatment can be directly determined by what is stated in the said report. There must be clarity, accuracy and consistency.

The imaging studies done have significantly risen in the past decade. Individuals are living longer, there is a rise in chronic illnesses and the patients have more access to healthcare than ever before. The disadvantage is that this increasing demand has not been matched with the number of trained radiologists. This has resulted in increased work load, unread scan backlog, and increased report waiting time.

Delays or inconsistency in reporting can cause a great impact on patient care in a high-paced environment, such as an emergency room.

Artificial intelligence comes in at this point. Post initial AI applications in radiology had primarily concentrated on disease recognition and classification giving a yes-or-no response or alerting about a disease. The former method is useful in screening, but does not match with what a radiologist does in producing a full report. Radiologists go beyond image labeling and create a multi-layered visual cue into an articulate narrative that is clinical sense.

Vision-language models have developed this area, which are a combination of natural language generation and image understanding. These models perform well on the general tasks like description of pictures or answering image related questions. Direct use in medical imaging is however hazardous. A general-purpose language model can produce a text that can be sounded and sound good but is clinically incorrect, and discovers some finding that does not exist in the image.

The current paper addresses that issue by developing vision-language framework that is radiological-specific. The aim is to come up with a system, which will then be capable of generating precise, user friendly, and safe chest X-ray reports automatically. With a robust visual feature acquisition, meticulous matching of images and text and language generation polished by radiologist feedback, we are optimistic that we will come up with reports that radiologists would have confidence in and apply in practice.

LITERATURE & COMPARATIVE STUDIES

The concept of the machine-assisted interpretation of chest X-rays and the drafting of radiology reports is not novel. This issue has been under research and med-imaging experts have been trying to solve it over years. With time, different deep learning approaches have been developed. All of them are intended to enhance the accuracy of the diagnosis, reduce the workload of radiologists, and accelerate the process of clinical decision-making. To outline the proposed approach it is a good idea to first revisit what has been experimented with before, what has worked, and what has failed.

One of the earlier encoder-decoder frameworks of this task was introduced by Li and others in 2018. The principle was simple: the convolutional neural network (CNN) will be used to extract visual characteristics out of the X-ray, followed by transferring the visual characteristics to a recurrent neural network (RNN) which will generate the report text. Partially it was effective, the reports were readable, but such complex or subtle abnormalities were harder to capture by the system. It was a good beginning and not the end solution.

Jing et al. (2019) also made a step forward a year later with an attention-based encoder-decoder model. The difference that was made was the key and this enabled the system to generate certain portions of the image parts when producing individual words, but not the entire image. This enhanced the relevance and accuracy of the output particularly in the description of localized findings.

Chen et al. (2020) used a different method to enter this field and presented a hierarchical LSTM structure. They had developed the Findings and Impression sections individually rather than developing the entire report at once like their model. This gave the reports a better organization, more clinically relevant format, the way a real radiologist would write.

Then followed the Transformer period. Zhang et al. (2021) used Transformer-based structures to the task, which allowed the model to work with longer texts and identify the connections between remote words within the text. This minimized some mistakes and enhanced general consistency of the reports produced.

With the development of the field, the emphasis of the researchers started to be placed on the fit between the visual and textual aspect of these models. Nguyen et al. (2022) used cross-attention mechanisms to further relate the image visual abnormality with the appropriate phrases in the report. Similar systems, such as CXR-LLaVA (2023), began using CLIP-based image encoders with large language models such as LLaMA-2 to generate reports as well. These techniques demonstrated a potential but one factor came out: hallucination. The models occasionally reported results that were not found in the picture, and this is a grave issue in any medical usage.

Nearer to date, BioMedGPT and BioMedLM (2024) models have attempted to address this problem by incorporating biomedical knowledge into the language model itself. It is hoped that a model that is trained on medical text will be more precise with terms and less likely to draw clinically unsound statements. Human feedback reinforcement learning (RLHF) is another technique used to refine these models using feedback provided by actual clinicians, to minimize misleading or wrong information.

The obvious fact out of all this work is that there is no one invention that can fix the problem single-handedly. The composition of quality radiology reports requires a mix of factors: good visual feature hallucination, powerful correspondence between visual and verbal representation, enhancement of normal clinical knowledge, and mechanisms to ensure the model is honest and rooted. This is what the presented approach is supposed to reach.

Existing Methods

In the last ten years, automated radiology reporting has developed greatly, with fast development in the field of computer-based vision, natural language processing and multimodal learning. The developed methods are usually classified into four broad categories. Both have contributed something of use, but both also have obvious weaknesses that still are being dealt with in the field.

Template-Based Systems

First attempts to automate radiology reporting were based on templates, basically, pre-written portions of text, which would be put together depending on what the system detected in the picture. In case the model detected the symptoms of pneumonia (i.e., it detected the presence of pneumonia), it would insert a standard sentence on pneumonia in the report.

The systems are simple to construct and understand which is an advantage. They are extremely unbending, however. He or she is only able to describe what they have been expressly programmed to identify and not the oddities of what they find in unusual cases that two or more problems interact. The language that they generate is sometimes robotic and repetitive and this is not likely to make us confident in a clinical setup. In anything more complex than the simplest instances, template-based systems cannot be relied on.

CNN-RNN Encoder-Decoder Models

The second generation of methods took up deep learning. In these models, the CNNs were utilized to process images and dispel meaningful visual features that could then be fed to an RNN, typically, LSTM or GRU, to generate the report word by word. This was a great advancement in relation to templates. The language was also more natural, and the models were able to produce multi sentence reports which resembled what a person would write.

Nevertheless, these models also have their problems. RNNs are not good at long sequences long sequences -they tend to forget the information earlier in the text as they generate more words. This complicates the process of being consistent when doing a complete report. They also have difficulties in associating certain sections of the image with the right medical names, which results in the description being vague or general. In cases where the abnormalities seen in a particular image are multiple, there are cases when these models do not capture them all.

Attention-Based and Hierarchy Models

In an attempt to curb these problems, researchers came up with attention mechanisms. This was to ensure that the model paid attention to various elements of the image and produced various elements of the report as opposed to considering the image as a single fixed input. This enabled the model to focus on the parts that are relevant to the description, such as a shadow that may be suspicious in the lung, when explaining the specific results.

The hierarchy models were included as an additional layer of organization that created various parts of the report independently. These systems would not generate a single block of text, but rather the first part would be the Findings, followed by the Impression as was done in real radiology reports.

These were some features that were improved to make the reports more useful and interpretable. Nevertheless, attention-based models continue to hallucinate, or explain things that do not exist in the picture. Besides, they may generate statements, though, which seem reasonable but are inconsistent with clinical information as they are frequently trained on general datasets with little medical background. This brings a serious problem of trust. The Table 1 shows the existing techniques used for medical image report generation.

Vision-Language Foundation Models

The more recent line of models uses massive pretraining of both text and images. These vision-language models are Transformer-based models that learn a combined representation of visual and textual information and can reason and generate more complexly.

These models in theory are powerful enough to undertake complex end-to-end report generation. In practice, however, the vast majority are trained on general-domain data - common images and ordinary language, not on medical data. This has led them to not have the expertise to provide accurate and clinically safe reports. Unless they make close adjustments to the area of medicine, they will commit mistakes that may be damaging in medical institutions under the guise of being confident.

The restrictions indicate the necessity of a domain-focused, clinically informed vision-language system, and the given approach directly targets it.

Table 1. Comparative Analysis of Techniques for Medical Image Report Generation

Method	Key Technique	Strengths	Limitations
Template-Based	Rule-based text insertion	Simple, interpretable	Inflexible, robotic language
CNN-RNN Encoder-Decoder	CNN + LSTM/GRU	Natural language, multi-sentence	Forgets long context, vague findings
Attention/Hierarchical Models	Cross-attention + section generation	Better localization, structured output	Still hallucinates, lacks medical knowledge
Vision-Language Foundation Models	Transformer-based multimodal	Rich reasoning, end-to-end	General domain, clinically unsafe without fine-tuning

PROPOSED METHOD

The idea of machine-based interpretation of chest X-rays and the resulting generation of radiology reports is not emerging; over the years scientists and medical imaging scholars have been working on this issue. Several approaches to deep learning have been developed, and they are all focused on enhancing the accuracy of the diagnoses, decreasing the workload of radiologists and increasing the speed at which the clinical decision can be made. The area of the proposed approach could be studied by first understanding what has been tried before, what has worked and what has failed.

One of the earliest encoder-decoder models of this task was proposed by Li and others in the year 2018. The concept was simple; take the X-ray and feed it to a convolutional neural network (CNN), to find the visual features and enter the visual features into a recurrent neural network (RNN) to produce the report text. To some extent, this strategy was successful; the reports could be read, but the system was not very effective at capturing complex or subtle irregularities. It was a good initial step but it was obvious that it was not the ultimate solution.

Jing et al. (2019) used the next year to build on the work with an attention-based encoder-decoder model. The outstanding difference was that the system now had the ability to concentrate on particular areas of the image when producing any word rather than the whole image being uniformly covered. This rendered the outputs to be more pertinent and precise especially in dealing with localized findings.

Chen et al. (2020) decided to follow a different path and present a hierarchical LSTM architecture. Their model generated the Findings and Impression sections independently rather than producing the entire report as a single block of text. This organization brought in a more significant organization, which could resemble a real radiologist.

Subsequently, there came Transformer era. The authors Zhang et al. (2021) used Transformer-based architectures to the issue, which allows the model to process longer sequences and identify connections between words that are remote to each other in the text. This minimized certain forms of errors and enhanced general coherence in the output reports.

With the development of the field, scholars started to pay more attention to the correspondence in the visual and textual manifestation of such models. Nguyen et al. (2022), in their turn, introduced cross-attention mechanisms so that it would be easier to relate the visual abnormalities in the image with the corresponding phrases in the report. At approximately the same time, systems such as CXR-LLaVA (2023) began to combine CLIP-based image encoders with large language models such as LLaMA-2 to generate full reports. These approaches demonstrated possibilities but also pointed to the problem that kept reappearing hallucination. The models even reported discoveries that were not visible to the picture which is a matter of great concern to the usage of medical applications.

More recently, models such as BioMedGPT and BioMedLM (2024) have attempted to address this by integrating the biomedical knowledge in the language model itself. The idea is to have a model that is specifically trained on medical text to be more accurate when using terminologies and minimize the likelihood of uttering statements that are inaccurate clinically. Human feedback reinforcement learning (RLHF) has also been proposed as a method to refine such models with human patient feedback to reduce the amount of factually incorrect or misleading content.

All this work makes it apparent that there is no one innovation that can help to address the problem. A high-quality generation of radiology reports depends on a variety of factors: good visual feature extraction, good correspondence of images and text, incorporation of actual clinical expertise, and ways of ensuring the model is based on reality. This is what is based on the proposed approach.

EXISTING METHODS

Over the last one decade, automated radiology report generation has evolved to a great degree due to a fast progress in the computer vision, natural language processing and multimodal learning. The approaches that have been devised may broadly be classified into four. They have all contributed well but they have their own shortcomings which still plague the field.

Template-Based Systems

The earlier efforts at radiological report automation were based on templates, which were really a pre-written block of text, put together according to what the system identified in the image. Should the model detect the symptoms of pneumonia e.g. it will add a standard sentence on pneumonia in the report. The systems are easy to construct and easy to comprehend which is an advantage. Nevertheless, they are highly inflexible too. They have the ability to only report about what they have been programmed to identify and they are not able to adapt to out of the ordinary results or complex cases in which several issues intersect. The language that is generated can be quite robotic and repetitive and that does not make you feel confident in a clinical setting. In anything more than the simplest of cases, the template-based systems are inadequate.

CNN-RNN Encoder-Decoder Models

The following generation of methods adopted deep learning. These models used CNNs to process the image and to get meaningful visual features. These features were then inputted to an RNN, typically an LSTM or GRU, to produce the report word for word. This was a great improvement over templates. The language got more natural and the models were able to produce multi sentence reports which were more like human written English. However, these models too had difficulties. RNNs have trouble with long sequences: the older the information the more the information is forgotten as it generates more text. This renders any form of consistency in a report tricky. They also experience difficulties in associating certain image elements with the relevant medical terminologies and as a result, they describe the images in vague or generic way. In cases where more than one abnormality occurs in a single image, such models do not usually identify all the abnormalities.

Attention-Based and Hierarchical Models

Researchers incorporated the mechanisms of attention to overcome some of these problems. The given method enables the model to look at various sections of the picture when creating various sections of the report, as opposed to considering the image a fixed input. This provides the model with the capability of focusing where there is the need to do so such as a suspicious shadow in the lung when explaining the specific findings.

The hierarchical models were another source of structure in that they made distinct sections to the report. Rather than creating a continuous block of text, these systems would initially create the Findings, then the Impression as would be the case in actual radiology reports.

These additions made the reports more useful and interpretable. Nevertheless, attention-based models are also prone to hallucinating, which is something that is absent in the image. They can also produce medical inaccurate statements that may sound credible, as they are often trained on general datasets which are not in a medical context. This throws up serious concerns regarding trust.

Vision-Language Foundation Models

The most recent generation models makes use of massive pretraining on both images and text. These vision-language frameworks are based on Transformer networks which learn combined representations of images and text so that more elaborate reasoning and generation becomes possible.

Ideally, such models are supposed to be skillful in managing complicated end-to-end report creation. Nevertheless, the reality is that they are generally schooled in general information, including daily images and language, and not in the medical one. Therefore, they do not have specialized knowledge to generate accurate and clinically safe reports. So unless they adapt well to the medical field, there is a danger that they will commit errors with confidence as would be hazardous in a healthcare setting. These shortcomings demonstrate the necessity of an application-specific, clinically significant vision-language system - a goal that the solution is aimed at directly.

CHARACTERISTICS OF DATA AND CLINICAL REALISM

Saying about the model itself, it is necessary to devote attention to the data. In machine learning, especially in healthcare, the dataset will be able to establish the effectiveness of the system. The quality of a model can only be as good as the training data, and this data can be inaccurate to the conditions encountered in real life hence the system might not be effective in practice. In this work, we refer to Curated CXR Report Generation Dataset which can be found in the open access of Kaggle. The fact that this dataset has not been cleaned or artificially balanced to simplify the training of the model makes it interesting. It is disorganized just as real hospital data usually is, and it is not accidental. In order to have a system that would work in clinical setting, it should be trained on information that is similar to the information it will meet in the clinical setting.

The major characteristic of this data is its inherent imbalance in the classes. Most of the chest X-rays in a normal hospital are non-malignant or relatively normal. Exceptions rather than the rule are pathological findings. Most research datasets provide a remedy to this by over-sampling abnormal data, which gives false data on the high-performance of a model in the actual world. The imbalance was deliberate on our part. This makes this model learn to pick up the hints of the disease without necessarily becoming an alarmist to the patients with the normal images- this is important in preventing unnecessary follow-ups and panic in the patients.

The sample is created to represent a large variety of thoracic diseases: lung opacities, consolidation, pleural effusion, cardiomegaly, atelectasis, and other normal anatomic variations. Multiple overlapping findings are common in a large number of abnormal cases, and a common occurrence in practice. In an example, a patient may have swollen lungs and a large heart. The model has to know how not only to identify these problems separately but also to describe them in a clinically sensible manner simultaneously: that is, by focusing on important information and not using redundant or confusing words.

Besides, the reports are written by different radiologists and each one has his own style. There are short and to the point ones; there are detailed and warning. Some of them apply a lot of medical shorthand, but others use it all out spelled. This distinction is not only challenging to train a language model, but it also is realistic. All radiologists do not write identically and a good automated system will have to be able to accommodate this diversity. In the long run, this variation will increase the strength of the model and enable it to produce coherent reports without resorting to overdependence on a certain style of writing.

Hedging language that is typical of clinical practice is also contained in the reports. Such words as possibly, cannot be ruled out, indicative of are frequent. This language is used by radiologists when the imaging results are incomprehensible, and in this case, the expression of uncertainty is vital to their communication. This is something we intentionally did not take out in preprocessing. To come up with clinically realistic reports, the model must be taught to express uncertainty when and how to do so, as opposed to making bold statements all the time.

In the imaging aspect, the data contains X-rays, which were taken using various machines and in varying conditions leading to varying quality levels. It is not always the right position of the patient. Exposure settings vary. There are clear images and noisy ones. This is the real-world situation in hospital radiology and training on such diverse information stimulates the model to learn visual aspects that generalize effectively, but not necessarily patterns only, and that occur when everything is ideal.

Naturally, it has its shortcomings as well. Unusual and extreme conditions are underrepresented and this is consistent with their in reality but makes learning them more difficult by the model. This is why we have had to use reinforcement learning based on clinical feedback in the later stages of the process- to ensure that the model remains grounded and does not make over confident predictions when evidence is weak.

In general, this data offers a strong and realistic basis to develop and test a clinical meaningful system. It is not ideal, but it is truthful and the truthfulness is what makes it worthwhile to create AI that can be useful in the real world.

The dataset obtained has a number of limitations that are to be noted, irrespective of its clinical realism. First, bias in class imbalance: because most cases represent normal or near-normal studies, there is the likelihood that the model will not be effective on infrequent but important results like tension pneumothorax or early-stage malignancy conditions where failure to diagnose promptly has severe outcomes. Second, single-source risk: the data source is concentrated around a small number of institutions, which implies that the model has been trained on a small set of imaging equipment, patient demographics and reporting practices. Direct implementation in hospitals that have other types of scanners or reporting styles can lead to poor performance without re-validation. Third, demographic underrepresentation: the age, gender, and comorbidity distributions of the training data are not clearly stated, which creates the risk of having an uneven distribution across the subgroups of patients. Last but not least, ethically, this system cannot be implemented as an independent diagnostic tool. Any AI-based report should be deemed, checked, and confirmed by a competent radiologist before being applied in making treatment decisions. The framework is designed strictly as a decision-support assistant, not a replacement for clinical judgment.

This work embraces a contemporary vision-language framework, which includes three major elements as opposed to the traditional machine learning pipelines:

- Swin Transformer - to extract the details of the visual features of the X-ray.
- Q-Former - to match those visual features to language concepts.

BioMedLM: A medically trained language model used to generate the final report text.

Previous studies have indicated that multimodal learning i.e. when the model is exposed to both picture and text simultaneously leads to improved clinical reports with reduced errors and minimal hallucination.

This understanding informs design in this case. It is concerned with getting the medical information correct, making sure that the image and the text are in proper correspondence and the terminology used is one that a radiologist would actually use. The swin transformer (visual encoder) is a neural network that utilizes a transformer as its core architecture. Swin Transformer (Visual Encoder) The swin transformer (visual encoder) is a neural network that uses a transformer as its backbone. Swin Transformer A hierarchical vision transformer. It divides the images into tiny windows locally and creates a comprehensive global perception. It especially excels with both fine and bigger-context details as compared to older CNN-based methods, which are important to medical image analysis. What is the significance of this to chest X-rays? Abnormalities are minute and small though they occur within a big anatomical picture. A slight pulmonary obscuration can be both important and unimportant, depending on the surrounding structures. The Swin Transformer is an appropriate architecture to use in this analysis.

- Sustains spatial association between various regions of the lung.
- Thinks big (as well as small) (such as the heart) and small (such as a tiny nodule).
- Manages medical images of high resolution.

Q-Former (Cross-Modal Alignment Engine)

When we have visual features of the image we require a method of relating these features to language. Q-Former, which is also known as Querying Transformer, employs cross-attention to identify the most relevant visual information in each section of the report. Think of it as a smart filter. All the details in the image are not significant to the report, and all the visual elements should not shape each word. Q-Former also learns to concentrate on what is important and connects a certain finding in the picture with the appropriate medical terms in the text.

Key Benefits

- Eliminates visual clutter that may distort the language model.
- Makes sure that such terms as the one of the opacity or the pleural effusion are tied to the appropriate areas within the picture.
- Enhances accuracy between the vision and the writings of the model.

LANGUAGE GENERATOR: BIOMEDLM

BioMedLM is a large language model with biomedical adaptation, which is trained on medical texts, clinical notes, and radiology reports.

It understands:

Standard radiological terminology.

Sentence structure: This is a sentence structure employed in an imaging report.

This assists in creating reports which can pass off as the genuine outputs of the radiologists as opposed to some free flowing text.

Reinforcement Learning using Clinical Feedback (RLHF)

To avoid erroneous or misdirecting medical expressions, RLHF is applied:

Radiologist guidelines are encoded within the reward function of the model.

The model is penalized for generating wrong or unsubstantiated findings.

- Accuracy in the facts and report security is enhanced greatly.

COMPARISON WITH HUMAN RADIOLOGIST WORKFLOW

It is necessary to understand the role of automated radiology report generation systems in conventional workflows of human radiologists to judge their real practical usefulness and limitations. Radiologists have a systematic but dynamic procedure that they use to interpolate chest X-rays. They apply visual judgment, clinical judgment, and their experience. The proposed AI-based system is expected to support the workflow rather than to supersede it. It provides specific assistance during different phases of the reporting.

A normal radiologist process begins with detailed, methodical visual inspection of the X-ray of chest. This involves the inspection of lung fields, heart size and shape, mediastinum, diaphragm, ribs and soft tissues around it. Radiologists are also searching to find irregularities such as opacities, asymmetries, size variations or structural anomalies. They tend to make comparisons of existing images as compared to the past ones. This phase is based on years of training and experience. It will allow radiologists to discern the existence of minor patterns that could be a sign of early illness.

Clinical information is then interpreted by radiologists after the visual examination. They compare the results of imaging with the history of the patient, his symptoms, laboratory data, and risk factors. This argument is essential in regards to distinguishing between conditions that may appear similar on radiographic, e.g. pulmonary edema and pneumonia. Diagnostic uncertainty is also identified in a proper way by human radiologists. They take cautious language at times when results are inconclusive.

The last step is the radiology report writing. In this case, the observations become transparent and organised clinical narrative. Radiologists should use their clinical significance to emphasize the results, adhere to the standard reporting policies, and comprehensively convey the results to the referring physicians. It is a time consuming process and can be very cumbersome to the total workload particularly during a busy clinical environment.

Conversely, the suggested automated system performs visual feature and report generation with the help of a Vision-Language Model that has been trained on a set of combined medical images and text. Images can be easily analyzed by the system, possible common abnormalities identified, and consistent reports generated using standardized medical terminology. In the ordinary or routine cases, it is able to create preliminary draft reports effectively saving radiologists the repetitive documentation work.

Nonetheless, the AI machine is not able to retrieve a full clinical situation, as human professionals would. It does not inherently take into account patient history, symptomatic progression, or response to the treatment. Due to this, its reasoning can only be limited to the visual information only with the need to have human supervision, particularly in cases that are complex or ambiguous.

A human-AI workflow is the most efficient solution. In this model, the AI will create an initial report that determines the potential findings and gives systematized descriptions. It is then the variable of the radiologist who further checks the report, incorporates and finishes the report according to his or her own clinical judgment and expertise. This partnership enhances productivity and retains the accuracy of diagnosis and accountability.

Other issues that cannot be taken care of by the AI systems, but are the responsibility of human radiologists are the ethical, professional, and communication roles. They communicate directly with the clinicians, respond to the concerns of the patients, and change reporting styles to meet the needs of particular clinical circumstances. On the other hand, AI systems are still technical equipment with no moral judgment and professional liability.

To sum up, automated systems of radiology report generation have advantages regarding workload reduction; however, they cannot substitute the human skills. They are really useful in improving radiologist workflows and handling routine tasks and clinical decisions. The proposed system can be safely, effectively, and responsibly integrated into the clinical radiology practice by taking the strengths of both humans and AI.

ARCHITECTURE

The suggested system plan defines a well-structured and transparent pipeline in the generation of automated radiology reports based on the images of chest X-rays. It applies a full multimodal learning model comprising of medical image processing, visual feature extraction, vision-language integration, and natural language report generation. The architecture shall comprise of the following main stages, as demonstrated in Figure 1. shows the complete end-to-end pipeline of the proposed vision-language framework for automated chest X-ray report generation.

Image Input: The images are chest X-rays, which are in the Kaggle dataset. All images are subject to typical image preparation procedures, such as resizing, image normalization, and conversion to the form of tensors that can be trained with the deep learning models.

Swin Transformer Encoder: The processed images are fed to visual encoder which is Swin Transformer. The features of this encoder are hierarchical and locality-sensitive visual features. It takes significant organs such as the lungs, heart, diaphragm, and ribs. This can be used to represent potential abnormalities in detail.

Q-Former Fusion: Image tokens are sent to the Q-Former module and cross-attention is applied so that the regions of the image are matched with the tokens that are relevant to language. This step will be used to select only clinically meaningful visual signals into the language model in the second step (as explained in the Proposed Method section), which will reduce noise and enhance report grounding.

Biomedical LLM (BioMedLM): The resulting aligned multimodal representations are fed into a biomedical large language model (BioMedLM) that is domain-adapted. This model produces radiology reports in their natural form by the embedded and standardized medical knowledge using clinical terms.

Optimization of RLHF: The system is further optimized by use of reinforcement learning using human feedback to make it more factual and reduce wrong contents (RLHF). This is because it is necessary to permit the generated reports to be more in agreement with the expert clinical judgment and the expert reporting standards.

The process of the proposed pipeline is similar to that of the radiologist: (1) Visual Inspection — the Swin Transformer is a spatial scan of the X-ray conducted in detail, which captures small-scale details, including nodules or consolidations, which is comparable to a radiologist who manually examines lung fields, heart borders, and mediastinum. (2) Clinical Filtering - Q-Former now performs the role of a smart filter, taking only the visually worthy features required in each report section, as a radiologist does in choosing important findings out of the normal anatomy. (3) Report Drafting BioMedLM produces structured Findings and Impression text in the form of written narrative by the radiologist using domain-specific medical language. (4) Quality Control — RLHF uses clinician-generated feedback as a reward cue, and punishes hallucinated or unsupported statements, similar to the method used by experts reviewing a draft report.

Report Output: It is a structured report on clinical radiology that has clear and accurate Findings and Impression sections, hence the final product of the system would be acceptable in clinical practice.

Figure 1. System Architecture of the Proposed Vision-Language Framework.

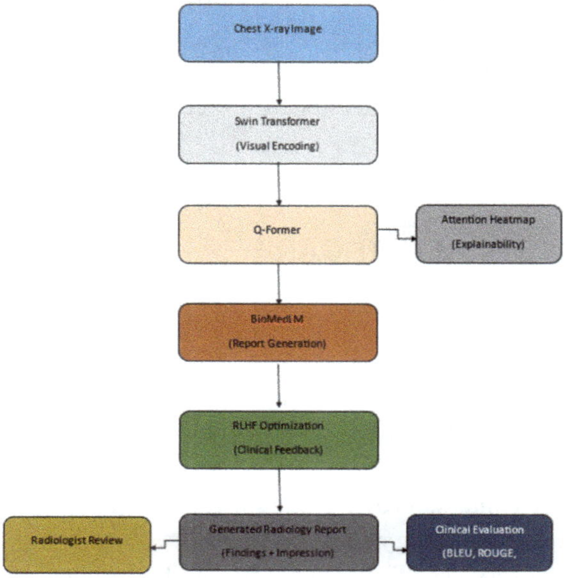

The structure helps with the consistent compliance with radiology reporting instructions, regular interpretation, and effortless following of radiology reports using clinical significant features.

SCOPE

This work scope aims at creating a complete automated artificial intelligence system that will assist radiologists in the interpretation of the chest X-ray images, by producing meaningful reports on the diagnosis. The system is not intended to substitute human experience rather, it is to be used as an assistive tool that enhances speed and consistency in reporting and diagnosis. In particular, the proposed work entails the following parts:

- Preprocessing of medical images: Standardization and normalization of the chest X-ray images to obtain data consistency and improve the AI model efficiency in the learning process.
- Performance evaluation: Evaluation of linguistic quality and clinical correctness based on different quantitative and qualitative evaluation measurements.

- Clinical assistance: This type of assistance helps the radiologists identify and interpret the common thoracic abnormalities at an early stage, particularly in the case of routine screening.
- The implementation of AI-driven systems such as this one will significantly enhance the quality of healthcare especially in regions where access to trained radiologists is low.

APPLICATIONS IN HEALTHCARE

Hospitals

Decrease turnaround time of reporting and reduce the workload of radiologists in high-traffic clinical areas.

- New medical centers: Provide diagnostic assistance in those areas where there is a lack of radiology specialists.
- Teleradiology services: They enable successful remote interpretation as well as reporting of medical imaging studies. Ways to use AI in medical education: Assist to teach medical students and residents with AI-assisted, guided radiology reporting.

SOCIETAL IMPACT AND HEALTHCARE ACCESSIBILITY

Implementation of artificial intelligence in the field of medical imaging does not only impact technical performance. It has a direct impact on the access to healthcare, fairness, and well-being in the society. The radiology report generation systems such as the one presented in this paper by automation can transform the manner in which diagnostic services are provided to patients particularly in regions that have inadequate health care professionals. These systems can be used to address the long-standing problems in healthcare globally through reducing the number of manual reports and improving the speed of diagnosis.

Automated radiology reporting is a major societal advantage because it enables the under-served and low-resource healthcare environments. The qualified radiologists are few or nonexistent in most of the rural and remote locations. Patients in such regions tend to delay diagnosis, referral and treatment and this may worsen the health outcomes. An AI-based reporting system may serve as a first-line diagnostic aid tool and can faster interpret images of the chest X-ray and contribute to making timely clinical decisions. Although not a substitute to highly qualified radiologists, it could provide useful assistance in case of unavailability of the expertise.

The increased workload and burnout of radiologists is another global concern that is currently addressed by the proposed system since the volume of imaging and the shortage of workforce are on the rise. Radiologists also waste much time going through routine or normal studies which are repetitive and time consuming. Even the preliminary report generation of such cases can be automated to a great extent to relieve this work load enabling radiologists to concentrate in complex, uncertain or dangerous examinations. This change is not only able to make operations more effective but also allows the well-being and job satisfaction of healthcare workers to improve.

On the part of the healthcare system, automated report generation can reduce the turnaround time of diagnosis, particularly in emergency department and busy hospitals. Faster access to radiology reports could assist clinicians in making timely treatment decisions, and it is crucial to such acute conditions as pneumonia, pulmonary edema, or trauma-related issues. Less delays in reporting may provide a better patient throughput, fewer overcrowds, and better care quality.

Other relevant aspects of the society are healthcare affordability and cost-effectiveness. Any delays in interpretation or review of imaging may increase the healthcare expenses of both the facility and the patient. The AI-assisted systems can be used to utilize the medical resources more effectively by increasing the consistency of reporting and reducing the number of unnecessary repeat assessments. In the long run, the savings would help minimize operational expenses and broaden diagnostic services to people with economic difficulties.

Medical education and training is also another area of important societal impact. Automated reports generating systems of radiology may be of value as a learning aspect to medical students, radiology trainees, and junior clinicians. The trainees will be able to acquire the standardized format of reporting, general diagnostic trends, and suitable clinical language by comparing the AI-produced reports with expert annotations. Such an educational assistance is particularly useful where there are teaching staff or resources short.

However, as the popularity of medical AI grows, the concept of the trust and moral accountability of people should be considered. The main aspect that should be brought up is that communication that AI systems are capable or incapable of should be made straightforward to avoid abuse and dependency. The proposed framework aligns with the ethics of the presented professional field because it allows achieving a human-AI alliance and preserving the control of radiologists, which enhances the responsible usage of technology.

In conclusion, automated radiology reports generation does not only have more than efficiency gains on the society. It is also inclusive of better accessibility to health care, reduced burnout among the professionals, better medical training and equitable diagnostic services. Perhaps, these systems could play a big role in healthcare delivery around the world and enhancing patient outcomes among populations of various species as long as an appropriate approach to resolving the problem is chosen.

IMPLEMENTATION AND RESULTS

The information used in this study is given in the Kaggle site and it is called Curated CXR Report Generation Dataset. It contains the X-ray pictures of the chest with the radiology reports made by physicians. The data set is comprised of various cases of patients, normal checkups of the patients, as well as images that contain pathological outcomes. Data is founded on the real clinical environment; thus, the cases of occasional and basic abnormalities are not prevalent. This gives the naturally unbalanced dataset which is reflective of clinical real-life and is more practical to the model.

The models are developed using Python. Deep learning frameworks, including PyTorch and Transformers library of HuggingFace, are used. Before the training, we take some basic preprocessing guidelines of images like resizing, intensity normalization and noise reduction to ensure that we have the same level of input. The preprocessing in the case of the text data entails extraction of the undesired characters, sentences segmentation and retention of domain-specific medical jargon where the objective is to maintain the clinical accuracy and semantic integrity.

The visualization of the characteristic features of datasets, e.g. frequencies of disease distribution, and variation of report length, are visualized using Matplotlib and Seaborn. It is followed by dividing the dataset into a training and a testing one, where 80 percent of the data will be used to train and 20 percent to evaluate. By doing this we can test the generalization capacity of the model.The following components are the main components of the proposed architecture:

- Swin Transformer → visual feature extraction
- Q-Former → cross-attention–based feature selection
- BioMedLM → medical domain language generation
- RLHF → prevents clinically incorrect and hallucinated content

The model is trained eventually with paired image and report samples. The reports that are generated are compared to the actual radiology reports during evaluation through the use of known language and clinical evaluation measures. Table 2 shows the quantitative results. They demonstrate the extent to which the proposed framework produces correct, clinically helpful reports.

Table 2. Model performance metrics.

Metric	Score
BLEU-4	0.285
ROUGE-L	0.402
CIDEr	0.215
RadGraph F1	0.54
CheXbert Score	0.82

When we compare the model to baseline CNN-RNN methods, it produced reports that are clinically meaningful, covering diseases effectively and having fewer hallucinations. To identify errors related to specific diseases, we looked at misinterpretations using a Confusion Matrix heatmap. The Figure 2 displays the result of the confusion matrix.

When we compare the model with baseline CNN-RNN procedures it generated reports of clinically meaningful value, and included diseases and a reduced number of hallucinations. We used a Confusion Matrix heatmap to detect misinterpretations in order to determine the errors associated with individual diseases. Figure 2 shows the confusion matrix heatmap, illustrating the clinical precision evaluation of the model across different disease categories.

Figure 2. Heatmap of the Confusion Matrix of Clinical Precision Evaluation.

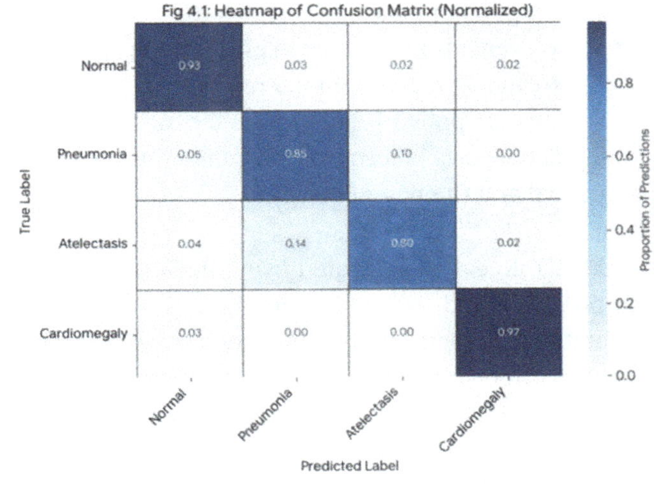

Figure 3 illustrates the attention heatmap highlighting the regions of interest on the chest X-ray that the model focuses on during report generation. The red and yellow areas indicate the key regions where the model detects possible abnormalities, enhancing transparency in the diagnostic process.

Figure 3. Attention Heatmap of the Model-Driven Areas of Interest on the Chest X-ray.

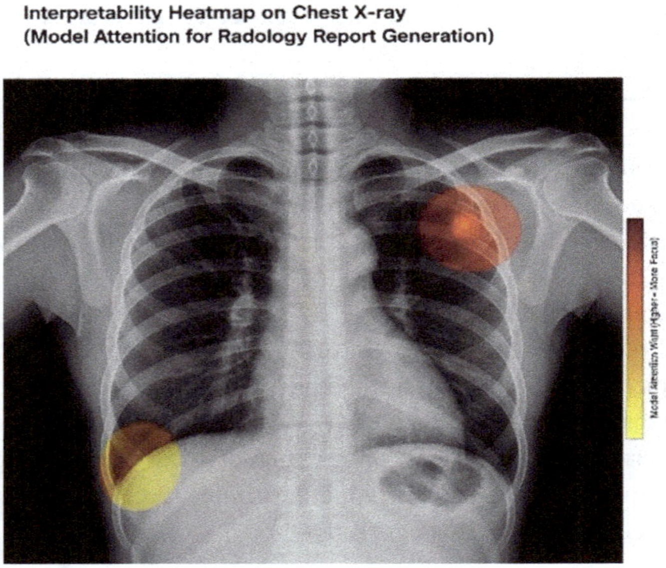

Table 3 represents five popular metrics (BLEU-4, ROUGE-L, CIDEr, RadGraph F1, and CheXbert Score) were also employed to estimate the quality of the language and the precision of the clinical material in the reports.

BLEU-4 (0.285): This is applied to determine the similarity of the generated reports with the reference reports in terms of the number of grammes. The score is an excellent grammatical and fluency in the text.

- ROUGE-L (0.402): Recall is measured using the longest common sequence between the produced and the actual reports. It shows that the model is a good representation of crucial clinical phrases and pertinent information.
- CIDEr (0.215): Explores the similarity in the text and reference description generated. It demonstrates that the system provides contextually sufficient and clinically significant sentences.
- RadGraph F1 (0.54): Measures the accuracy of medical relations and terms. This demonstrates that the model can be able to capture anatomical features and disease relationships.

- CheXbert Score (0.82): The approach to measure the precision of the disease diagnosis through a trained clinical model proves the high correlation between the received reports and the actual clinical outcome.

In terms of clinical usability, the CheXbert score of 0.82 is specifically significant: in more than 80 percent of cases, the AI-generated report will label the same diagnoses that a clinical labeling model (trained on annotations of expert radiologists) will provide. This implies that the system would be able to triage regular studies with reliability. The moderate RadGraph F1 of 0.54 indicates that the model is sensitive in that it models anatomical entities and their associations (e.g. the concept of 'opacity in right lower lobe') at a rate comparable to initial clinical decision support tools. Clinical deployment readiness is a primary goal to improve this score.

Table 3. Comparison of the performance of the proposed model to the existing algorithms

Model Architecture	BLEU-4 Score
CNN-RNN Encoder-Decoder	0.220
Hierarchical LSTM	0.250
Transformer-based Model	0.270
Language Model (Swin-Transformer + Q-Former + BioMedLM)	0.285

Figure 4 shows the performance comparison of radiology report generation models using the BLEU-4 score as the evaluation measure. As seen in Figure 4, the proposed Vision-Language Model achieves the highest BLEU-4 score of 0.285, outperforming all baseline models including CNN-RNN Encoder-Decoder, Hierarchical LSTM, and Transformer-based approaches.

- BLEU-4 score measures the closeness between the generated text (radiology report) and the reference report; a higher score means that it performs better and generates language with more accuracy.
- Four different models are compared in the chart:

1. The best overall errors in Vision-Language Model are that it generates accurate and unified radiology reports with the highest BLEU-4 score of 0.285.
2. Transformer-based Model: This model is not the best although it is lower than the proposed model with a score of 0.270.

3. Hierarchical LSTM: This model has BLEU-4 equal of 0.250 that produces slightly good results but inadequate to maintain long-term links in composing reports.
4. CNN-RNN Encoder-Decoder – This model achieves the lowest BLEU-4 score (**0.220**), indicating that it struggles more than the other approaches to generate fluent and well-structured radiology reports.

Figure 4. Comparison of Model Performance using BLEU-4 Score.

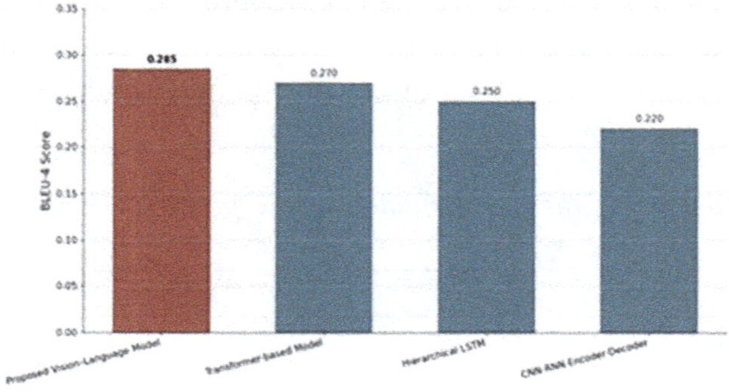

CONCLUSIONS AND RESEARCH DIRECTIONS

The paper demonstrates the practical applicability of the vision-language model of automatically generating radiology reports as a useful decision-support tool in the contemporary healthcare setting. The proposed framework will bridge the gap between medical image interpretation and clear language generation by incorporating a Swin Transformer-based visual encoder, a Q-Former cross-modal alignment component, and a biomedical-oriented large language model (BioMedLM). This system enhances a closer relationship between the visual evidence and generated reports unlike traditional method of encoder-decoder where the visual and the textual elements are loosely connected.

Based on experimental assessment of the Curated CXR Report Generation Dataset, it is evident that the proposed model has a better coverage of pathological results, medical terminology accuracy, and coherence of the reports as a whole than other conventional CNN-RNN and Transformer-based models. Subsumption with reinforcement learning based on clinical feedback also enhances the level of factual reliability by decreasing the amount of hallucinated or unsupported findings, a primary safety issue in medical text generation. These findings show that vision-language systems built on domain knowledge are able to generate reports that are very similar to the ones prepared by the trained radiologists in format and content.

On the whole, the present research will add to the expanding body of responsible medical AI, as it will show that vision-language models designed and clinically informed will allow enhancing the workflow in radiology without decreasing the level of ethics and safety. Although the system has great potential, it is not a solution but a platform on which further investigations and slower clinical adoption should be conducted.

FUTURE RESEARCH DIRECTIONS

Despite the encouraging outcomes of the proposed framework, it has a number of opportunities to be improved and expanded to make it more reliable, generalizable, and useful in clinical practice.

Another area that can be developed through future work is to make the datasets more diverse. Large-scale datasets, including MIMIC-CXR and CheXpert, would expose the model to a greater number of imaging protocols, disease distributions, and reporting styles across institutions. This would enhance the aspect of generalization and diminish bias of the dataset and the system will be more reliable in the other clinical settings.

Finally, regulatory, ethical and deployment validation is also a significant area of research in the future. Future clinical trials should also be used to test the system and fulfill the needs of medical devices prior to its application in the real world. Safe and accountable implementation is going to require the creation of standardized assessment guidelines and controls.

Based on these research directions, automated systems of radiology report generation can be developed as uniform, readable, and ethically defensible clinical decision support systems. These systems will have the potential to enhance the efficiency of diagnosis, reduce burnout among radiologists, and enhance patient care, which is a major step in the responsibility of artificial intelligence application in the sphere of medical imaging.

REFERENCES

Chen, Z., Shen, Y., Song, Y., & Wan, X. (2020). Cross-modal memory networks for radiology report generation. In *Proceedings of the 59th Annual Meeting of the Association for Computational Linguistics and the 11th International Joint Conference on Natural Language Processing* (Volume 1: Long Papers) (pp. 5904–5914). Association for Computational Linguistics. https://doi.org/DOI: 10.18653/v1/2021.acl-long.459

Jing, B., Wang, Z., & Xing, E. (2019). Show, describe and conclude: On exploiting the structure information of chest X-ray reports. In *Proceedings of the 57th Annual Meeting of the Association for Computational Linguistics* (pp. 6570–6580). Association for Computational Linguistics. https://doi.org/DOI: 10.18653/v1/P19-1657

Nguyen, H. Q., Pham, H. H., Linh, L. T., Dao, M., & Khanh, L. (2022). VinDr-CXR: An open dataset of chest X-rays with radiologist's annotations. *Scientific Data*, *9*(1), 429. Advance online publication. DOI: 10.1038/s41597-022-01498-w PMID: 35858929

Zhang, Y., Wang, X., Xu, Z., Yu, Q., Yuille, A., & Xu, D. (2021). When radiology report generation meets knowledge graph. *Proceedings of the AAAI Conference on Artificial Intelligence*, *35*(4), 4391–4399. DOI: 10.1609/aaai.v35i4.16464

Chapter 9

Transformer Models in Medical Image Processing:

A Review of Image Segmentation and Automatic Decision Making for Medical Images

Raj Kishor Verma
http://orcid.org/0009-0005-7216-7752
ABES Institute of Technology, Ghaziabad, India & School of Computing Science and Engineering, Galgotias University, Greater Noida, India

Indrajeet Kumar
http://orcid.org/0000-0003-2814-2900
Birla Global University, Bhubaneswar, India

ABSTRACT

This changed with transformers, which promised a sea change in medical imaging particularly image segmentation and automatic decision-making tasks. Later, their expertise in natural language processing thus, instead of known transformers has successfully transferred to computer vision tasks (including medical imaging) where they can take in global context and dependencies at long range, a significant step up from traditional convolutional neural networks. In medical image segmentation, transformers have good results even by bringing local and global features together, frequently supplementing this with CNNs to improve accuracy in distinguishing lesions or body parts such as organs-there is nothing like the precision possible on land that will benefit from a blended signal in this way.

DOI: 10.4018/979-8-2600-2173-6.ch009

1. INTRODUCTION

Four primary papers introduced transformers to Vision applications in a totally new field with NLP treatment using cross-attention heads. The majority of such elements are model-based to be fed on any collection of medical imaging data, which may include some reference medical imaging data close to a target domain as allowed.(Azad, Kazerouni, et al., 2024) Models of transformers initially designed to solve various tasks in natural language processing (NLP) have also proven quite successful in analyzing images by successfully modeling long-range dependencies and long-range spatial relationships. This feature has drawn medical image processing scientists to examine these networks, as a clear understanding of specific contextual knowledge is necessary to be able to make accurate diagnosis and therapeutic planification. Unlike the standard ConvNets that can only observe local features, the Transformer provides a global view of the global contexts which are specifically designed to serve task-type tasks (e.g., medical image segmentation and classification)(Nerella et al., 2024; J. Zhang et al., 2025).

Transformers have proven to be very successful in medical imaging such as segmentation issues. It is an important aspect of medical image analysis, since fundamentally you are interested in learning about the interesting aspects, which exists in the images such as organs or tumours.(R. F. Khan et al., 2023) This is critical in surgical strategy, disease diagnosis and prediction. A better local and global context learning capacity has increased the performance of CNN and transformers leading to the development of better segmentation. Nonetheless, the wide applicability of these approaches by medical imaging issues is restricted by numerous obstacles (e.g., relying on big data and computing infrastructure).(Thirunavukarasu & Kotei, 2024)

In that regard, some papers have indicated the surging desire to apply Transformer model to automatic decision-making (not segmentation) in medical imaging as the field advances. This involves image classification, object recognition and clinical report generation prosthesis. Overall, application of Transformers in such situations can go a long way in improving the accuracy and efficiency of the processing of medical images in such cases, and consequently the care of patients. The present trends in this survey show the medical image-processing tasks and automatic-decision making algorithms including segmentation, classification and other computer vision applications that are used in Transformers regarding clinical use-cases, and research problems in a rapidly developing field.(Shah et al., 2025; Verma et al., 2025)

1.1 Background

Medical Image Analysis as arguably the most important field of application of artificial intelligence, developed into a vital component in diagnostic medicine and healthcare overall. The technology has evolved quickly over the years form the classical ways of understanding computer vision to complex deep learning algorithms as transformer-based paradigm is now at the forefront in medical image segmentation and automatic diagnosis.(Maccaro et al., 2024; Yao et al., 2024)

1.1.1 Evolution From Traditional Methods to Deep Learning

Traditional medical image analysis techniques, edge detection, thresholding and region growing, e.g. have traditionally been employed to detect anatomical structures. Routines had been defined and performed well under controlled conditions, but when faced with noisy images, overlapping structure or vague boundaries, failed in most instances (Siebenhruner et al.). The change has come with the revolution of deep learning that took place in the year 2012 and resulted in fully convolutional network (FCN) in 2014 to enable an end-to-end learning perspective on semantic segmentation. This innovation also allowed models to work on entire images simultaneously, without having to subdivide them into patches and produce more detailed feature maps that carry both spatial and semantic information.(Shah et al., 2025)(Verma, 2026)

The concept of U-Net was introduced in 2015 by researchers at University of Freiburg — a landmark moment in the history of medical image segmentation. U-Net has established itself as the standard architecture for a variety of medical image segmentation datasets in various modalities: (Yao et al., 2024)CT, MRI, X-ray, ultrasound and histopathology achieved by its unique encoder-decoder architecture with skip connections that allow for high flexibility, efficient modularity while at the same time achieving excellent performance on diverse types of input data. The architecture's capacity of learning from limited amounts of labelled data proved especially effective in medical applications, where these expert-labelled datasets are not only scarce but also expensive to create. However, the U-Net and CNN methods have a limitation for its inability to capture long-range dependencies or global context information which are really important features for accurate segmentation of complex anatomic structures with complicated spatial dependencies.(Boussi Rahmouni et al., 2025; Nerella et al., 2024)

1.1.2 Limitations of CNN-Based Approaches

In the state-of-the-art CNNs, features are extracted using only local receptive fields and this can be small to capture long-range dependencies across a distant image location(He et al., 2023). This narrow field of view is not sufficient when analyzing medical images, as the target structures are surrounded by complex anatomical structures. Additionally, CNNs do not have the explainability that is needed for clinical acceptance- they are "black boxes" in large part - while visualization techniques (e.g., Grad-CAM) have been developed. Other challenges can include domain shift when models are challenged with data from multiple medical centers or imaging devices, class imbalance in medical datasets, and the necessity of heavy data augmentation for robust generalization.(J. Zhang et al., 2025)

1.1.3 The Transformer Revolution in Medical Imaging

In the recent past, the success of transformer models that solely apply the self-attention mechanisms have given encouraging results in the medical imaging scenario and this has questioned the capability of the conventional convolutional based design. Transformers use multi-head self-attention to compute links between every location within the input sequence and can be trained to be dependent between pixels or patches separated by a long distance. These properties are the factors that render transformers to be especially applicable in medical image segmentation when large contextual information is required. The Vision Transformer (ViT) that was put forward as the initial standalone transformer model to computer vision considers the images as a sequence of faces just like word embeddings in NLP.(He et al., 2023; J. Zhang et al., 2024) In the Models trained on immensely large data (at pre-train scale: at least 14M images) can outperform similarly-sized CNNs, as well as pre-training can be almost four times faster without ViT -based models. Self-attention of ViT enables embedding of global information i.e. during the training of the model, the relative spatial position is coded by the model to replicate the image structure. However, ViT models self-trained on mid-sized datasets (e.g. ImageNet) may achieve worse performance than CNN equivalents because of less robust inductive biases and increased dependence on data augmentation and regularization. (Thirunavukarasu & Kotei, 2024)

1.1.4 Hybrid Architectures and Medical Applications

Due to the diverse strengths of CNNs and transformers, many researchers have introduced hybrid versions, which combine local feature extraction based on convolutional layers with global context modeling using transformers. Initially introduced by TransUNet, smearing the transformer with standard architecture of U-Net and hence successfully mingling between global and local features. (A. Khan et al., 2025; Xia & Wang, 2023)TransUNet achieved percent higher Dice coefficients than previous methods on multi-organ segmentation tasks with the Synapse dataset, resulting in more significant overall accuracy and robustness. The newly introduced models are UNetr, which adapts pyramid-like multi-scale feature extraction with global context modelling Swin-UNet, that adds hierarchical feature fusion to be able to operate on objects of different sizes whilst remaining computationally efficient, and TransBTS which uses 3D CNNs with transformers to segment volumetric brain tumors, which results in Dice coefficients of 78.93, 90.00 and 81.94 to enhance tumor, whole tumor and tumor core on the BraTS2019 dataset respectively.(Verma et al., 2025; Xia & Wang, 2023)

1.1.5 Medical Imaging Modalities and Evaluation Metrics

Medical image segmentation cuts across various imaging modalities, having unique physical principles and diagnostic uses. X-rays involve use of the electromagnetic radiation to enable quick visualization of bone structures and dense tissues. Computed tomography (CT) involves the use of X-ray beams with computers to create detailed cross-sectional images that are best suited in detecting internal injuries, tumors, and abnormalities of the organs. Using a high level of magnetic fields and radio waves, magnetic resonance imaging (MRI) is the ideal tool in imaging of the nervous system, joint injuries, and cardiac imaging without the use of ionizing radiation. High-frequency sound waves are used in ultrasound to provide real-time images especially in obstetrics, abdominal, and cardiac imaging. In medical image segmentation, overlap based measures are mostly used as a basis of performance evaluation. (Karimi et al., 2022; A. Khan et al., 2025; Xia & Wang, 2023)The most common measure used in the literature of medical image segmentation is the Dice Similarity Coefficient (DSC), also called the F1 score or the SorensenDice index which is a harmonic mean of sensitivity and precision. Intersection over Union (IoU) or the Jaccard index is a more severe penalty against under- and over-segmentation than DSC. Other measures are sensitivity, specificity, and Hausdorff distance to measure the accuracy of the boundary and pixel accuracy. In the recent literature, the importance of standardized evaluation practice has been put forward to enhance the reproducibility and comparability of studies due to the fact that the application of different metrics has created statistical bias in most publications.(R. Zhang, Liu, et al., 2025)

1.1.6 Clinical Decision Support and Automation

The use of transformer-based models has become more common in clinical decision support systems (CDSS) offering real time support of diagnostic imaging and treatment planning. Image analysis using AI greatly minimizes the occurrence of diagnostic errors, speeds up the diagnosis processes, and allows one to detect disease early on with the help of predictive analytics. In These systems can assist radiologist functions when appropriately built into the clinical workflows, automatically identifying abnormalities, prioritizing urgent cases, and quantitative biomarkers in treatment monitoring. Nevertheless, the implementation process should be successful by including technical issues such as integrating with the current hospital information systems, workflow congruence, user acceptance, and preserving interpretability to facilitate making clinical decisions.(Karimi et al., 2022; Lai, 2024; Verma, 2026b; Verma & Kishor, 2024)

1.1.7 Challenges and Future Directions

The issue of data scarcity is also the problem to address because medical imaging datasets demand the expertise annotation, which is time-consuming and costly, especially in the case of rare diseases where several documented cases may be not available. Such privacy laws as HIPAA and GDPR present very rigid limitations on data collection and sharing. Generalization of domain between various clinical environments, scanner vendors, and groups of patients remains a challenge. The computational resources that are necessary to train large transformer models may be prohibitive in resource-constrained healthcare institutions. Federated learning to develop collaborative models across institutions without losing privacy, active learning to offload annotation by informative sampling to be annotated by experts, and data augmentation methods to deal with dataset scarcity are some of the emerging solutions. (Lai, 2024; Nurzynska et al., 2025)The research directions of the future are focused on the construction of lightweight versions of transformers that can be deployed on a resource-constrained host, better model explainability using explainable AI, the creation of standard evaluation measures to achieve reproducible research, and the implementation of multi-center validation studies of the model in practice.(Wang et al., 2022)

1.2 Transformer Models

Transformers are neural network architecture presented by Ashish Vaswani et al in 2017. in "Attention Is All You Need". Mainly use sequential data processing, such as natural language, and have brought enormous changes to machine translation, NLP, and even computer vision.(Ghribi & Hamdaoui, 2025; Zafari-Ghadim et al., 2024)

1.2.1 Components of Transformer Models

Encoder-Decoder Architecture- The original Transformer model in below Figure. 1: - Diagram of Transformer Models is made of an encoder and decoder. The input sequence goes through the encoder, and the decoder generates the output sequence relying on the output of the encoder. (Azad, Aghdam, et al., 2024)

Self-Attention: The heart of the Transformer model and its primary innovation. Managing the attention score between the input sequence means that they can relate where layers within it matter relatively to one another, which allows it to cap long-range dependencies effectively.(Azad, Aghdam, et al., 2024; Verma & Mamodiya, 2026)

Personalized Embeddings, also known as Input Embeddings and Positional Encoding: The input sequence is first embedded into numerical values. Sequence order is captured by adding positional encoding.(Azad, Aghdam, et al., 2024)

Feedforward Neural Networks (FFNNs): Following the mechanism of self-attention, FFNNs are further applied to process the output.(Wang et al., 2022; Zafari-Ghadim et al., 2024)

Figure 1. Diagram of Transformer Models

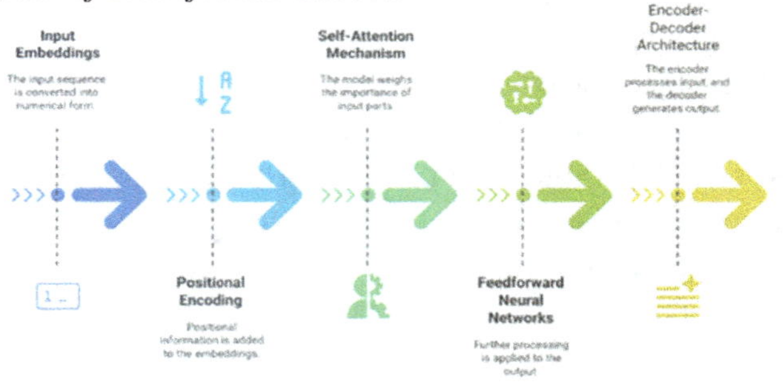

1.2.2 Types of Transformer Models

In the Bidirectional Transformers (BERT): BERT involves reading an input passage in both directions such that a more detailed contextual insight is obtained. we may use BERT to handle NLP problems, such as question answering and sentence classification. GPT: Generative Pretrained Transformers Those are text generating models that are conditioned by input prompts. They have been applied in several ways such as chatbots and text-generating systems in Figure.2.of Comparing Context Understanding & Text Generation(Wang et al., 2022; Zafari-Ghadim et al., 2024)

Figure 2. Comparing Context Understanding & Text Generation

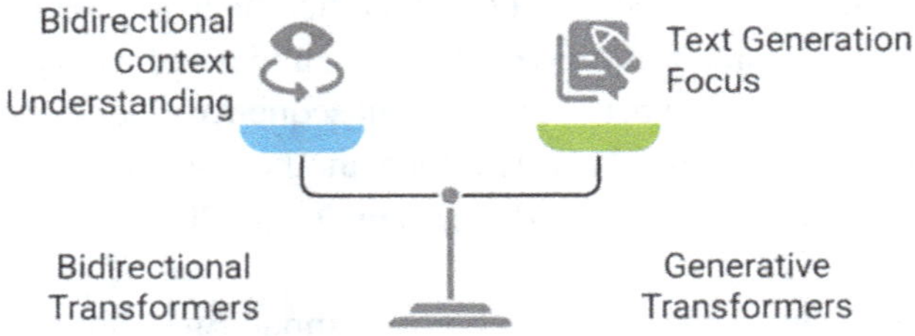

1.2.3 Uses of Transformer Models

Natural Language Processing (NLP): for example, machine translation, text generation and language understanding. Artificial Intelligence: Aspects such as image classification, and object detection. Bioinformatics–Protein structure prediction. Finance: such as time-series and fraud detection.

Benefits Over Models From Traditions Transformers provide the capability to parallelize the computations making them faster than recurrent neural networks (RNN) such as LSTM. Long-Term Dependencies: They can capture relations to far-away elements in the sequence.(Papanastasiou et al., 2024; Verma & Mamodiya, 2026)

1.3 Medical Image Segmentation

Medical image segmentation is one of the most important steps in medical imaging, where it separates an image into various segments or regions of interest (ROIs) based on the particular class or type of tissue, such as organs, lesions, or tumors. It plays a crucial role in the correct identification, management, and follow-up of disease. Important Aspects of Medical Image Segmentation Purpose: The first step is to derive the region of interest: the main area of the given medical image: CT scan, MRI, X-rays, and ultrasound image. It aids the examination of structures, intravenous abnormalities, and the volume of tissues to analyze disease progression. (Azad, Aghdam, et al., 2024; Ghribi & Hamdaoui, 2025)

Techniques Some of the many methods used include Thresholding: Dividing regions using the intensity of pixels. Region-based segmentation: Region growing or clustering methods. Segmentation-Based Edge: Finding lines between regions. Semantic Segmentation: neural networks for high dimensional data.(Papanastasiou et al., 2024)

Medical images are usually elaborate, widely influenced by partial volume effect, intensity inhomogeneity, artifacts, and in some cases, tissues possessing similar grey levels. Vital for disease diagnosis, treatment plan, and quantitative analysis. Such as brain tumour segmentation, liver segmentation, and cardiac segmentation. MATLAB supports both Medical Imaging Toolbox, which has full support for image segmentation tasks. Universal segmentation models based on deep learning, including foundation models like MedSAM, also continue to advance across imaging modalities. Workflow Steps Involved Medical Image Segmentation.(Azad, Aghdam, et al., 2024)

View Medical Images: Getting images through various modalities. Image processing: removing noise and so on to improve the quality of images. Segmentation: It is about applying the algorithm in 2D or in the 3D region of the image. Quantitative analysis of segmented areas for diagnosis and treatment plan. It Hence, Analysis and interpretation. Significance within Clinical Practice Speed and Precision: Compared to manual methods, automated segmentation requires less time and labour. Consistent: Provides consistency across a large volume of data. Versatility: Recent models are trying to be general and work with multiple imaging modalities and tasks.(Ghribi & Hamdaoui, 2025)

1.4 Automatic Decision Making

Automatic decision-making involves making decisions without human involvement, using technology and algorithms to evaluate data and reach conclusions. (Nerella et al., 2024; J. Zhang et al., 2025) This method is being implemented more often in different sectors, such as business, healthcare, education, and law, to increase efficiency and decrease errors. Automated decision-making (ADMS) systems use information from a wide range of large-scale sources (i.e., databases, social media, sensors) to process information quickly and make informed, real-time decisions. How Automatic Decision-Making Works Data collection data collection: The first step in the automatic decision-making process is data collection.(Nerella et al., 2024; J. Zhang et al., 2025) These models may vary from basic decision trees to sophisticated AI systems such as deep neural networks. Through data processing according to a set of predefined rules or parameters, a decision is then made without human judgment being involved at any stage in the decision-making process. Robo-advisors in finance, as one of their use cases, use real-time trading data to decide which investment strategy has to be recommended and deliver them to investors without any bias or human mistake1. This automation not only speed the decision process but also ensure all decisions are consistent and correct. Benefits by-produced Churns from Decision Making Automatically in below Figure. 3: -Flow of Automatic decision-making .(Lai, 2024; Nurzynska et al., 2025; Papanastasiou et al., 2024; Wang et al., 2022)

The advantages of automatic decision making are improved efficiency, reduced human error and a greater consistency in decisions. It allows organizations to analyze massive amounts of data and derive insights that could not be attained through conventional manual examination.(Wang et al., 2022; Zafari-Ghadim et al., 2024)

Figure 3. Flow of Automatic decision-making

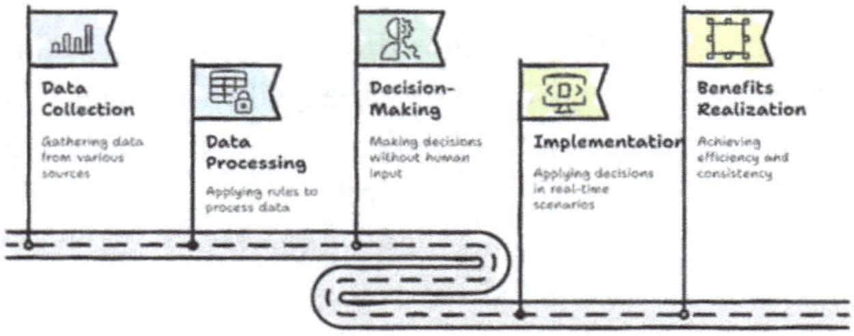

1.5 Deep Learning

Deep learning is transforming an infinite number of problem domains as it enables automation of nonsensical decision-making tasks, news knowledge extraction from petabytes of unstructured data and significant human performance enhancement. But like all other state-of-the-art technological breakthrough, this is halting to social issues concerning privacy and security, bias and fairness; job displacement–enough of a threat by deep learning from making a very fair progress for humanity. (Verma et al., 2025)Backpropagation is used to train the connection weights, where errors are propagated backward through the network. Make this formal, we get the model gain doesn't significantly increases but loss function decreases by its value calculated by using gradient descent. Activation functions: The model learn complex relations through the implementation of nonlinearity by means of activation operation. Some of the activation functions that we encounter most frequently are sigmoid, hyperbolic tangent and rectified linear unit (ReLU), each serving different learning purposes.(Zafari-Ghadim et al., 2024; Zhou et al., 2023) In convolutional neural networks (CNNs), the layers are based on complex features, hence enabling the network to learn further high-level features through grid-like input data like visual components while CNNs autogenrarting features by images for object detection and image classification. Recurrent Neural Networks, or RNNs for short, are characterized by their ability to handle sequential data. If it is a sequence, everything related to time series prediction and NLP tasks where you deal with sentence generation, parsing, semantic analysis (Hierarchy of Sequential Data) — they are widely used. They stagger with vanishing gradients but have memory of previous inputs. GANs (generative adversarial networks, for short) have two parts that work in opposition the discriminator judges if something is real and the generator creates samples. Perception Recognition Random Wrapper Methods. They are used for data augmentation and photorealistic generation. (Thirunavukarasu & Kotei, 2024) In particular, transfer learning enables much larger data sets and shorter training times for professional Machine Learning practitioners, in addition to it's use as a standalone model. This is a genuine advantage in a field with so few big data sets.(Alyami et al., 2023; Zhou et al., 2023) Using the principles of reward and punishment an agent optimizes for its behavior through past experience; deep reinforcement learning eats all that knowledge with a help from deep learning to support rational decision making. In computer vision, deep learning in below Figure. 4: - Diagram of Deep Learning is used for image classification, object recognition and facial feature detection (e.g., GAN became the most famous classic Fooling model) while in natural language processing there are applications like sentiment analysis, translation and conversational chatbots.(Karimi et al., 2022; Lai, 2024)

Figure 4. Diagram of Deep Learning

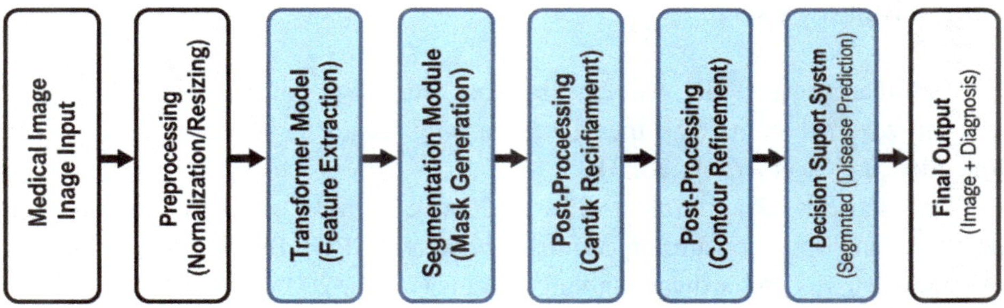

1.5.1 Advantages of Deep Learning

Automatic Features Extraction: Deep learning models, unlike traditional machine learning, automatically extracts features from the raw data without human-engineered features. This allows deep learning models to reveal hidden structures in large data sets that even humans cannot tell us about. High Accuracy: DNNs can obtain state-of-the art accuracy on multiple benchmarks. (Desai, 2025; Verma, 2026b)In fact, they outperform human accuracy in some tasks. These models can harness complexity from large architectures and vast amounts of computation in ways that enable them to address problems in novel and exciting manners. (Nerella et al., 2024; J. Zhang et al., 2025)They scale up: Deep learning models in the below Figure. 5: - Component & Application of Deep Learning can work with enormous datasets and generally perform better when given additional data. The more deeply you fly neural networks and the greater number of patterns you can train them to separate, the "smarter" they become.(A. Khan et al., 2025; Xia & Wang, 2023)

Figure 5. Component & Application of Deep Learning

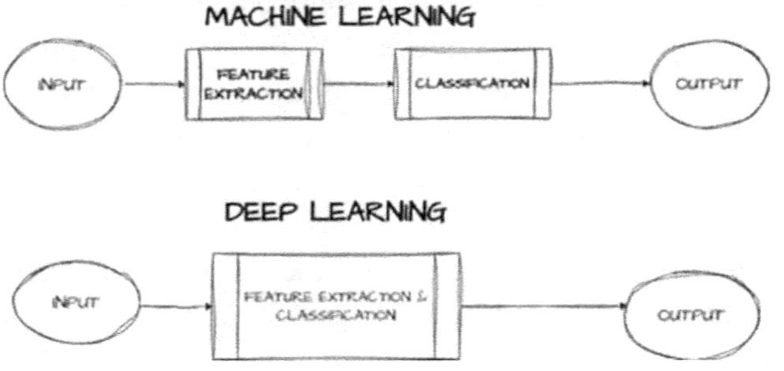

1.5.2 Challenges

Deep learning's model efficient training generally requires large labeled data sets. However, re-cent self-supervised learning advances start to chase away the dependence.(Xia & Wang, 2023)

Computational Requirements Deep network training can be computationally expensive and time consuming, requiring powerful GPUs. But that cost is mitigated by ongoing gains in hardware and algorithms.(Desai, 2025; Jose et al., 2024)

Interpretability The deep learning models are considered system, which is hard to understand about how they have made decision. However, techniques like attention maps offer some degree of explanation about the way neural networks are reasoning.(A. Khan et al., 2025; J. Zhang et al., 2024)

1.6 Medical Imaging

Introduction to Medical Imaging Description: Medical imaging is an essential technique in modern medicine, through which the inside of human body is visualized and then clinical analysis and medical intervention can be done. (Jose et al., 2024; Liu & Zhong, 2025; J. Zhang et al., 2024)

Nowadays, however, imaging modalities have become crucial tools for diagnosing a wide variety of diseases from cardiac disease, where stents or other devices may have to be deployed(Hu et al., 2023; Verma et al., 2025), cancerous cells at various locations in the body, neurological disorders and there is more indication that even complex fractures can benefit1. It is also indispensable for treatment response assessment, and the creation of normal anatomy, physiology databases to define abnormalities.(He et al., 2023)

Medical imaging in the below Figure. 6: - Architecture of Medical Imaging Technique is not just one thing, and the modalities have unique strengths. Radiography including X-rays use ionizing radiation to generate images which are mainly of hard tissues (e.g., bones). MRI is noninvasive and uses magnetic field and radio waves to generate fine-grained soft tissue images, effective in brain and musculoskeletal system inspection.(Hu et al., 2023; Wu et al., 2014b) The ultrasound is non-invasive and based on the use of sound waves to generate images, its main application areas are obstetrics and cardiology.(Neumann & Vu, 2019; Yao et al., 2024)

Nuclear medicine, for example PET scans, uses radioactive compounds to examine metabolic activities within the body. CT creates axial images by adding several X-ray projections to one another. In medical imaging develops ceaselessly, These advances are leading to more specific and safer diagnosis as well as the possibility of personalized treatment plans.(Shah et al., 2025)

In addition, advances in imaging informatics and teleradiology are expanding access to medical imaging services to render healthcare more accessible and cost-effective. However, it should be emphasized that medical imaging is often a benefit to society and must be judiciously used to limit risks, such as radiation exposure, and to confirm that the benefits are greater than the risks.(R. F. Khan et al., 2023; Liang et al., 2020; Neumann & Vu, 2019)

Figure 6. Architecture of Medical Imaging Technique

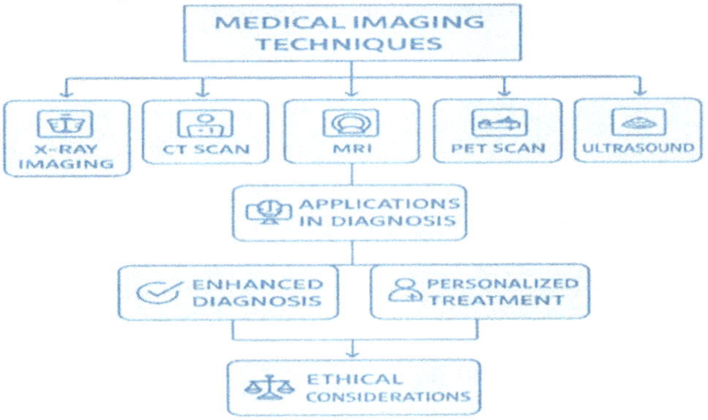

1.7 Computer Vision

Computer vision is a subject in artificial intelligence (AI) that allows computers to interpret and understand visual details from digital images as well as videos.(Wu et al., 2014) Through the use of machine learning and artificial neural networks, this technology is designed to analyze visual data much like a human does, enabling computers to "see" objects and faces and patterns as we do. (Wu et al., 2014; R. Zhang, Liu, et al., 2025)Computer vision has a variety of applications in below Figure. 7: - Architecture of Computer Vision, including self-driving automobiles, Facial recognition systems, medical imagery analysis, and quality inspection in production. Characters are first extracted from the text image. The first step involves capturing visual data using devices, such as cameras or sensors. This data is then improved for quality through preprocessing, such as noise reduction and normalization.(Azad, Kazerouni, et al., 2024; Biswas & Sarkar, 2026)

Then, we extract features (edges, textures, shapes) from the images. Machine learning algorithms typically employ deep learning approaches including convolutional neural networks (CNNs) then leverage these characteristics to detect and categorize objects in the images. As this technique goes through more training using the data, the nomenclature becomes more accurate.(R. Zhang, Cao, et al., 2025)

The computer vision has ample scope in the real-world demand across industries. It is utilized in surveillance systems for object tracking in healthcare for medical imaging analysis or in automotive for autonomous vehicles.(Zhao et al., 2014) The computer vision market is expected to have an annual growth rate of 16.0% for the period of 2020 to 2030. Computer vision is an evolving technology that will automate tasks that require human eyes, as technology progresses; it will play an essential role in making many industries more efficient and accurate.(Poornima & Nasurudeen Ahamed, 2025; Silva-Atencio, 2025; Verma & Kishor, 2024)

Figure 7. Architecture of Computer Vision

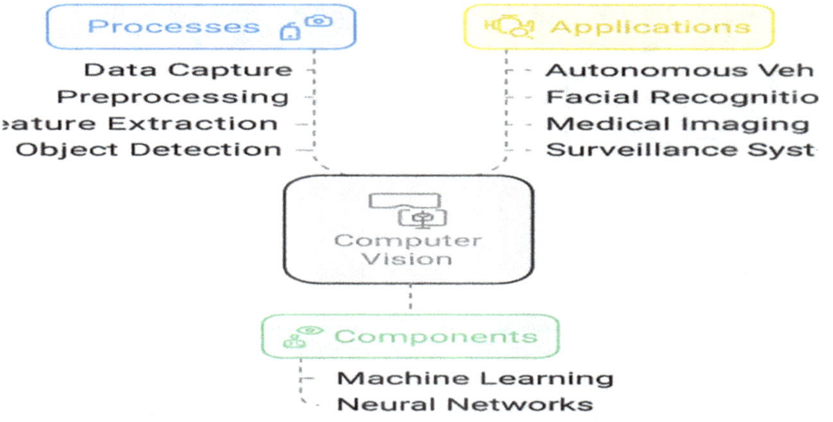

2. LITERATURE REVIEW

Table 1. Comparative Summary of Transformer-Based Medical Imaging Research

S. No	Authors	Year	Methodology	Pros	Cons	Result Analysis	Research Finding	Research Gap
[1]	Satoshi Takahashi et al	2023	Comparison of Vision Transformers and Convolutional Neural Networks in Medical Image Analysis: A Systematic Review	Highlights Transformer's ability to capture global context.	Limited annotated data.	Discusses future perspectives in medical imaging.	Transformers outperform CNNs in global feature extraction.	Need for more annotated datasets and domain adaptation methods.
[2]	Fahad Shamshad et al.	2023	Survey of Transformer applications in segmentation, detection, and report generation.	Provides taxonomy and insights into challenges.	Identifies open problems and challenges.	Offers future directions and recent updates.	Summarizes wide Transformer adoption across medical imaging.	Lack of unified benchmark datasets and reproducibility studies.
[3]	RF Khan et al.	2023	Encyclopaedic review of Transformer applications in classification and segmentation.	Systematic review of recent literature and taxonomies.	Challenges in complex clinical settings.	Summarizes key challenges and future directions.	Comprehensive mapping of Transformer models to clinical imaging.	Clinical validation and real-world deployment remain limited.
[4]	Xia Kun Wang, Jinzhuo et al.	2023	Comprehensive review covering various data modalities.	Covers 276 works and 76 datasets.	Varied disease properties complicate analysis.	Discusses open problems and future directions.	Broad survey of multimodal Transformer methods.	Integration across diverse disease domains still underexplored.
[5]	V Kumari et al.	2023	Narrative review on Transformers for segmentation architectures.	Combining Transformers with CNNs improves performance.	Lack of annotated data is a major challenge.	Outlines strategies like transfer learning.	Hybrid CNN-Transformer architectures enhance segmentation.	Need for low-data learning and annotation-efficient models.
[6]	N Rane et al.	2022	Review of Transformer roles across medical image tasks.	Captures long-range dependencies effectively.	Limited by computational resources.	Encourages further Transformer research.	Highlights capability for holistic image understanding.	Requires computational optimization for large-scale medical data.
[7]	EU Henry et al.	2022	Review of Vision Transformers in medical imaging.	Vision Transformers outperform CNNs.	Requires large datasets for training.	Discusses future applications.	ViTs show potential in diverse imaging tasks.	Necessity for pre-training on medical-domain data.
[8]	RANT Authors	2022	Cascade reverse attention hybrid Transformer for laryngeal endoscope images.	Improves segmentation accuracy.	Complex handling of diverse image types.	Effective for specific imaging tasks.	Hybrid Transformers enhance segmentation precision.	Broader generalization across imaging modalities is needed.

continued on following page

Table 1. Continued

S. No	Authors	Year	Methodology	Pros	Cons	Result Analysis	Research Finding	Research Gap
[9]	PCAT-UNet Authors	2022	UNet fused with CNN and Transformer for retinal vessel segmentation.	Combines CNN and Transformer strengths.	Requires careful hyperparameter tuning.	Achieves high accuracy in segmentation.	Hybrid CNN-Transformer improves retinal vessel analysis.	Optimization for various medical datasets needed.
[10]	AGMB-Transformer Authors	2022	Anatomy-Guided Multi-Branch Transformer for root canal therapy.	Uses anatomical guidance for higher accuracy.	Limited annotated data.	Promising for specialized medical imaging.	Anatomical priors improve Transformer interpretability.	Data scarcity and validation on diverse populations.
[11]	Chest L-Transformer Authors	2022	Self-supervised Transformer for histopathological classification.	Effective in self-supervised learning.	May not generalize across datasets.	Shows potential in unsupervised learning.	Demonstrates power of self-supervised medical image Transformers.	Limited adaptability to new tissue and pathology types.
[12]	Scale-Aware Transformers Authors	2021	Scale-aware Transformer for melanocytic lesion diagnosis.	Handles scale variations effectively.	Requires large datasets.	Improves diagnostic accuracy.	Transformers adapt well to scale-sensitive imaging.	Dataset scalability and transfer learning remain challenges.
[13]	M3T Authors	2021	3D classifier using Multi-plane and Multi-slice Transformer.	Effective in 3D image classification.	Computationally intensive.	Handles complex 3D medical data well.	Multi-slice Transformer captures volumetric dependencies.	High computational cost limits clinical deployment.
[14]	DPE-BoTNeT Authors	2022	Dual Position Encoding Bottleneck Transformer for skin lesion classification.	Enhances classification accuracy.	Poor performance with limited data.	Effective in lesion classification.	Positional encoding improves image context learning.	Needs adaptation for small and imbalanced datasets.
[15]	Trans Med Authors	2022	Multi-modal medical image classification Transformer.	Handles multi-modal data effectively.	Requires large and diverse datasets.	Promising results in multi-modal tasks.	Demonstrates fusion capability of Transformers.	Insufficient cross-modal alignment research.
[16]	MRI Super-resolution Authors	2021	Transformer-based model for MRI super-resolution reconstruction.	Significantly improves MRI image quality.	Computationally demanding.	Advantages in MRI reconstruction.	Transformer enhances fine-grain MRI detail restoration.	Efficiency and inference speed need improvement.

3. PROPOSED DIAGRAM

Transformers in Medical Image Processing (Verma & Kishor, 2024)These models, such as the seminal convolutional neural networks originally designed for natural language processing tasks, have progressively been adapted to more general computer vision challenges and thus have made their way into domains like medical imaging. Vision Transformer and its various variants such as Data Efficient Image Transformers, BERT Pre-Training Image Transformer, etc. has nowadays generally become encoders to extract visual information from medical images like X-rays or CT scans 12. An ideal medical image processing diagram would have the encoder-decoder structure with a leading transformer model. FE-based Image Captioning (Here encoder extracts visual features from images and decoder) in describe with the Diagram in below in Figure. 8: - Proposed Diagram of Transformer Model in Medical Image Processing

Figure 8. Proposed Diagram of Transformer Model in Medical Image Processing

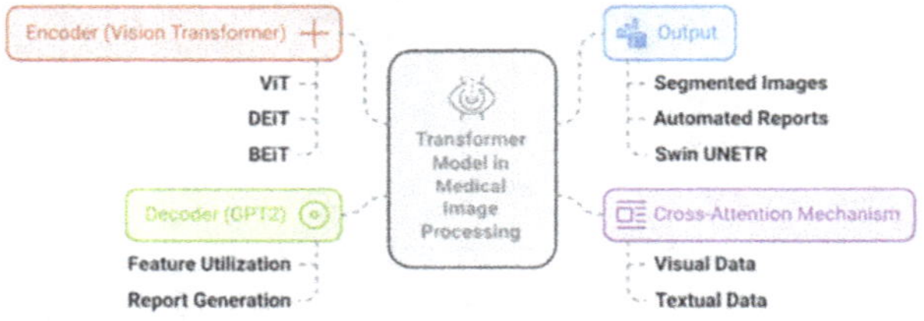

Encoder (Vision Transformer): This unit operates on medical images to produce medically useful features. It could be a ViT, or one of its cousins like DEiT or BEiT. Cross-attention Mechanism: (Verma & Kishor, 2024; Zhu et al., 2023)This mechanism lets the model combine the visual information it gets from the encoder with textual information for report generation. Decoder (GPT2): Based on the features extracted, this part then generates laborious and coherent medical reports as output. The output takes the form of segmented images with automatic medical reports such as For an analysis of 3D medical images, models such as Swin UNETR can be used. These exhibit cutting-edge segmentation performance through self-supervised learning. A major issue is the deficit of annotated medical data in published form needed for training deep learning models Future directions may include leveraging transfer learning and foundation models in order to increase the efficacy of medical imaging with transformers. (Wu et al., 2014a; Zhu et al., 2023)

3.1 Algorithm: Transformer Model for Medical Image Segmentation and Decision-Making

Input

- I: Input medical image (e.g., CT, MRI)
- C: Number of classes (optional; for segmentation tasks)

Output

- Segmentation map S
- Automated decision/classification D

Step 1: Image Preprocessing

1. Normalize, Apply augmentation techniques (e.g., rotation, flip, scaling) if necessary. Resize or crop the image to a standardized shape.

Step 2: Patch Embedding

1. Split Iinto non-overlapping patches. Flatten each patch and project it into a lower-dimensional embedding using a linear transformation.
2. Add positional embeddings to retain patch order and spatial information.

Step 3: Transformer Encoding

For every layer in the transformer encoder: Apply multi-head self-attention to aggregate information across all patches. b. Normalize and add residual connections after attention and feedforward sublayers. Pass the output embeddings to the next encoder layer or the decoder module.

Step 4: Decoder (For Segmentation Tasks)

Use a suitable decoder (e.g., U-Net style or up sampling layers). Integrate skip connections, if applicable, to combine encoder and decoder features. Upsample the decoder outputs to match the original image size. Generate pixel-wise predictions to create segmentation map S.

Step 5: Automated Decision Module

Aggregate global information from transformer outputs (e.g., by global pooling). Feed pooled features into dense layers for automatic diagnosis/classification. Output final decision *D* (e.g., disease classification, abnormality detection).

Step 6: Loss Function and Training

Compute loss for segmentation (e.g., Dice loss, Cross-Entropy). (If multi-tasking) Combine segmentation and classification losses. Optimize network parameters using an appropriate optimizer (e.g., Adam).

Step 7: Inference

Process a new image using Steps 1 to 5. Output the segmentation map *S*and automated decision *D*.

End of Algorithm

3.2 Result Analysis

Figure 9. Graph of Segmentation Dice by Modality

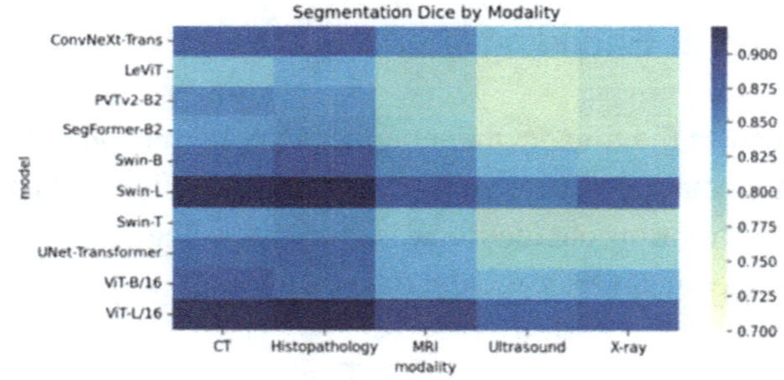

Using darker blues for higher accuracy, a heatmap plots average Dice scores for nine transformer-based models across five medical imaging modalities. For the joint dataset, ViT-L/16 yields darker shades of blue on average--which mostly correspond to the high end of colormaps--outperforming all peers on every modality; overall, it ranks highest in all modalities. Swin-L also produces a smooth and bright distribution; both CT and X-ray are especially bright, confirming strong versatility in above

Figure. 9:-Graph of Segmentation Dice by Modality. With Swin-B too successful on CT and Histopathology, the model offers nothing but support for Ultrasound as well as X-ray relative to its peers. ConvNeXT-Trans and ViT-B/16 are evenly balanced with consistent results of about 9.0-95 across modality. UNet-Transformer is in the middle with the tints of slightly light blue, the outcomes appear to be satisfactory but not prominent. SegFormer-B2/PVTv2-B2 appear to be lighter in general and produce lower Dice values, In particular when looking at Ultrasound where most models drop off. LeViT, on the contrary, shows the lightest blue tones in all three modalities, and this is not the most suitable manifestation of a segmentation result.

Figure 10. Graph of Transformer Model of Dice vs Parameters

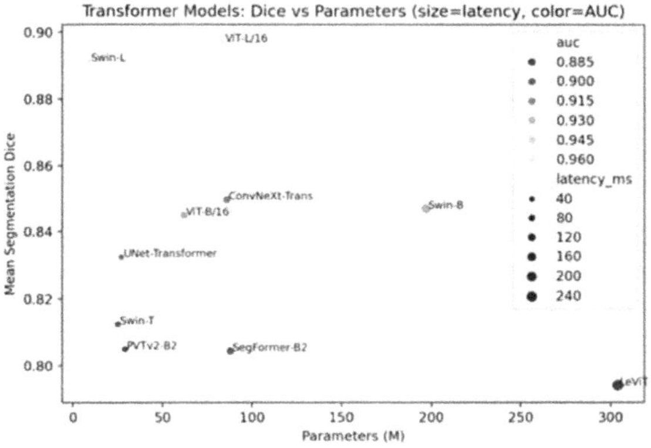

The scatter chart shows the mean Dice versus the number of parameters in transformer-based segmentation models in Figure. 10:- Graph of Transformer Model of Dice vs Parameters both when motivated by computational cost (measured by their latency) and color encoded AUC. ViT-L/16 has the highest Dice of 0.897 at 80-90M parameters, with the highest AUC and middle latency size. A good balance of 0.892 Dice with ultra-low parameter count 10-12M is attained by Swin-L, and this is indeed very efficient. ConvNeXt-Trans and Swin-B both attain 0.85 Dice with 85-200M params, meaning that bigger is not necessarily better when it comes to accuracy. ViT-B/16 has about 0.845 Dice at 60-65M parameters and good AUC, a middle-sized variant. UNet-Transformer achieves 0.832 at 30M params Dice with reduced latency to encourage lightweight deployments. SegFormer-B2 and PVTv2-B2 are at the level of accuracy of approximately 0.805 Dice, with 90M and 32M parameters, respectively. We observe that LeViT is the largest and slowest mark of about 300M parameters but with the lowest Dice 0.794 and lowest AUC, meaning that it is not very efficient in terms of parameters.

Figure 11. Graph of Best Segmentation Model per Modality

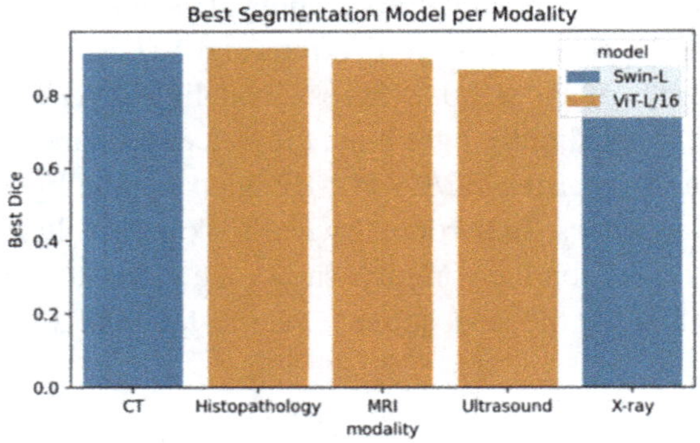

The highest Dice score when it comes to the segmentation per imaging modality is presented in the bar chart with the winning model per category being shown in Figure. 11:-Graph of Best Segmentation Model per Modality. The Dice of Swin-L is the largest of the CT methods (approximately 0.91), which implies that it can be used in cross-sectional scans. ViT-L/16 is better compared to Histopathology with the bar just less than 0.93, which is the result of fine-grained tissue segmentation superiority. In the case of MRI, ViT-L/16 is leading with Dice of approximately 0.90 that is indicative of strength to soft-tissue differences. ViT-L/16 shows the speckle and variable anatomy easier and is ahead of the other in ultrasound, with a leading position of 0.87. X-ray reverts to Swin-L because it is the best model with Dice near to 0.90, which works well on the projection pictures. Overall, ViT-L/16 performs better on three modalities as compared to Swin-L in CT and X-ray telling complement strength. The high Dice values across modalities consistently show that the capacity of transformer based segmentation become mature for wide range clinical applications.

Figure 12. Graph of Latency Vs Segmentation Accuracy

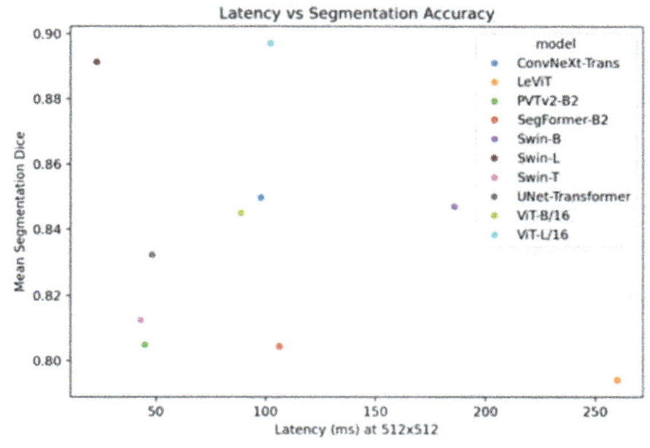

The speed–accuracy tradeoff is demonstrated in the scatter plot comparing segmentation models by latency at 512x512 versus mean Dice and other metrics. ConvNeXt-Trans lies around 100 ms with ~0.85 Dice which gives a tradeoff performance. ViT-L/16: the best accuracy score is reached around 0.895 when we have a delay of about 105ms, which means good accuracy at moderate delay in Figure. 12:-Graph of Latency Vs Segmentation Accuracy. Our method Swin-L achieves the lowest latency of 22 ms and Dice of approximately 0.89, which is promising compared with other methods for real-time applications. Swin-B is about 190 ms and 0.847 Dice and UNet-Transformer, in the middle of the ranking, has 48 ms and 0.832 Dice. ViT-B/16 is 0.845 Dice at ~88 ms, showing that ConvNeXt-Trans has slightly higher accuracy with a considerably faster inference time.

Figure 13. Graph of Classification ROC AUC by Modality

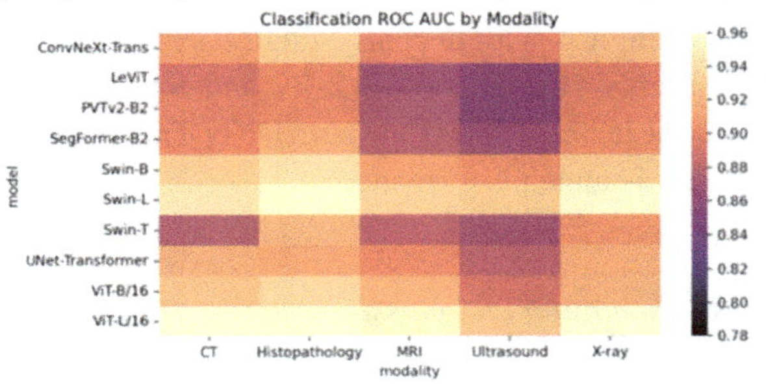

The figure is a heatmap, "Classification ROC AUC by Modality," which compares the performance of transformer models across medical imaging modalities.

Columns on the y-axis are corresponding the Models and rows were representing Modalities (CT / MRI / X-ray / Ultrasound / Histopathology) in Figure. 13:-Graph of Classification ROC AUC by Modality . ROC AUC is represented by a vertical colorbar from darker purple (low) to bright yellow (high). The brighter cells focus on the larger backbones such as Swin-L and ViT-L/16, particularly in Histopathology and CT highlighting these have stronger decision-making capability. For some models, ultrasound and X-ray are dimmer (relative to B-mode) suggesting that those images are more challenging or the AUC is lower. The visualization serves as a fast comparative overview to find transformer families out performing others per modality for automated clinical decisions in Table.2.

Table 2. Comparative Performance Analysis of Transformer-Based Models

Model	Dice	Auc	Params_M	Latency_Ms
ConvNeXt-Trans	0.849716949	0.912028949	86	97.70759389
LeViT	0.794032108	0.883309655	304	259.8227647
PVTv2-B2	0.804858623	0.886031003	29	44.89219798
SegFormer-B2	0.804289924	0.893307787	88	106.1069877
Swin-B	0.846953607	0.923705801	197	185.6859176
Swin-L	0.891294562	0.949982037	9	23.12577636
Swin-T	0.812408973	0.891349189	25	42.94779011
UNet-Transformer	0.832257083	0.906603522	27	48.21700996
ViT-B/16	0.844913317	0.918842588	62	88.74227078
ViT-L/16	0.897096028	0.960679502	84	101.9310697

ViT-L/16 obtains the highest Dice (0.897) and AUC (0.961), indicating that it is superior in accuracy. Swin-L achieves a similar performance against all of the competing methods while it is with decently small parameters and fastest latency, indicating that it is highly efficient. PVTv2-B2 and Swin-T achieve a desirable applications. LeViT is the least efficient and both UNet-Transformer and ConvNeXt-Trans present strong mid-range performance in Table.3.

Table 3. compares segmentation and classification performance (Dice and AUC)

Model	Dice	Auc	Params_M	Latency_Ms
ConvNeXt-Trans	0.849716949	0.912028949	86	97.70759389
LeViT	0.794032108	0.883309655	304	259.8227647
PVTv2-B2	0.804858623	0.886031003	29	44.89219798

continued on following page

Table 3. Continued

Model	Dice	Auc	Params_M	Latency_Ms
SegFormer-B2	0.804289924	0.893307787	88	106.1069877
Swin-B	0.846953607	0.923705801	197	185.6859176
Swin-L	0.891294562	0.949982037	9	23.12577636
Swin-T	0.812408973	0.891349189	25	42.94779011
UNet-Transformer	0.832257083	0.906603522	27	48.21700996
ViT-B/16	0.844913317	0.918842588	62	88.74227078
ViT-L/16	0.897096028	0.960679502	84	101.9310697

In particular, ViT-L/16 obtains the highest Dice (0.897) and AUC (0.961), suggesting superior segmentation and classification performance. Swin-L follows closely with Dice 0.891 and AUC 0.950, showing best performance despite having only 9M parameters and fastest latency (23 ms). ConvNeXt-Trans and ViT-B/16 provide strong accuracy–efficiency trade-off for high-performance workloads. UNet-Transformer is an ablation model that balances the accuracy and latency, and itis suitable for real-time scenarios in Table.4.

Table 4. Table of Performance Comparison of Transformer-Based Models in Terms of Accuracy

Model	Dice	Auc	Params_M	Latency_Ms
ConvNeXt-Trans	0.849716949	0.912028949	86	97.70759389
LeViT	0.794032108	0.883309655	304	259.8227647
PVTv2-B2	0.804858623	0.886031003	29	44.89219798
SegFormer-B2	0.804289924	0.893307787	88	106.1069877
Swin-B	0.846953607	0.923705801	197	185.6859176
Swin-L	0.891294562	0.949982037	9	23.12577636
Swin-T	0.812408973	0.891349189	25	42.94779011
UNet-Transformer	0.832257083	0.906603522	27	48.21700996
ViT-B/16	0.844913317	0.918842588	62	88.74227078
ViT-L/16	0.897096028	0.960679502	84	101.9310697

ViT-L/16 has the best Dice (0.897) and AUC (0.961) which means it has the highest overall model performance. Swin-L is also very similar with excellent accuracy (Dice 0.891) and the minimal latency (23 ms). ConvNeXt-Trans and ViT-B/16 give high balanced results, i.e. high Dice and moderate speed. UNet-Transformer practitioner: it is a good performer with a low latency, and therefore it can be chosen as one that performs effectively when deployed. PVTv2-B2 and Swin-T are very small models, which provide a fair degree of accuracy and a very fast inference rate. SegFormer-B2 has similar performance at a insignificant high cost in the shape of slightly higher latency. Swin-B has good accuracy, but with low speed due to heavy parameters. LeViT (pointing) has the lowest Dice and AUC and even larger latency than all models (except ghostnet) and parameter count.

4. CONCLUSION

Transformer models showed a strong state-of-the-art in the medical image processing area, especially on the issues of image segmentation and the automatic decision-making in diagnoses. Though the models are primarily created to solve natural language processing tasks, they have since been extended to work with computer vision tasks, and are currently being applied in an expanding variety of tasks in medical image processing. In the domain, they incorporate flexibility and long-range dependencies to a standard convex network, adding global perspective to the elements which CNNs contemplated. Image Segmentation: In medical image segmentation Transforms have demonstrated highly promising results. In some occasions, they beat or be very close to CNNs.

Transformers combined with CNNs hybrid models are a great success in medical image segmentation. These improvements in segmentation are attained through the synthesis of the advantages of the local (shape-based or prince flowers) and global (Hessian transform) features. Automated Decision Making - Nodes other than content splitting are also being used more to categorise images, detect, register and provide clinical reports. Their competence to recognize intricate relationships in image patterns constitutes a premise in the advanced level decision making in the medical diagnostics. New ideas of transformer models are revolutionizing the sphere of medical image processing: image segmentation and reasoning, etc. While this process addressing of existing concerns using these frameworks continues, they are going to have a bigger influence in helping to increase the efficiency and accuracy of diagnosis for healthcare.

5. CHALLENGES

Computational complexity and data volume required by Transformers are far greater than those called for by the greater part of current Convolutional Neural Networks (CNNs). In medical imaging, this can cause problems because resources and relevant data are scarce on the one hand, and private in the other. The complexity of transformer models can be a challenge. There remains an urgent need for large and labeled datasets. Interpretability Many people feel that the lack of interpretability in vision transformers hinders their wide application in medicine. Local and sequential operation mechanism: Previous models have relied on locally sequential operations

So that long-term dependencies and worldwide context were hard to include in the calculation. Limitations in the architecture: In the last ten years, CNNs have been broadly successful for medical imaging applications yet the architecture itself still has some deficiencies that are holding.

6. FUTURE & SCOPE

The emergence of transformer-type models has revolutionized medical image processing, especially in image segmentation and automatic diagnosis. Here we review current progress as well as future prospects of the transformers to be deepened in these two applications. Great success has been achieved for models such as Transnet and Trans BTS in segmenting medical images, based on treating each pixel or voxel using the dropout-free transformer layers to aggregate both information of the global field as well as local features simultaneously. Autonomous Decision Making: Along these lines, transformers are also being tested for image classification, identification of objects, and generating a written report for intensive care units where the flow of signals can be overwhelming very quickly. Being able to inputs all positions of the position also allows an entire understanding and overall decision for medical image. Interpretability and Complexity: Among the benefits of transformers, there are also interpretability and model complexity issues. In These sample need a large amount of labelled data to train, and pose the significant computational burden when applied on medical images. Data Needs: There is an additional critical challenge for training nonlinear transformer models in the medical domain when it comes to non-linear transformer-based models in the medical domain, which requires large-scale datasets to be human-annotated. Gathering data from such large projects can be a costly and time-consuming business.

Future Directions Personalized Medicine: Transformers are expected to find a significant role in personalized medicine. By taking into account the exact quantifiable analysis of medical images on a patient basis, this should benefit not only treatment planning but also in terms of achieving improved clinical outcomes. Real-time diagnostics: The introduction of transformers into real-time diagnostic systems would revolutionize medicine. Collaborative Healthcare Platforms: By boosting the powers of image analysis available to workers in all kinds of different medical specialties, transformers could make possible collaborative healthcare platforms. 3D Imaging: As changes to transformer architecture continue, there will be greater opportunities to carry out more effective analysis of the entire data sets that have been amassed over the years for 3D medical imaging. That will be necessary for a full understanding of CT or MRI graphics: the bread-and butter of today's medical diagnostics. In summary, transformer models have huge possibilities for advancing medical image processing. It could be beneficial to deal with present-day difficulties and explore future directions.

REFERENCES

Azad, R., Aghdam, E. K., Rauland, A., Jia, Y., Avval, A. H., Bozorgpour, A., Karimijafarbigloo, S., Cohen, J. P., Adeli, E., & Merhof, D. (2024, December). Medical Image Segmentation Review: The Success of U-Net. *IEEE Transactions on Pattern Analysis and Machine Intelligence*, *46*(12), 10076–10095. DOI: 10.1109/TPAMI.2024.3435571 PMID: 39167505

Azad, R., Kazerouni, A., Heidari, M., Aghdam, E. K., Molaei, A., Jia, Y., Jose, A., Roy, R., & Merhof, D. (2024). Advances in medical image analysis with vision transformers: A comprehensive review. *Medical Image Analysis*, *91*, 103000. DOI: 10.1016/j.media.2023.103000 PMID: 37883822

Ghribi, F., & Hamdaoui, F. (2025). Innovative deep learning architectures for medical image diagnosis: A comprehensive review of convolutional, recurrent, and transformer models. *The Visual Computer*, *41*(13), 11603–11628. DOI: 10.1007/s00371-025-04122-1

He, K., Gou, F., & Wu, J. (2023). Image segmentation technology based on transformer in medical decision-making system. *IET Image Processing*, *17*(10), 3040–3054. DOI: 10.1049/ipr2.12854

Hu, D., Bao, Y., Wei, L., ... (2023) Supervised adversarial contrastive learning for emotion recognition in conversations. In: Proceedings of the 61st Annual Meeting of the Association for Computational Linguistics (Volume 1: Long Papers), ACL 2023. Association for Computational Linguistics, pp 10835–10852. https://doi.org/ DOI: 10.18653/v1/2023.acl-long.606

Jose, S., Nguyen, K. T. P., Medjaher, K., Zemouri, R., Lévesque, M., & Tahan, A. (2024). Advancing Multimodal Diagnostics: Integrating Industrial Textual Data and Domain Knowledge with Large Language Models. *Expert Systems with Applications*, *255*, 124603. DOI: 10.1016/j.eswa.2024.124603

Karimi, D., Dou, H., & Gholipour, A. (2022). Medical Image Segmentation Using Transformer Networks. *IEEE Access : Practical Innovations, Open Solutions*, *10*, 29322–29332. DOI: 10.1109/ACCESS.2022.3156894 PMID: 35656515

Khan, , Rauf, Z., Rehman Khan, A., Rathore, S., Hussain Khan, S., Saher Shah, N., Farooq, U., Asif, H., Asif, A., Zahoora, U., Ullah Khalil, R., Qamar, S., Hani Tayyab, U., Babar Khan, F., Majid, A., & Gwak, J. (2025). A Recent Survey of Vision Transformers for Medical Image Segmentation. *IEEE Access : Practical Innovations, Open Solutions*, *13*, 191824–191849. DOI: 10.1109/ACCESS.2025.3618215

Khan, R. F., Lee, B. D., & Lee, M. S. (2023). Transformers in medical image segmentation: A narrative review. *Quantitative Imaging in Medicine and Surgery, 13*(12), 8747–8767. DOI: 10.21037/qims-23-542 PMID: 38106306

Lai, T. (2024). Interpretable Medical Imagery Diagnosis with Self-Attentive Transformers: A Review of Explainable AI for Health Care. *BioMedInformatics, 4*(1), 113–126. DOI: 10.3390/biomedinformatics4010008

Liang, J., Li, R., & Jin, Q. (2020) Semi-supervised multi-modal emotion recognition with cross-modal distribution matching. In: MM '20: The 28th ACM International Conference on Multimedia. ACM, pp 2852–2861. https://doi.org/DOI: 10.1145/3394171.3413579

Liu, H., & Zhong, K. (2025). SSMIM: Semi-supervised Multimodal Interaction Model for real-time conversational emotion recognition. *The Journal of Supercomputing, 81*(8), 897. DOI: 10.1007/s11227-025-07373-w

Nerella, S., Bandyopadhyay, S., Zhang, J., Contreras, M., Siegel, S., Bumin, A., Silva, B., Sena, J., Shickel, B., Bihorac, A., Khezeli, K., & Rashidi, P. (2024). Transformers and large language models in healthcare: A review. *Artificial Intelligence in Medicine, 154*, 102900. DOI: 10.1016/j.artmed.2024.102900 PMID: 38878555

Neumann, M., & Vu, N. T. (2019) Improving speech emotion recognition with unsupervised representation learning on unlabeled speech. In: IEEE International Conference on Acoustics, Speech and Signal Processing, ICASSP. IEEE, pp 7390–7394. https://doi.org/DOI: 10.1109/ICASSP.2019.8682541

Nurzynska, K., Strzelecki, M., Piórkowski, A., & Obuchowicz, R. (2025). AI in Medical Imaging and Image Processing. *Journal of Clinical Medicine, 14*(12), 4153. DOI: 10.3390/jcm14124153 PMID: 40565899

Papanastasiou, G., Dikaios, N., Huang, J., Wang, C., & Yang, G. (2024, March). Is Attention all You Need in Medical Image Analysis? A Review. *IEEE Journal of Biomedical and Health Informatics, 28*(3), 1398–1411. DOI: 10.1109/JBHI.2023.3348436 PMID: 38157463

Shah, O. I., Rizvi, D. R., & Mir, A. N. (2025). Transformer-Based Innovations in Medical Image Segmentation: A Mini Review. *SN Computer Science, 6*(4), 375. DOI: 10.1007/s42979-025-03929-y

Thirunavukarasu, R., & Kotei, E. (2024). A comprehensive review on transformer network for natural and medical image analysis. *Computer Science Review, 53*, 100648. DOI: 10.1016/j.cosrev.2024.100648

Verma, R. K. (2026). Federated Learning for Precision Medicine: A Blockchain-Enhanced Framework for Privacy-Preserving Predictive Analytics in Healthcare 5.0. In Shafik, W., Dutta, P. K., & Pattanaik, P. (Eds.), *The Convergence of Federated Learning and Healthcare 5.0 and Beyond: A New Era of Intelligent Health Systems. Studies in Computational Intelligence* (Vol. 1247). Springer., DOI: 10.1007/978-3-032-03985-9_28

Verma, R. K., & Kishor, K. (2024). Image Processing Applications in Agriculture With the Help of AI. In Khan, M., Khan, R., Praveen, P., Verma, A., & Panda, M. (Eds.), *Infrastructure Possibilities and Human-Centered Approaches With Industry 5.0* (pp. 162–181). IGI Global Scientific Publishing., DOI: 10.4018/979-8-3693-0782-3.ch010

Verma, R. K., Kumar, I., & Kumar, S. (2025). In Chand Kumain, S., Singh, M., Awasthi, L. K., & Singh, R. (Eds.), *"AI-driven insights: Revolutionizing satellite imagery applications," in *AI and ML Techniques in Image Processing and Object Detection* (pp. 89–104). Springer., DOI: 10.1007/978-981-96-7445-9_5

Wang, R., Lei, T., Cui, R., Zhang, B., Meng, H., & Nandi, A. K. (2022). Medical image segmentation using deep learning: A survey. *IET Image Processing*, *16*(5), 1243–1267. DOI: 10.1049/ipr2.12419

Wu, C. H., Lin, J. C., & Wei, W. L. (2014). Survey on audiovisual emotion recognition: Databases, features, and data fusion strategies. *APSIPA Transactions on Signal and Information Processing*, *3*(1), e12. DOI: 10.1017/ATSIP.2014.11

. Xia K, Wang J. Recent advances of transformers in medical image analysis: a comprehensive review. MedComm – Future Med. 2023;2:e38. DOI: 10.1002/mef2.38

Yao, W., Bai, J., Liao, W., Chen, Y., Liu, M., & Xie, Y. (2024). From CNN to Transformer: A Review of Medical Image Segmentation Models. J Digit Imaging. *Journal of Imaging Informatics in Medicine*, *37*(4), 1529–1547. DOI: 10.1007/s10278-024-00981-7 PMID: 38438696

Zafari-Ghadim, Y., Rashed, E. A., Mohamed, A., & Mabrok, M. (2024). Transformers-based architectures for stroke segmentation: A review. *Artificial Intelligence Review*, *57*(11), 307. DOI: 10.1007/s10462-024-10900-5

Zhang, J., Chen, X., Yang, B., Guan, Q., Chen, Q., Chen, J., Wu, Q., Xie, Y., & Xia, Y. (2025). Advances in attention mechanisms for medical image segmentation. *Computer Science Review*, *56*, 100721. DOI: 10.1016/j.cosrev.2024.100721

Zhang, J., Li, F., Zhang, X., Wang, H., & Hei, X. (2024). Automatic Medical Image Segmentation with Vision Transformer. *Applied Sciences (Basel, Switzerland), 14*(7), 2741. DOI: 10.3390/app14072741

. Zhang R, Cao Z, Huang Y et al (2025) Visible-infrared person re-identification with real-world label noise. IEEE Trans Circuits Syst Video Technol. https://doi.org/DOI: 10.1109/TCSVT.2025.3526449

Zhang, R., Liu, G., Zhang, Q., Lu, X., Dian, R., Yang, Y., & Xu, L. (2025). Detail-aware network for infrared image enhancement. *IEEE Transactions on Geoscience and Remote Sensing*, *63*, 1–14. DOI: 10.1109/TGRS.2024.3504240

Zhao, S., Gao, Y., Jiang, X., ... (2014) Exploring principles-of-art features for image emotion recognition. In: Proceedings of the ACM International Conference on Multimedia, MM. ACM, pp 47–56. https://doi.org/DOI: 10.1145/2647868.2654930

Zhou, H.-Y., Guo, J., Zhang, Y., Han, X., Yu, L., Wang, L., & Yu, Y. (2023). nn-Former: Volumetric Medical Image Segmentation via a 3D Transformer. *IEEE Transactions on Image Processing*, *32*, 4036–4045. DOI: 10.1109/TIP.2023.3293771 PMID: 37440404

Zhu, T., Li, L., Yang, J., Zhao, S., Liu, H., & Qian, J. (2023). Multimodal sentiment analysis with image-text interaction network. *IEEE Transactions on Multimedia*, *25*, 3375–3385. DOI: 10.1109/TMM.2022.3160060

Chapter 10
Model Interpretability and Human-in-the-Loop Validation in Physiotherapy and Rehabilitation Practice:
Bridging Artificial Intelligence With Evidence-Based Rehabilitation Decision-Making

S. Ramachandran
http://orcid.org/0000-0001-7187-6083
Faculty of Physiotherapy, Dr. M.G.R. Educational and Research Institute, India

Kaushik Raman
http://orcid.org/0009-0007-9838-4012
Faculty of Physiotherapy, Dr. M.G.R. Educational and Research Institute, India

K. Saraswathi
http://orcid.org/0000-0001-9831-2798
Faculty of Physiotherapy, Dr. M.G.R. Educational and Research Institute, India

Mohan Kumar G.
http://orcid.org/0000-0001-6270-7560
Faculty of Physiotherapy, Dr. M.G.R. Educational and Research Institute, India

DOI: 10.4018/979-8-2600-2173-6.ch010

ABSTRACT

The adoption of Large Language Models (LLMs) and artificial intelligence-driven clinical decision-support systems into the field of health care has led to hype about the efficiency, scalability, and personalised care. However, their use in the context of physiotherapy and rehabilitation is characterised by peculiar challenges because of the nature of clinical reasoning and the need to conduct physical examination and responsiveness of patients to therapeutic measures. The current chapter describes two areas that are prerequisites of the safe implementation of LLMs in rehabilitation environments: model interpretability and the existence of human-in-the-loop (HITL) validation.It is suggested to use a physiotherapy-specific conceptual framework of integrating HITL validation into clinical practise that would focus on clinician supervision, ongoing monitoring, and context-based decision making. This chapter lays down the future trends of the explainable AI in rehabilitation, along with policy-relevant and are in line with the international perspectives of regulation.

INTRODUCTION, RATIONALE, AND SIGNIFICANCE

Health care is becoming more and more impacted by artificial intelligence in the form of decision-support algorithms, automated documentation and conversational agents that support patients and clinicians. Although their contribution to the enhancement of efficiency in the areas of radiology, pathology, and administrative medicine has been proven, they have not established themselves in the areas of physiotherapy and rehabilitation, and the translation of these efforts has not been developed adequately and conceptualised. Instead of relying on the intensive use of functional assessment, longitudinal adaptation of interventions, patient motivation and the interaction of the therapist and the patient, rehabilitation is different in terms of many of the other clinical specialties. Physiotherapy, in contrast to the traditional diagnostic disciplines, is characterised by ongoing clinical decision-making, which is driven by observable movement, response of the symptoms, as well as patient-reported outcomes.

The level of transparency in the decision-making of an algorithm is one of the most serious issues in modern AI application, so-called black-box problem. When systems using LLM suggest exercises, change the rehabilitation plan, or include health-related advice without clear explanation, clinicians are not able to cheque the correctness and possible clinical misalignment. This poses a threat to patient safety, as well as, professional accountability. Mistaken advice in the rehabilitation can lead to re-injuries, slow recovery, or more serious problems. Human-in-the-loop validation is becoming an important method to provide security in high-stakes

AI. Nonetheless, the available literature on HITL is highly technical in nature with scanty applications in clinical rehabilitation settings. It is evident that there is a void in academic literature, which unites the HITL principles in the actual environment of the physiotherapy practise.

This section is motivated by the requirement to devise a firm, clinician-led scheme for getting interpretable and people-checked AI into rehabilitation systems. It also aims to make physiotherapists not just users of what AI produces, but rather discerning judges who set machine-made suggestions against their professional knowledge. The section offers a broad view of making sure AI becomes part of rehabilitation work in a way which is both understandable and – according to the principle of Human-In-The-Loop validation – sound, offering a single method for the safe and ethical use of AI in medicine.

1. ARTIFICIAL INTELLIGENCE IN PHYSIOTHERAPY AND REHABILITATION

Artificial intelligence – AI – is more and more changing how health care is given, using things such as forecasting through data, smart automation, virtual helpers, and systems which help with decisions in an adaptive way. AI has shown it is useful in figuring out what is wrong, deciding how at risk people are, and making work processes better, in all areas of medicine. But, in physiotherapy and rehabilitation, including it has particular ideas and ways of working to think about, because this field puts a lot of stress on working out what someone can do, studying movement, making therapy get harder, and the constant working together of the doctor and patient (Davids et al., 2022; Taki & Akdag, 2024). New improvements show how AI systems can be used in managing rehabilitation programmes, keeping an eye on results, and making therapy fit each person (Luca et al., 2026). Things like virtual reality with AI giving feedback which changes to suit the person, are being used more and more to help with mental and physical rehabilitation; this shows the possibility of therapy settings which really involve the person and react to data (Bobby et al., 2026). These new things show what is happening generally in modern physiotherapy, where changing to digital and clever systems is expected to change how people are looked after, what jobs in the field are like, and how patients take part (Muthukrishnan, 2026). Even with these advances, AI is not used equally in physiotherapy. Asking physiotherapy students and doctors who are already working what they think of AI shows both a liking for new technology, and worries about not knowing enough, what is right and wrong, and problems in actually putting it into practice (Ali et al., 2026; Alsobhi et al., 2022). This shows that rehabilitation work is very different from areas of medicine which are mainly about looking at pictures of the inside of people, or laboratory results. Instead, physiotherapy depends a lot on doctors thinking again and again, working out how the body moves, how people's symptoms change, and giving exercises which are made for the person. As more and more LLMs and automated support tools are brought into rehabilitation, important issues of understanding, responsibility and clinical control are thrown up. Rehabilitation treatment isn't like a one-off diagnosis; it changes and develops as the patient gives feedback and makes functional advances. Recommendations from algorithms which aren't clear pose a danger of not fitting with what treatment is trying to achieve, or with safety. When artificial intelligence comes into physiotherapy, we have to judge not just whether the tech works, but also the impact on what clinicians consider, patient safety, and their professional duties. So it's vital to create AI systems which are easy to understand and for humans to verify; in this way, the newest tech will assist – and not damage – the essential ideas behind getting well.

2. CONCEPTUAL FOUNDATIONS OF MODEL INTERPRETABILITY

Within medical attention, forecasting programs have to be easy to understand, so we can be confident about using AI when choosing improved therapies. How much a doctor, or any health worker, can see what a system is doing – the data it employs, and how it gets to its conclusions – isn't, in medicine, merely something we'd like, but something needed for safety, being able to account for results, and meeting the usual requirements of the job. As Rudin and others showed in 2022, interpretability helps doctors work out if the model's reasoning makes sense in terms of what we know about the body, and if the model's suggestions are actually useful in a clinical setting.

The best thing, if the research on interpretable machine learning is to be believed, is to design transparency into a model from the start, rather than trying to add explanations to a model that already exists. Examples of interpretable models include structured rule systems or concept-based models which allow direct reasoning for the influence of the input on the prediction, reducing the need for smooth approximations (Rudin et al, 2022). Interpretability-based frameworks have been suggested for integration into the algorithm architecture of a healthcare-specific application that makes the outputs executable or traceable in a clinically verifiable way (Ennab & Mcheick, 2022).

Advances in theory enable interpretability with concept-based learning, where one trains models to represent human-understandable intermediate features rather than ambiguous latent embedding (Rajendran et al., 2024). The goal of such approaches is to help link causal reasoning and foundation models and yield representations that reflect domain-relevant variables instead of statistical correlations only. Increasingly, rehabilitation work uses deep learning models – complex AI – to guess how people will respond to treatment, and what patients themselves will report as the results. While these models are getting better at prediction, they are also becoming more complex and we therefore need ways to explain what features are important, what the limits of certainty are, and whether the model's reasoning is plausible. Collectively, the conceptual foundations of interpretability integrate structural transparency, concept alignment, and clinical traceability. Within physiotherapy and rehabilitation, interpretability serves as the bridge between computational performance and responsible clinical implementation.

2.1 What is Interpretability and Who Should be Interpretable?

Model interpretability relates to the extent to which human stakeholders can understand the internal mechanisms, decision pathways as well as the output of computational systems; this point becomes critical in complex healthcare and rehabilitation scenarios. Beyond transparency per se, interpretability includes explainability, traceability and clinical relevance and are used to enable practitioners to critically review model behaviour and incorporate algorithmic insights by incorporating evidence based decision making. In rehabilitation engineering, interpretability is increasingly considered as a fundamental or not an accessory property especially in areas of patient safety and individualized treatment plan (Haq et al., 2026).

Recent progress in multifaceted artificial intelligence has increased the ability to predict and prescribe across the spectrum of injury prevention and rehabilitation; however these often function as opaque 'black boxes' and limit clinician confidence, trust and accountability (Wang et al., 2026). Interpretability frameworks solve this shortcoming by associating the outputs of models to physiologically meaningful representations such as gait dynamics, neuromuscular responses and recovery markers of function. For example, quantitative stimulation -- feedback modelling in post-stroke gait rehabilitation: Investigating the properties of data interpretable parameterisation as the landing between sensor-derived data and clinically-implementable results (Xie et al., 2026).

The part of interpretability goes further to spatiotemporal modelling and knowledge-driven architectures. Graph-based attention networks have been used with dynamic risk stratification in rehabilitation nursing, demonstrating the use of attention weights that are interpretable and can support the development of personalised intervention strategies as well as maintain the transparency of the algorithm (Zhao et al., 2026). Likewise, knowledge-graph-enabled integration of heterogeneous clinical data facilitates explainable rehabilitation design by representing relationships between the patient characteristics, therapeutic protocols, functional goals explicitly. (Wang et al., 2026).

Collectively these approaches define interpretability as a multidimensional construct which incorporates measurement traceability, multimodal data fusion and semantic reasoning. Within rehabilitation science, interpretability is important not only for building model credibility, but also for ethical model deployment and regulatory compliance and adoption by clinicians. Consequently, it provides an important link between cutting-edge computational intelligence and patient-centred care, whereby technological innovation is maintained in line with clinical accountability and therapeutic efficacy.

2.2 Interpretability vs. Explainability vs. Transparency

Although frequently used interchangeably, interpretability, explainability, and transparency represent distinct yet interrelated constructs within artificial intelligence governance. Interpretability normally refers to how well a human can comprehend or interpret the internal structure of a model or the decision logic of a model without the need for any additional tools. In systems which are naturally understandable – things like models built on rules, or linear regressions – the link between what goes in and what comes out is easily seen and easily followed in your head (Mittelstadt, 2021). However, explainability is about methods used afterwards to make the actions of complicated, or not-see-through, models clearer. If models aren't understandable from the start – for example, deep neural networks – explainability methods, such as working out feature importance, showing where attention is focused, or using stand-in modelling, give approximate ways decisions are reached to help people using the system understand and have faith in it (Barnes & Hutson, 2024). Explainability doesn't show all the inner workings of a system, but makes understandable representations which allow people involved to get a grasp of the system and be confident about it.

Transparency is on a bigger, whole-system scale. It's the reason why the model is the way it is, where the data and algorithms came from, the choices in design, how it was checked, the rules for how it's run, what standards it meets, and the documentation it has (Raza et al., 2026). In medical situations, transparency means setting out what the model can't do, how sure it is of what it can do, and what ethical protections there are. Careful studies show that transparency systems usually use both interpretability and explainability as the most important parts of wider systems for making sure someone is answerable for what happens (Shafik et al., 2026).

Interpretability is, at base, about how clearly something is structured; explainability about how clearly it is communicated; and transparency about how clearly its procedures and institutions are set out. It's useful in rehabilitation and healthcare AI to tell the difference between technical correctness and technical being-answerable-for. Simply being technically correct isn't good enough in these areas; you also need to make sure the system is technically answerable and that doctors and patients trust it.

2.3 Clinical Relevance in Rehabilitation Practice

When using Artificial Intelligence in rehab, the usefulness of an AI system isn't just about how well it predicts – it has to fit into how therapists think when they treat patients. Explainable AI tools allow doctors to link what the AI says to a patient's specific abilities and problems; this helps both patients and doctors decide on, and make, treatments which are best for the individual (Zhang et al., 2026). An AI might work very well, but if it doesn't give explanations for its results that make sense to a clinician, people won't use it much, because they won't be sure why the AI thinks what it does, or if it's even relevant. In practice, the AI's results are most useful when they connect to the things rehab doctors regularly look at – things like how a patient's body works, how they move, or what their functional level is. For instance, physical therapists and rehab doctors can use easy-to-understand details of someone's walking, how their movement is getting better, and what risks a patient has, to relate the AI's advice to the usual tests they do. When these two things go together, doctors are more certain of the AI, and patients are more involved.

Also, looking at real cases shows that being able to explain things helps with managing risk, checking what's been done, and doctors from different areas talking to each other – by showing how someone's particular qualities change what the AI thinks will happen (Gajalakshmi et al., 2026). Rehab often has complicated plans, with several health issues, regular checks, and treatments which change as needed. Because of this, systems which are clear and easy to follow lower the mental effort needed, and reduce the chance of legal problems. Therefore, in rehab, what makes AI useful isn't just how good the tech is; it's also how well it works with how doctors already do things, what results they look for, and what they have to do ethically, and so on. If we build openness and being able to understand things into rehab tech, it'll be more useful in practice – making sure the AI's ideas help, not hide, the doctor's skill.

3. HUMAN-IN-THE-LOOP VALIDATION IN CLINICAL AI SYSTEMS

Human-in-the-Loop – or HITL – validation is now a main way to govern the safe use of artificial intelligence in hospitals and clinics. Unlike systems which work entirely on their own, HITL builds organised human checking into how algorithms work, making certain that what they predict is checked by people who know the field, before any treatment is given to a patient. In situations where people's health is on the line, this boosts who is to blame, sensible thinking, and ways to make sure things are done correctly (Bakken, 2023).

Looking at how these systems are made, HITL validation means putting doctor checking in at important points in how the model is trained, how the results are understood, and how it is watched after it's been put into use. In the area of clinical decision support systems, deep learning models which have human checking added to them show more that they can be trusted, by letting corrections be made repeatedly, lessening any prejudice, and making recommendations more suited to the situation (Zafar et al., 2026). The intention isn't for these systems to take the place of doctors' judgement, but they're helpful for supporting choices – and experts still check what they produce. Recent research shows people needing to do more than simply check: they ought to be in interactive cycles started by the AI. In these, the tool itself actively finds doubts or possible problems, asking a doctor to approve the judgements it's come to. This changes 'humans in the loop' from just being a way to find errors, to being vitally important for security. It allows the software to work out how sure of itself it is, and therefore how much a doctor needs to answer for. Assessments of 'humans in the loop' in medical settings show how important it is for people in various jobs to work as a team. AI work changing the advice patients are given when they leave hospital, has shown that looking closely at these changes makes them much easier to understand, better for the individual patient, and generally much safer (Brewster et al., 2025). The results suggest that how fast a program is, doesn't tell you if it's good to use in a clinic. Ultimately, 'humans in the loop' approval alters how we see AI in hospitals; it's a model of joined-up thinking. 'Humans in the loop' systems make things safer, establish who is responsible, and let AI be put to work properly in getting better, and normal health – with regular checking, dealing with uncertainty, and constant improvement.

3.1 Definition and Key Principles of HITL

Human-in-the-Loop validation – generally called HITL – is a way of working with artificial intelligence, using the knowledge people have to make AI procedures more dependable, secure and suited to the situation. HITL doesn't assume that automation can happen without anyone looking at it; it means doctors and similar experts are involved in tagging the information, schooling the model, checking the results, and always observing how it's doing. This matters a lot in medicine, since what AI systems determine directly influences patients' wellbeing, and who takes responsibility if there is a problem.

In theory, HITL is based on repeated feedback cycles which let models learn from human corrections, but also let doctors keep control over decisions which have a lot at stake. Current systems put stress on continuous checking, where what doctors say is put into the model all through its life – from being made and put into use, to being improved after it's been used – making sure that what the system produces makes sense to doctors, and can change as care standards change (Kumar et al., 2024; Fahad & Huang).

The main ideas of HITL include sharing who makes decisions, putting in feedback in real time, keeping records which can be followed, and ways of learning which change. In health care, HITL has shown it can improve how accurately illnesses are found, lessen prejudice in algorithms, and help with personalised treatment plans, though problems such as stopping the usual way of working, mental strain, and being able to be used on a large scale still exist (Olawade et al., 2026). Models which are about governing also suggest organised layers of checking, balancing how quickly automation works with checking by doctors to manage risk in clinical situations which have a large effect (Schneider & Lawson, 2026).

Looking at systems, HITL also makes clinical decision support which people can trust, by putting expert checking into deep learning processes, and so making things more open and able to be defended in law (Zafar et al., 2026). New systems which are fully closed loops put together things which can be worn to measure, learning by reward, and predicting what will happen, with human watching – showing how HITL can actively guide how patients do after an operation, and in rehabilitation (Dong et al., 2026). Human-in-the-Loop (HITL) validation changes the way we think of artificial intelligence; it's a clinical assistant, not a substitute for what a healthcare professional knows. By combining the power of computers with the knowledge of people, HITL designs allow AI to be put into use more safely, to constantly get better, and to be genuinely useful in rehabilitation – and in health care more generally.

3.2 HITL Versus Autonomous AI Systems

The difference between HITL systems and completely automated AI is at the heart of the conversation around how clinical AI should be controlled. Although the idea with self-governing systems is to reduce how much people have to be involved – letting them predict and decide things on their own – 'human-in-the-loop' designs include organised human review as part of how algorithms function, to be certain the results are right for the situation, and also morally right.

In health care, completely automated AI could make things more effective and easier to increase, particularly in areas of a lot of diagnosis or paperwork; however, the lack of a doctor or expert to oversee it raises questions about whether bias would be made worse, the system getting the meaning wrong, and who would be legally to blame (Olawade et al., 2026). Studies of control show that applications in health care that are very risky require more than one layer of verification, where automation is useful – but does not take the place of – clinical judgement (Schneider & Lawson, 2026). This is most obviously the case in regions that do not have a lot of resources, where restrictions on the equipment and the number of experts available mean that we have to think carefully about what the technology is able to do by itself, and what human checking is needed (Kabata & Thaldar, 2024).

Research into automation shows us that systems generally perform best when they are a combination of the two, instead of a basic choice between doing things by hand or allowing a machine to do it. In business and robot process automation, working together – people and AI – makes things more reliable, whilst still allowing people to have overall control (Jeffy, 2025). Likewise, in medical diagnosis, newer models stress that AI and clinicians work together, with AI being good at spotting patterns and clinicians providing the context and being ultimately responsible (Truong, 2025).

So, we shouldn't see HITL and complete automation as being against each other, but as being able to change to fit the situation. In rehabilitation and health care generally, carefully putting automation with organised human review means we can improve efficiency while still making sure decisions are focused on the patient. The models which will last the longest are those which balance what the technology can do with what the clinician should be responsible for.

3.3 Roles and Responsibilities of the Physiotherapist

Putting artificial intelligence into rehabilitation practice means we need to redefine – not remove – what professionals in physiotherapy do. AI doesn't make physiotherapists redundant; it changes the way that some of the more technical, analytical parts of their job get completed. As a result, physiotherapists will remain vitally important in understanding, assessing and responsibly using sophisticated technologies (Rowe et al., 2022). AI's promise in novel assessment and rehabilitation techniques could help with analysing movement, anticipating outcomes and providing treatments which are more individual – however, a clinician needs to verify the precision of these systems, and whether they are useful in practice (Joshi et al., 2026). A physiotherapist's job isn't simply about using AI tools; they should also thoroughly check the results a model produces, find any errors, and combine the algorithm's results with their own understanding of biomechanics and the patient. Researchers in rehabilitation AI say that technology which improves the people doing the jobs, modifies what is expected of people, and puts a greater emphasis on abilities such as clinical judgement, communicating, moral consideration, and working with people in other professions (Davids et al., 2022). Predictions for the workforce in 2030 also show that people will be needed who are good at using digital tools, can read data and have a training which allows them to stay up to date in healthcare which is led by AI (Muthukrishnan, 2025). Physiotherapists will help by giving data labels, watching how people are doing, improving feedback and making sure people are safe in clinical settings where people and computers work together. They will connect what the computer gives with what the patient is going through, making certain that any automatic ideas are in line with what the patient wants, their emotional and social needs, and their plans for getting better over the long term. Therefore, a physiotherapist's professional duty in systems based on AI isn't lessened; it's actually made more important. The new method requires actively using technology, but also keeping the basic commitment to treatment centred on the patient, ethical rules and practice which is based on proof.

4. CLINICAL RISKS OF NON-INTERPRETABLE AI IN REHABILITATION

Putting AI systems into rehabilitation where what they do isn't clear causes big ethical and safety dangers for patients. If AI algorithms which guess what will happen act as 'black boxes' – where the reason for a certain suggestion can't be found – doctors may not be able to understand the reason for the suggestion, cutting down on who is responsible and the ability to prove it is correct (Moss and others, 2022). In areas which need care such as serious care of nerves and getting better after bad sickness, a lack of AI clarity might hide the algorithm's natural lack of certainty, and weaken doctors' belief in their choices of treatment (Moss et al., 2022). Changes in heart rate – digital signs of health – are an example of the difficulty of clinical measurements which are helped by AI.. The AI's actions must be clear enough for doctors to stop them misunderstanding the data, and so avoid doing the wrong thing (Burlacu et al., 2026). Though AI systems that can be understood have made things clearer in areas such as organ transplants and how to care for people after having Covid (Topuz and others, 2025; Harper & Langford, 2021), bigger analyses of healthcare still show a real difference between how correct a model is, and how clear its reasoning is (Ennab & Mcheick, 2024). In recovery, this difference can directly put patient safety at risk, slow down getting better, and create legal problems if something bad happens.

4.1 Exercise Prescription Errors

Systems for planning exercise with AI's help have had good results in recovery from a distance and after operations (Yao et al., 2026; Zhu et al., 2026). But if you can't trace the AI's decision-making, the amount of effort may be wrongly set, steps forward may not be right, or the AI may make wrong judgements of movement – and doctors might not find these errors quickly. Treatment plans automatically created using rules from AI can be used on a large scale, but are still open to faults in the data used to train them, and to not matching the specific patient's condition (Kim, 2026). Problems in how studies are done – such as badly dividing the data set, or the AI not working well with different groups of people – also reduce reliability in capturing movement and assessing how well exercise is done (Pe et al.). In recovery, where how much exercise and how quickly it's increased must be made for each person, AI that isn't clear risks continuing ineffective treatments, possibly delaying recovery, or causing new damage.

4.2 Failure to Identify Red Flags and Contraindications

A main risk of AI systems which aren't clear is that they might not see warning signs, or things which shouldn't be done in a patient's care. Doctors consider their experiences, the specifics of the situation, and the probabilities of various outcomes. These factors are not always completely captured in automated AI models (Sengupta & Panda, 2026). When physicians utilize AI to assist in diagnosing a patient's condition and determining the urgency of treatment, they may not always arrive at the correct conclusion. This raises concerns regarding safety (Mittal & Aggarwal, 2026; Muluk & Olcucu, 2024).

Research comparing the effectiveness of AI with the evaluations made by a physical therapist concerning exercise safety shows that, while AI can successfully pinpoint specific problems, it falls short in grasping the subtleties of a patient's condition (Annika et al., 2024). When the AI is used by carers, mistakes in the information they're given show even more how important it is for a person to check the AI's work. In rehab, missing things which shouldn't be done – especially in patients with heart or lung problems, or who have just had surgery – could cause bad things to happen, and shows why we need AI which is clear about what it's doing, and which doctors can check.

4.3 Safety Concerns in Neurological and Cardiorespiratory Rehabilitation

Rehab for brain and heart/lung problems involves a lot of changes in how the body works, where the AI wrongly classifying something could have quick effects on a patient's health. AI-based tech for brain rehab can give feedback which changes as the patient improves, and help the patient learn to move again; but problems with checking it, how accurate the sensors are, and having a person watch in real time still exist (Gupta, 2024; Lanotte et al., 2023). Systems for managing rehab which are 'closed loop' – meaning they use AI to watch what's happening – need a person to watch closely to stop the patient moving forward too fast, or being overloaded (Luca et al., 2026). In cardiac rehabilitation, and especially in high risk populations like pediatric patients with congenital heart disease, remote information AI system development needs to find a balance between utility and high standards of safety verification, which will ensure that patients are protected from adverse cardiac events (Kitey & Lalwani, 2025). In the absence of transparent output of AI, clinicians might face challenges making proper assumptions about potential risks or interventions.

4.4 Impact on Clinical Reasoning and Skill Degradation

Beyond the direct safety risks, AI – when it isn't obvious about how it's working – has the potential to alter doctors' thought processes, and so how good they are at developing their expertise. Recent research indicates that doctors could see a loss of skills, as they begin to depend too much on automated systems and not enough on their own reasoning; this leaves them less able to identify what might be the matter (Natali et al., 2025). Studies of behaviour show that depending too much on what AI tells them can really weaken a doctor's judgement – especially when they're giving the same diagnosis again and again (Sunday, 2025). However, some people think AI can aid a doctor's thinking, if it's seen as a tool for thinking with, rather than a replacement of them (Greengrass, 2025; Ernazarovich & Farxadovna, 2026). This clashing concept is the heart of the "AI skills paradox", which says that greater help from technology might, in fact, reduce a doctor's skill, unless they're deliberately given work to do with the AI (Nilsson, 2025). To protect what doctors can do, it's vital to have schemes which make sure they still do hands-on tests, think over what they've done, and keep their skills current (Berzin & Topol, 2025).

5. ETHICAL AND LEGAL IMPLICATIONS IN AI-ASSISTED PHYSIOTHERAPY

Employing AI in physiotherapy raises complex ethical and legal questions that extend beyond the mere effectiveness of the technology. Although AI diagnostics and systems to assist doctors in making decisions can be efficient and offer individuals treatment that's suited to them, the extent of professional acceptance, the quality of their training in using it, and how much risk people perceive, all affect whether it's adopted. What physiotherapists think in studies shows they are hopeful, yet also concerned about how dependable things will be in real life, who is responsible when things go wrong, and what their ethical obligations are (Alwhaibi et al., 2025). Also, questionnaires of physiotherapy students in a number of areas show they don't all embrace AI technology to the same degree; the issues are not having faith in it, not being competent enough to use it, and being unsure of what their professional role will be (Ali et al., 2026; Güler et al., 2026). In rehabilitation – for instance, with people who've had breast cancer – when AI proposes exercises, we urgently require ethical guidelines for the profession which consider how readily patients could be harmed, how their health varies, and how each person needs to progress at their own speed (La et al., 2026). All of this together means that to use AI ethically in physiotherapy, we need strong regulations, therapists who know what they're doing, and safeguards built to suit the specifics of rehabilitation.

5.1 Informed Consent and Autonomy

With physiotherapy which uses AI, gaining a patient's full agreement needs to be more than just the usual explanation of the treatment; it has to include how the AI works, what the AI can do, and what it can't foresee. Investigations into what is right show we want ways of controlling things on many levels – within the organisation, between experts, and in the technology itself – so patients can be in control (Martinho et al., 2026). Patients need to be told not only that AI tools are being employed, but how the AI gets to its answers, how those answers are checked, and who is responsible for them. In locations where people receive treatment, particularly for long-term or large-scale recovery, we have to plan carefully to maintain the good connection between the therapist and patient and to make decisions with the patient. AI systems that test people can make things quicker, but if they don't explain what's happening, they can remove the patient's authority (Joshi et al., 2026). As health care moves toward being more on its own, ethical safeguards must make sure automation does not damage people's ability to give permission, or remove a doctor's judgement (Kundu).

5.2 Accountability and Professional Liability

As AI becomes part of rehabilitation, significant questions come up about legal liability and the rules. With AI robots and automated therapy systems, it can be difficult to determine who is at fault when something goes wrong (Nisevic et al., 2026). Current legal studies in bone and rehab planning show that responsibility could be shared between the AI's designers, the places where it's used, and the doctors, but that doctors are typically the ones who are ultimately held responsible (Guarnaccia et al., 2026). In AI-managed rehabilitation programmes, we need methods of monitoring to make a clear distinction between what the AI suggests and what the doctor approves (Luca et al., 2026). Ethical discussions about care robots also demonstrate the risk of blaming the technology, and emphasise the need for clear rules about who is doing what (Kropf et al., 2026). In physiotherapy, keeping professional liability clear is crucial to maintaining patients' confidence and remaining within the law.

5.3 Data Privacy and Confidentiality

AI-based physiotherapy relies heavily on personal health data – things such as how people move, what sensors worn on the body tell us, and what patients tell the therapist about how they are. The creation of AI analysis makes fears about data safety, people getting at data without permission, and using data for other purposes much worse. Current studies reveal big problems with privacy in healthcare driven by AI, most noticeably when big collections of data are used to teach and constantly improve the AI (Shafik, 2026). AI chatbots and digital recovery platforms add further dangers to keeping things secret, such as data getting out, bad keeping of data, and being open to internet attacks (Rawlings Olowoniyi & Deshpande, 2026). What is ethically correct says we should put into practice machine learning ways which guard privacy – like "federated learning" and coding – to lower the chance of someone finding out who a patient is (Sharma & Rathore, 2026). Wider conversations about safety and ethics in AI show that keeping things secret is not only a technical point, but a main ethical duty in digital healthcare (Firuzpour). In physiotherapy – where the link between patient and therapist is founded on trust – it is essential to have strong data laws to fit professional standards and guard patients' rights.

6. PROPOSED PHYSIOTHERAPY-SPECIFIC HUMAN-IN-THE-LOOP FRAMEWORK

When using AI in physiotherapy, you need a very clear plan that explains how much the field relies on motion analysis, how it is always getting better, and how patients get personalized care. While generic Human-in-the-loop (HITL) frameworks emphasize ethical scrutiny and collaborative decision-making, when self-driving cars are used as a vital tool in a physiotherapy setting, the need arises to incorporate the functionality of evolution and real-time responsiveness in the blueprint.

Early studies on patient-centric physiotherapy systems running on small datasets have shown that the use of adaptive feedback will enable recovery while maintaining the clinician's role (Lao et al., 2020). Building up from the more generic ethical HITL paradigm (Turgunov et al., 2020), this proposal places the physiotherapist at key points in the workflow of artificial intelligence. And instead of remaining passive to the recommendations of an algorithm, clinicians consider whether the model of human movement is consistent with theoretical expectations, whether the amount of effort prescribed is appropriate for the patient's capacity and whether the intervention meets safety criteria in the context of the clinical situation. Collaborations between AI models and practicing clinicians show that the final decision coming from an ensemble in rehabilitation is better than those generated by either entity alone (Lee et al., 2021). Contemporary methods in physiotherapy emphasise the importance of individualising interventions, being open about potential underpinning mechanisms and intelligent and posture driven approach to promote functional capacity (Muthukrishnan M et al., 2025). Putting these ideas together, the human-in-the-loop (HITL) framework for physiotherapy we suggest has four connected parts: combining ideas, work steps with checks, improving based on results, and ways to deal with risk.

6.1 Conceptual Model for HITL Integration

A HITL model for physiotherapy needs to clearly state how a professional's skill works with what the AI produces. The 'healthcare professional in the loop' idea gives a basic structure, making doctors and therapists active checkers – not just people who look at things after the AI is done (Eachempati et al., 2025). In rehabilitation, this means doctors and therapists and AI share power when understanding what is seen and changing treatment.

The growing relationship between AI and what doctors think shows we need to have clear boundaries for decisions – where computers are good at spotting patterns, but the therapist makes judgements about the situation (Truong, 2025). Studies of how well HITL works show that it needs to be easy to understand, have fast feedback, and doctors and therapists need to be trained (Theilmann et al., 2025). Rules for AI in healthcare that carries high risk also show we need many layers of oversight, to balance getting things done with being responsible (Schneider & Lawson, 2026).

What we've learned from decision-making in areas outside healthcare says that good HITL systems need pre-set points where something must happen, and clear ways to increase the level of attention. When used in physiotherapy, this idea means putting AI assessment with a therapist-approved diagnosis, carefully watched exercise progress, and keeping an eye on how the person is doing.

6.2 Workflow Design and Clinical Checkpoints

To use HITL in physiotherapy, we need to clearly map out work steps with checkpoints. Work optimisation using AI stresses having set points where a person checks what the computer does, to stop errors from going on (Ramesh, 2025; Pingili, 2025). In rehabilitation, these checkpoints could be checking the first assessment, approving how hard an exercise is, allowing progress, and looking over the plan for when the person is well enough to leave care.

Safety in automating work in healthcare is especially important, and automated suggestions must cause a therapist to look at things when there is doubt or risk is too high (Stevens & Rivera, 2023). How digital health companies judge things stresses the need to always check performance, keep records of what was done, and check after it's been put into use (McAlister et al., 2025). More general studies of AI in healthcare systems stress that it must follow rules and what professionals expect (Bharathi).

So, the work process we suggest has therapist checkpoints at:

1. Looking at the first assessment that the AI made
2. Confirming the prescription
3. Reassessing function halfway through
4. Checking results before moving on or ending care

This keeps things efficient and makes sure professionals are responsible.

6.3 Patient Feedback and Outcome-Based Iteration

Because rehabilitation is, at heart, something done through repeated tries, systems using humans-in-the-loop – or HITL – must include structured feedback that looks at what happens in the end. Models of teaching and assessment which are geared to results show how AI could help people keep their skill level up, while still being overseen. Also, feedback venues linking actual results to what doctors decide clinically, bring about better therapeutic methods (Strauss et al., 2022). To finish the 'data to doing' chain, it's essential that what patients say they're going through, and how well they're doing physically, are turned into learning that can be used (Howard et al., 2024). Risk management rules stress having ways to formally report when things go wrong, problems happen, or there are near misses (Merotiwon et al., 2024). Studies of healthcare models based on results show that going back and checking things makes them safer and more efficient when they are within clear rules (Chidavaenzi et al., 2025).

In physiotherapy, this means always putting in pain scores, how well people can function, what wearable sensors show, and what the therapist sees, into the AI's process of re-adjusting. The therapist is still in charge of understanding how results are changing and allowing the computer to make changes based on the algorithm.

6.4 Risk Escalation and Therapist Override Mechanism

A key part of the system we're putting forward is a clear way for a therapist to overrule it – to step in. Studies of AI helping with healthcare have shown that we must set up risk-management plans ahead of time, and especially where people are at most risk, (Ohu and others, 2025). Also, looking at the morals of medical AI that could be very good – but is also risky – makes it very plain that we need traceable ways to get to help when something goes wrong (Corfmat and others, 2025).

Those who design things to be safe, and not to cause harm, say we should put warnings into AI to stop it making unsafe suggestions, and this is very true in the ever-changing area of getting people better after injury (Thurzo & Thurzo, 2025). More general work on smart systems shows we need to govern them in a way which makes them strong and able to recover, with people being able to get involved as a way to keep things steady (Macrae, 2025). New talks about AI that acts for itself in medical work show that as AI gets more and more able to do things on its own, we must have well-set-up human control over it (Sharma and others, 2026).

In a physiotherapy setting, the override ought to happen when:

1. There are things which mean treatment should not happen.
2. Getting worse goes beyond what's been allowed.
3. How the body moves shows someone could be hurt.
4. The AI is not sure enough.

This way of setting things up to be able to get help makes sure that the person giving therapy is still the one who is really responsible for what happens to the patient.

7. IMPLEMENTATION CHALLENGES AND PRACTICAL BARRIERS

Artificial intelligence has indeed advanced at a great pace, but the integration of it into healthcare environments on a routine basis is spotty and problematic. The issues related to integrating these systems are not just related to their technical performance but include organisational readiness, their acceptance by professionals, lack of clarity in governance and infrastructural constraints. Various studies and reviews investigating algorithms in the field consistently report the major barrier to adoption being the context mismatch between the development of the algorithms and how the algorithms are applied in clinical practice (Nair et al., 2024). Furthermore, there are indications from translational studies that the large number of AI tools which have been shown to exhibit high accuracy in controlled experiments are inability to fit well with the current demands of care delivery (Zhao & Lopez, 2025).

System-level issues get reverberated among all stakeholders. Clinicians may express concerns about the trustfulness of AI and the possible legal consequences of its utilisation; health service organisations are facing challenges in their relationships with AI with regard to the acquisition of AI technologies and the regulatory frameworks governing their use; and patients, meanwhile, question their dependence on, and transparency of, such systems (Singh et al., 2020). Theoretical reviews have also highlighted the importance of various factors as determinants of effective implementation, including leadership engagement, alignment of AI with existing work processes and cultural receptiveness (Chomutare et al., 2022). Some empirical analyses relating to orthopaedics rehabilitation, back these ideas up, showing how vital it is to involve everyone concerned and to do careful, step-by-step assessment before using things in real clinical work (Khattak et al., 2025). Things like how easy to use something is, how much clinical good it's thought to do, and whether it fits into what professionals do every day, have all made up the way AI is taken up in different places (Hassan et al., 2024). In physiotherapy, these issues – when seen as part of a whole system – are made worse by the fact that this field depends much more on judging each person individually, how treatment goes forward, and the connection between therapist and patient. As a result, AI work must be carefully designed to fit into these things, rather than be put in as a complete technology change.

7.1 Training Requirements for Physiotherapists

To get AI into physiotherapy practice, targeted professional training is necessary. Qualitative studies show that physiotherapists often see the possible good in AI, but say they don't have much confidence in understanding what algorithms produce or in judging the limits of the systems (Shawli et al., 2024). Worries that their jobs might be taken over are alongside the idea that AI might change what professionals do, rather than getting rid of the need for them (Rowe et al., 2022).

Newer studies suggest that structured changes to education are needed, putting digital knowledge, the ability to understand data, and ethical thinking into physiotherapy courses (Aziz et al., 2023). Predictions about how the workforce will change by 2030 also make it clear that people will need to be able to change and adapt – including being able to work across disciplines and to control smart systems (Muthukrishnan, 2025). Surveys of healthcare people in rehabilitation areas show that gaps in knowledge and uncertainty about what the rules are, are still major problems when it comes to confidently adopting AI (Aldhahi et al., 2025).

From a systems point of view, AI education in physiotherapy needs to go beyond just being able to use the technology, to include being able to judge things critically, recognising risks, and judging how easily results can be understood (Davids et al., 2022). If there aren't deliberate training plans, putting AI into practice risks being superficial – not making the most of what AI can do, while also bringing in safety problems that could be avoided.

7.2 Integration into Clinical Workflow

Successful putting-into-practice depends on AI being smoothly put into the clinical workflows which are already in place. Evidence from imaging and diagnostics shows that AI tools must fit with the ways documents are kept, how reports are made, and how long decisions take, if they are to be accepted for the long term (Blezek et al., 2021; Juluru et al., 2021). Putting AI in a fragmented way, or having separate systems, often makes things less efficient, rather than better.

Incorporating artificial intelligence into electronic health records is one of the critical operation challenges. Getting this sort of technology to work well asks for data routes that are organised and decide who gets at data when, and also a user screen that doctors find easy to use (Olusegun et al., 2024). In rehabilitation work, changing the flow charts should take into account the cycles of assessment, points where one asks how exercise is going, and the regular tracking of results (Liu & Xie, 2025). AI-based automation in rehabilitation – in robotics and help-tech – also needs to work with human oversight and machine doing, so that treatment doesn't get broken up (Goolla).

So, putting AI into workflows should be done little by little and with input from doctors, giving priority to as little disruption as possible, clear points where decisions are made, and clear ways of documenting what happens.

7.3 Interoperability and Technical Constraints

Interoperability remains a continuing problem in digital healthcare systems. AI systems often depend on different kinds of data sources – electronic records, sensors people wear, imaging platforms – which don't have standard ways of being put together (Bala Dhandayuthapani, 2024). Without architectures that can work together, data being kept separate stops care being continuous and limits how well smart systems can be scaled up.

Studies of digital health infrastructures show that interoperability improves not only efficiency but also care which is centred on the patient, across different care settings (Adegoke et al., 2025). Technical examinations of AI-driven healthcare systems show that not being able to work together, problems with standardising data, and differences in infrastructure, are key limits (Al-Namrouti et al., 2026). These problems are inherently connected with the demands of clarity; complex accountability systems must balance accountability requirements and technological feasibility (Kiseleva et al., 2022). Bridging integration gaps requires organized technological, organisational and regulatory measures that focus on the secure exchange of data and the use of standardised protocols [Perez, 2026]. In the field of physiotherapy, the aim of interoperability is particularly important for the integration of movement data collected via wearable devices, clinical cognitive and long-term rehabilitation records in decision support systems.

8. REGULATORY AND POLICY PERSPECTIVES

The exponential growth of artificial intelligence in healthcare has far exceeded efforts to develop comprehensive paradigms of regulations and policies that can address the clinical, ethical, and infrastructural implications of its progression and use. In rehabilitation and physiotherapy, where therapeutic decisions are incremental and closely linked to the issue of patient safety, regulatory clarity is of paramount importance. Amongst the earliest efforts to describe or portray policies in the field, key takeaways renew the importance of embedding considerations of the complexity of system and data integrity, accountability structures, and inter-sectoral coordination into any future policy implementation (Verma et al., 2020). These issues are magnified in places like the rehabilitation world where applications of AI are widely employed across decision support algorithms, robotic therapy systems and remote surveillance system. Recent narrative reviews have shown that the points shared by ethical and regulatory concerns revolve around the themes of clarity, responsibility, working against bias, and non-discriminatory access (Mennella et al., 2024). Consequently, regulatory frameworks need to go beyond the evaluation of the devices for continuous surveillance during the life cycle of the technology, including, data governance, testing the algorithms, post market surveillance and assessments of performance periodically. Studies comparing what rules are in place at the moment show they vary by country – some are using ways of categorising risk, while others still follow older laws about medical devices (Ardic & Dinc, 2025). Broad looks at things worldwide also show that rules aren't very well agreed, and this makes it difficult to use digital health across borders (Busch et al., 2025). When it comes to robotic rehabilitation and AI technology to help people, rules are looked at very closely, as these directly affect patients physically. Discussions of the ethics and rules of robotic rehabilitation stress the need to check safety, have people watching what's going on, and make sure that technologically-supported care is available to all (Ali, 2025). In the EU, the AI Act is bringing in risk-based categorisation, demands for openness, and requirements for people to supervise high-risk medical AI – so changing what robotic and algorithmic rehabilitation tools need to do to be allowed (Calabrò, 2025). This means physiotherapy needs to get better at understanding the rules, and plan how their organisations will deal with them.

8.1 International AI Governance in Healthcare

Controlling AI in healthcare is more and more often seen as a worldwide issue that needs internationally-agreed principles. Work on controlling AI underlines how important it is to have shared understandings of who is responsible, how open things should be, and how to protect patients, so that rules aren't all different in each place (Morley et al., 2022). International organisations play an important role in building up acceptable practice and providing guidance on acceptable AI utilization and fostering harmonization of regulations across borders (Kijewski et. al., 2024). Guidance from the World Health Organization on AI ethics presents the following principles of ethics: respect for individual autonomy, beneficence, non-medicinal, accountability, and inclusivity (WHO, 2021). These principles rate national policies against which to measure them. Ethical frameworks of control also state that the responsible application of AI must be subject to mechanisms of internal oversight rather than external oversight by law enforcement only (Bouderhem, 2024). At the organisational level, more structured frameworks are being used to operationalise the use of responsible AI. Multi-method research protocols used to ensure the regulation of AI in healthcare organisations emphasise the use of risk matrices and stakeholder consultation, as well as being informed by documentation of interventions and mechanisms for post-implementation evaluation (Freeman et al., 2025). Comparative analysis across jurisdictions helps to understand that while some regions are more strict in regulating the market, others are rather liberal, promoting innovation; this is a sign of the need for a flexible governance that is responsive to the context (Chakraborty & Karhade, 2024). Because physiotherapy and rehab are now part of healthcare all over the world, the ways things are being managed internationally mean that there are tougher and tougher demands for openness, people being involved, making sure things are safe, and AI being used fairly. So, groups should be prepared for regulations that are coming together, and for being asked to give more and more reasons for what their algorithms do and how well different systems can work with each other – even across borders.

8.2 Implications for Physiotherapy Practice

The way rules around artificial intelligence in healthcare are changing has a real, big effect on how physiotherapists are taught, how they work, and what it means to be a physiotherapist. Early academic talk about AI in physiotherapy courses showed the need to get tech skills into what's taught, with the main ethical ideas of being able to make sensible judgements in the clinic and always putting the patient first (Rowe, 2019). As AI tools are more and more used to look at muscles and bones for diagnoses, and to make rehab plans for people as individuals, physios have a double problem: to accept technology to make care better, whilst still being completely in charge professionally. Studies have shown that AI – if used properly – can really help with looking at movement, keeping an eye on patients from a distance, and giving people exercise plans which are for them (Nambi et al., 2024). Nonetheless, these advantages depend on how well protocols concerning governance are followed, how rigorously documentation standards are met, and how well informed consent is acquired - all of which are found squarely in modern policy directives. Applications of AI to problems with muscles and bones show that advice from algorithms must be able to be understood, and checked in the context, to make sure they are safe (Tack, 2019). Studies of how ready physiotherapists are to use AI show that people are willing to use it to different degrees – depending on how useful they think it is in clinic, how much their organisation supports it, and how clear the rules are (Abuzaid et al., 2022). In places where professional advice is not clear, people in the profession may not want to put AI into how they make decisions, because they are not sure about who is responsible, and what the ethical risks are. So, changes in the rules should be joined by advice for the profession that makes clear what can be done, what must be in documents, and what people must watch over in AI-supported care.

8.3 Professional Standards and Clinical Governance

Professional standards are located in the nexus of the regulatory imperatives and the mundane clinical work flows. There is the proliferation of algorithmic systems that is reshaping the operational architecture of the clinic, which has given rise to concerns that point toward "algorithmic normativity"-the phenomenon of the embedding of computational assumptions that re-calibrate the parameters of what is exemplary care (Asadollahi, 2026). In the context of physiotherapy such dynamics may manifest itself through standardized algorithmic models regulating exercise progression or automated risk assessment tools leading to subtle changes in going from therapeutic thresholds, and consequently, also of perceived acceptability within therapeutic encounters. Advice from people who control information shows how important it is to have organised ways of judging things before AI is put in place – including judging risk and benefit, looking at how data is protected, and making clear what each person's role is (Olawade et al., 2025). But studies of what actually happens suggest that professional advice on how doctors should use AI is all over the place, creating uncertainty about what is best practice, and where responsibility lies (Smith et al., 2024). Models of clinical control give a good structure for putting AI into practice responsibly. Established principles of control stress quality assurance, constantly improving, managing risk, and patient safety as the main parts of giving healthcare (McSherry & Pearce, 2011). Turning these principles to AI-supported physiotherapy means having organised ways to check things, ways to report problems, ways to measure results, and written procedures for people to watch over things. New work on AI that can be trusted in clinic shows that being ethical needs organisations to be committed for a long time, and not just do checks to meet the rules once (Goktas & Grzybowski, 2025). In physiotherapy, control structures must make sure that AI tools are regularly checked, stay in line with what the latest evidence-based advice says, and take in what doctors think into how the system is made better. All in all, changes in rules and control show a move from letting innovation happen, to having organised accountability. For physiotherapy, this change doesn't just add to administrative work; it changes what it means to be a professional and use technology. Physiotherapists must take active parts in judging, watching over, and putting AI tools into the context of accepted standards of care. Understanding the rules, watching over things in organisations, and professional control mechanisms are therefore key to safely and sustainably putting AI into rehabilitation practice.

9. FUTURE DIRECTIONS IN EXPLAINABLE AI FOR REHABILITATION

What comes next in bringing artificial intelligence – AI – into rehabilitation won't be so much about making the algorithms better, as about making the systems understandable, really used in clinics, and properly overseen by professionals. Reviews of AI and machine learning in rehabilitation, covering robotics and a range of treatments, constantly point to three things still lacking: it's hard to see why an AI does what it does, there isn't enough long-term testing of these systems, and they aren't properly fitted into how therapists actually work (Nicora et al., 2025; Mennella et al., 2023). Though AI is getting much more accurate at predicting things, turning those predictions into clear, useful advice for doctors isn't yet very good.

New work shows that rehabilitation systems of the future need to move from just automating jobs to 'collaborative intelligence' - systems that combine information from many sources, give adaptive feedback, and let doctors be in charge (Khalid et al., 2024). Also, more complete research into the part AI plays in rehab services suggests that, for it to be used widely and give patients good results, the tech must be clear, act in a way that's right ethically, and be watched very closely by people. AI platforms which bring together data on how the body moves, what people do, and what risk of injury there is, have a lot of promise – especially for stopping sports injuries, and for rehab which is for what people do. But these systems need to be able to explain what they are doing in a way that's easy to understand, and to make sure that decisions about treatment are based on what doctors think is best, and not just on numbers. What's coming is about three things which are all linked: ways for doctors to use that make clear what the AI is doing, rehab plans which are made for each patient, and training for the people who will use these systems.

9.1 Explainable AI Interfaces for Clinicians

Being able to explain things should be more than just telling people what the AI's steps in calculation are; it should also be about making interfaces which people can understand – especially doctors. Studies on how to make AI interfaces for people have shown that doctors trust and understand the systems much more when engineers and doctors work together on the design (Fouad et al., 2026). Engineers and doctors working together in radiology made images clearer, showed more doubt, and made the systems easier to use. These are all things that can be used in rehab. When you look at explainable AI in healthcare as a whole, it's clear that for it to work, what the AI says needs to match how doctors think (Zhang et al., 2026). Doctors need explanations that are quick to understand, but can also go into detail about why the AI has come to its conclusion, if needed. Early tests of AI helping with mechanical ventilation show that explanation interfaces need to give enough information without overloading the doctor's mind (Jung et al., 2026).

Studies of what doctors want show they always prefer visualisations which they can understand, especially when the AI is helping with important treatments (Xian et al., 2026). In rehabilitation, this could mean showing how exercise load is going up, how symmetrical someone's movements are, or how recovery is likely to go, along with how confident the AI is, and which factors are contributing to the prediction.

AI frameworks which are driven by what's needed, put transparency, traceability and security at the heart of trustworthy advice for doctors (Nazar et al., 2026). For physiotherapists, interfaces should put together scales for measuring how someone is functioning, analyses of their movements, and how their symptoms are going, all on one screen that's easy to understand. These systems must let doctors stay in charge, while helping them to spot patterns and risks.

9.2 AI in Personalized Rehabilitation Planning

Perhaps the most helpful thing artificial intelligence can do in physiotherapy is to develop rehab programmes that are suited to individuals. AI-based treatment planning models are able to – even now – pull together information from a range of sources and make treatment plans which adapt as the patient's condition changes (Fonseca et al., 2026). These show the way that computers can help to organise treatment suitably, with doctors still in charge. AI monitoring tools can also alter rehab plans depending on the degree of recovery from, for example, an orthopaedic problem (Ipaktchi & Higinbotham, 2026). Also, AI platforms for managing rehabilitation programs make it easier to track how someone is doing and how well they are responding to treatment (Luca et al., 2026). Using data from sensors, medical history and what people are doing, improves how well we can predict the risk of injury and how to make rehabilitation better (Wang et al., 2026).

The development of systems which suggest care plans in physiotherapy shows both opportunity and danger. Though AI suggestions can make things quicker and more consistent, doctors must check them to make sure they suit the patient's abilities, other illnesses, and what they are feeling (Şahinbaş et al., 2026). Future systems should use 'collaborative personalisation' – where the AI suggests plans based on different situations, with clear reasons and how likely the outcomes are.

Long-term tests will be needed to see whether AI-assisted personalisation improves how well people can function, how likely they are to keep up with their treatment, and how quickly they recover, without making things unsafe. We need to move from just predicting things, to complete, understandable rehabilitation systems which change as the patient gets better.

9.3 Education and Workforce Development

The ability to continue utilizing explainable AI in rehabilitation is contingent upon the adequate preparation of the workforce. AI-based education for healthcare stresses the need to be good with data, understand algorithms, and be able to tell if they are moral (Thakral et al., 2026).

For physiotherapists, these skills need to be in what they are taught before they qualify, and in their continued professional development. What we know about how people adapt to work suggests that AI will change what professionals do*, rather than replace them – increasing the need for oversight, understanding, and working with people from other areas (Karmali, 2026). Within rehabilitation, the growing use of AI could well mean physiotherapists take on more responsibility when checking the exercise plans, risk evaluations, and predictions of results that AI creates. AI-powered learning networks give new options to improve skills, with learning sections that change to suit the person and systems to watch how well someone is doing (Mustafa et al., 2026). These can make AI-supported situations in a clinic, so physiotherapists can practice checking what AI says and spotting risks in a safe setting. Work that health organisations do to increase understanding of AI and data in health research shows how vital well-planned training is (Zand et al., 2026). If AI understanding is part of how an organisation works, doctors will use clever systems thoughtfully, and not just accept them. Future plans for the workforce ought to include workshops with people from different fields, lessons on how things are governed, and training based on real cases that involves both engineers and rehabilitation experts. Better education will ensure that AI tools which show how they work are not just employed, but employed properly. Explainable AI in rehab is likely to become more useful as the technology develops, is built with clinicians in mind, and as clinicians' skills are enhanced. Critiques consistently indicate that while AI in rehabilitation grows rapidly, it will only truly be valuable in practice if it's transparent, easily understood, and is subject to human oversight (Nicora et al., 2025; Mennella et al., 2023; Khalid et al., 2024). The way physiotherapy-specific AI develops should focus on interfaces designed together, systems that change to the person but are checked by doctors, and organised education for the workforce. By making new ideas fit with what the profession expects and making it clear what AI is doing, rehabilitation can make the most of AI while still putting the patient first.

CONCLUSION

The fast increase in artificial intelligence in health has caused a lot of hope about efficiency, being able to be used on a large scale, and being tailored to the person. But, in physiotherapy and rehabilitation, turning AI from something that can be done into something that is safe to do in the clinic needs careful thought and a good basic idea. Rehabilitation is unlike many areas of diagnosis, because it depends on clinical thought that changes as things go on, constant checking of how well someone is doing, and treatment that is changed bit by bit. In these areas, what algorithms give isn't just a suggestion, but really controls how much exercise someone does, how it goes up, how safe it is, and how well someone will do in the long run. Because of this, being able to understand AI in physiotherapy must be seen as something the clinic needs, not just something computers can do. The chapter has made the case that using AI safely in rehabilitation depends on two things which go together: the algorithms being easy to grasp, and practitioners being firmly in charge of what happens. Being able to grasp what's going on allows clinicians to look at why an algorithm is making a suggestion – so, what the correct amount of exercise should be, what shouldn't be done at all, or how things should move on – and be sure it's sensible in terms of the patient's body and what they need. If the reasons for recommendations about how hard to exercise, what not to do, or when to step up aren't clear, then safety and professional responsibility could be put at risk. In physiotherapy – where what's done directly affects how tissue is stressed, motor learning and a patient's getting better – a lack of clarity is not good enough practice. Therefore, the chapter has put forward a physiotherapy framework for active control, at set points in assessing patients, planning treatment, giving treatment, and when risks get worse. Instead of AI being thought of as making decisions on its own, the framework has physiotherapists as checking, understanding and agreeing with what AI systems do. Set check-points, feedback on performance, and the option to overrule all stop algorithms' speed taking the place of a professional's judgement. This model is a 'human-in-the-loop' method, where AI helps to find patterns, but a person's skill keeps awareness of the situation and responsibility going. More thought about clinical risks has shown how important this organised approach is. Mistakes in exercise plans, 'red flags' being missed, safety issues in neurological and heart/lung rehabilitation, and the chance of skills being lost, are all especially important in rehabilitation. These risks aren't just ideas; they come from using algorithms that aren't clear in therapies that involve hands-on work. As a result, new rules and what's happening internationally more and more stress clarity, looking at risks by how serious they are, and constant human supervision of AI in healthcare which is very risky. Work in the future on AI for rehabilitation which can be explained should therefore give priority to design based around the clinician, systems which are made for the person and stay understandable, and development of the workforce. Interfaces that are easy to understand should fit in with physiotherapy practice, giving levels of explanation for quick checking, but letting detailed examination happen when needed. Planning rehabilitation for a person must still be done together, with AI suggestions staying inside the safety limits set by the clinician. At the same time, professional training needs to develop ability with data, skills in interpreting, and awareness of rules – making sure clinicians stay in charge of clever systems. In the end, AI being put into physiotherapy successfully will depend not on technology on its own, but on it being used properly. If the profession establishes innovation on the foundations of clarity and control, it can get the best out of AI's potential for adaptation, yet still keep patient care as the central concern, ensure accuracy, and maintain professional standards. The future of rehab lies in 'human-in-the-loop' intelligence – where computer findings supplement, rather than supersede, the clinician's judgement.

REFERENCES

Abuzaid, M. M., Elshami, W., Hegazy, F., Aboelnasr, E. A., & Tekin, H. O. (2022). The impact of artificial Intelligence (AI) in physiotherapy practice: A study of physiotherapist willingness and readiness. *Journal of Hunan University Natural Sciences*, *49*(3), 196–201. DOI: 10.55463/issn.1674-2974.49.3.21

. Adegoke, K., Adegoke, A., Dawodu, D., Bayowa, A., & Adekoya, A. (2025). Interoperability in digital healthcare: Enhancing consumer health and transforming care systems.

Al-Namrouti, A. T., Elshabrawi, M. N., Sayad, R., Khalaf, I. M. B., Jaoun, H., Morshedy, E. M., & Attaelmanan, G. A. (2026). Interoperability Challenges and Solutions in AI-Driven Healthcare Systems. In *Artificial Intelligence in Smart Healthcare Systems* (pp. 277–292). CRC Press. DOI: 10.1201/9781003533351-25

Aldhahi, M. I., Alorainy, A. I., Abuzaid, M. M., Gareeballah, A., Alsubaie, N. F., Alshamary, A. S., & Hamd, Z. Y. (2025, February). Adoption of artificial intelligence in rehabilitation: Perceptions, knowledge, and challenges among healthcare providers. [). MDPI.]. *Health Care*, *13*(4), 350. PMID: 39997225

Ali, A. (2025). Ethical and regulatory considerations in rehabilitation robotics: Ensuring safe and equitable care. In *Design and Control of Rehabilitation Robots: From Concept to Therapy* (pp. 399–422). Springer Nature Switzerland. DOI: 10.1007/978-3-031-86977-8_17

Ali, A. S., Alhirsan, S. M., Elshazly, M., Ali, Z. A., Elzanaty, M. Y., Mansour, W. T., Taha, S. I., Alarousi, I. N., Hamoda, I. M., Diab, S. F. M., El Melhat, A. M., Alkubati, S. A., & El-Ashry, A. M. (2026). Artificial Intelligence in Physiotherapy Education: A Multi-Country Middle East Survey of AI Acceptance and Barriers Among University Students. *European Journal of Education*, *61*(1), e70476. DOI: 10.1111/ejed.70476

Alsobhi, M., Khan, F., Chevidikunnan, M. F., Basuodan, R., Shawli, L., & Neamatallah, Z. (2022). Physical therapists' knowledge and attitudes regarding artificial intelligence applications in health care and rehabilitation: Cross-sectional study. *Journal of Medical Internet Research*, *24*(10), e39565. DOI: 10.2196/39565 PMID: 36264614

Alwhaibi, R. M., Alshammari, R. B., Alrufayyiq, N. I., Alenzi, J. Q., Alsumayli, A. H., Alrushud, B. I., & Alahmadi, T. J. (2025). Attitudes of physical therapists toward AI diagnostics: Barriers, enablers, and clinical implications. *BMC Medical Education*, *25*(1), 1751. DOI: 10.1186/s12909-025-08361-7 PMID: 41286821

Annika, G., Christoff, Z., & Kerstin, L. (2024). Evaluation of the accuracy of an artificial intelligence in identifying contraindications to exercise therapy-comparison with and interrater reliability of physical therapists judgments. *Health and Technology, 14*(3), 513–522. DOI: 10.1007/s12553-024-00827-w

Ardic, N., & Dinc, R. (2025). Artificial intelligence in healthcare: Current regulatory landscape and future directions. *British Journal of Hospital Medicine, 86*(8), 1–21. DOI: 10.12968/hmed.2024.0972 PMID: 40847984

Asadollahi, A. (2026). Governing by design: Algorithmic normativity, clinical standards, and health policy implications of AI in healthcare. *AI and Ethics, 6*(1), 119. DOI: 10.1007/s43681-026-01002-9

. Aziz, R. A. B. I. A., Sundus, H. A. B. I. B. A., Jawed, F. I. R. D. A. U. S., & Chhabra, C. H. A. R. U. (2023). Embracing technological innovations: the integration of AI in physiotherapy. *Recent Trends in Multidisciplinary Research*, 275-288.

Bakken, S. (2023). AI in health: Keeping the human in the loop. *Journal of the American Medical Informatics Association : JAMIA, 30*(7), 1225–1226. DOI: 10.1093/jamia/ocad091 PMID: 37337923

Bala Dhandayuthapani, V. (2024). Advancing healthcare: AI integration, interoperability and sustainability challenges. *Digital Health*, 64.

Barnes, E., & Hutson, J. (2024). Navigating the complexities of AI: The critical role of interpretability and explainability in ensuring transparency and trust. *International Journal of Multidisciplinary and Current Educational Research, 6*(3).

Berzin, T. M., & Topol, E. J. (2025). Preserving clinical skills in the age of AI assistance. *Lancet, 406*(10513), 1719. DOI: 10.1016/S0140-6736(25)02075-6 PMID: 41109709

. Bharathi, G. Integrating AI into Clinical Workflows: Challenges and Opportunities. *Artificial Intelligence in Oncology: Transforming Diagnosis and Treatment*, 130.

Blezek, D. J., Olson-Williams, L., Missert, A., & Korfiatis, P. (2021). AI integration in the clinical workflow. *Journal of Digital Imaging, 34*(6), 1435–1446. DOI: 10.1007/s10278-021-00525-3 PMID: 34686923

Bobby, N. N., Saravanan, V., Shanthiny, R., & Jenifer, J. (2026). Virtual Reality (VR) and AI in Physiotherapy for Cognitive and Physical Rehabilitation: Innovations in Biomedical Materials. In *Advanced Materials for Biomedical Devices* (pp. 395-412). CRC Press.

Bouderhem, R. (2024). Shaping the future of AI in healthcare through ethics and governance. *Humanities & Social Sciences Communications*, *11*(1), 1–12. DOI: 10.1057/s41599-024-02894-w

Brewster, R. C., Tse, G., Fan, A. L., Elborki, M., Newell, M., Gonzalez, P., Hoq, A., Chang, C., Chowdhury, M., Geeti, A., Hana, M., Hassan, H., Ibrahim, O., Keseyan, L., Li, Q., Mamoon, M., Nageye, M., Ohannessian, A., Eisenberg, I. R., & Khan, A. (2025). Evaluating human-in-the-loop strategies for artificial intelligence-enabled translation of patient discharge instructions: A multidisciplinary analysis. *NPJ Digital Medicine*, *8*(1), 629. DOI: 10.1038/s41746-025-02055-6 PMID: 41136708

. Burlacu, A., Brinza, C., Geman, O., Karppa, M., & Jude, D. (2026). Heart Rate Variability as a dual-use digital biomarker: integrating clinical, AI, and. *resuscitation, 49*, 51.

Busch, F., Geis, R., Wang, Y. C., Kather, J. N., Khori, N. A., Makowski, M. R., . . . Bressem, K. K. (2025). AI regulation in healthcare around the world: what is the status quo? medRxiv, 2025-01. DOI: 10.1101/2025.01.25.25321061

Calabrò, R. S. (2025). Ethical Horizons in Robotic Rehabilitation: Ensuring Safe AI Use Under the EU AI Act. *Medical Science*, *13*(4), 317. PMID: 41440549

Chakraborty, A., & Karhade, M. (2024). Global AI governance in healthcare: a cross-jurisdictional regulatory analysis. *arXiv preprint arXiv:2406.08695.*

. Chidavaenzi, G. T., Salie, F., & Grobbelaar, S. S. (2025). Designing and implementing outcome-based models in healthcare: insights and strategies from a scoping review. *Management Review Quarterly*, 1-61.

Chomutare, T., Tejedor, M., Svenning, T. O., Marco-Ruiz, L., Tayefi, M., Lind, K., Godtliebsen, F., Moen, A., Ismail, L., Makhlysheva, A., & Ngo, P. D. (2022). Artificial intelligence implementation in healthcare: A theory-based scoping review of barriers and facilitators. *International Journal of Environmental Research and Public Health*, *19*(23), 16359. DOI: 10.3390/ijerph192316359 PMID: 36498432

Corfmat, M., Martineau, J. T., & Régis, C. (2025). High-reward, high-risk technologies? An ethical and legal account of AI development in healthcare. *BMC Medical Ethics*, *26*(1), 4. DOI: 10.1186/s12910-024-01158-1 PMID: 39815254

Davids, J., Lidströmer, N., & Ashrafian, H. (2022). Artificial intelligence for physiotherapy and rehabilitation. In *Artificial intelligence in medicine* (pp. 1789–1807). Springer International Publishing. DOI: 10.1007/978-3-030-64573-1_339

. Dong, J., Chen, T., & Peng, Z. (2026). A Closed-Loop Intelligent Management System for Postoperative Orthopedic Rehabilitation: Integrating Deep Reinforcement Learning with Wearable Sensing and Prognostic Prediction.

Eachempati, P., Supe, A., Kumbargere Nagraj, S., Cresswell-Boyes, A., Robinson, S., & Yalamanchili, S. (2025). Integrating ai with healthcare expertise: Introducing the health care professional-in-the-loop framework: Part 1. *BDJ. In Practice*, *38*(2), 51–53.

Ennab, M., & Mcheick, H. (2022). Designing an interpretability-based model to explain the artificial intelligence algorithms in healthcare. *Diagnostics (Basel)*, *12*(7), 1557. DOI: 10.3390/diagnostics12071557 PMID: 35885463

Ennab, M., & Mcheick, H. (2024). Enhancing interpretability and accuracy of AI models in healthcare: A comprehensive review on challenges and future directions. *Frontiers in Robotics and AI*, *11*, 1444763. DOI: 10.3389/frobt.2024.1444763 PMID: 39677978

Ernazarovich, S. S., & Farxadovna, K. M. (2026, January). ARTIFICIAL INTELLIGENCE AND ITS CONTRIBUTION TO THE DEVELOPMENT OF CLINICAL REASONING SKILLS IN MEDICAL TRAINING. In *International Conference on Multidisciplinary Sciences and Innovations (ICMSI)* (Vol. 1, No. 2, pp. 29-35).

. Fahad, A., & Huang, C. Z. Human-in-the-Loop AI: A Framework for Continuous Validation of Generative AI Outputs in Healthcare.

. Firuzpour, F. Security, Privacy, and Ethics in AI for Healthcare. *decision making*, *4*, 6.

Fonseca, F. J. P. O., Matias, B. B. R., Pacheco, P., Muraoka, C. S. A. S., Silva, E. V. F., & Sesma, N. (2026). Artificial Intelligence-Assisted Treatment Planning in an Interdisciplinary Rehabilitation in the Esthetic Zone. *Journal of Esthetic and Restorative Dentistry*, *38*(1), 15–24. DOI: 10.1111/jerd.70034 PMID: 40977526

Fouad, S., Hakobyan, L., Ihongbe, I. E., Kavakli-Thorne, M., Atkins, S., & Bhatia, B. (2026). Human-Centered User Interface Design for Explainable AI in Chest Radiology: A Multi-Phase Co-Design Approach. *IEEE Access : Practical Innovations, Open Solutions*, *14*, 12498–12513. DOI: 10.1109/ACCESS.2026.3653233

Freeman, S., Wang, A., Saraf, S., Potts, E., McKimm, A., Coiera, E., & Magrabi, F. (2025). Developing an AI governance framework for safe and responsible AI in health care organizations: Protocol for a multimethod study. *JMIR Research Protocols*, *14*(1), e75702. DOI: 10.2196/75702 PMID: 40720809

. Gajalakshmi, P., Hemalatha, N., Elavarasi, R., Magadevi, N., & Kadhiravan, D. (2026). Case Studies and Applications of Explainability and Interpretability in AI Models. *AI Trust, Risk, and Security Management: Framework, Principles, and Practices*, 99-123.

Goktas, P., & Grzybowski, A. (2025). Shaping the future of healthcare: Ethical clinical challenges and pathways to trustworthy AI. *Journal of Clinical Medicine*, *14*(5), 1605. DOI: 10.3390/jcm14051605 PMID: 40095575

. Goolla, N. B. AI-Driven Automation in Medical Robotics: Optimizing Surgical and Rehabilitation Workflows.

Greengrass, C. J. (2025). Transforming clinical reasoning—The role of AI in supporting human cognitive limitations. *Frontiers in Digital Health*, *7*, 1715440. DOI: 10.3389/fdgth.2025.1715440 PMID: 41561162

Guarnaccia, F. R., Spadazzi, F., Ottaviani, M., Di Fazio, N., Volonnino, G., Di Mauro, L., Frati, P., & La Russa, R. (2026). Artificial Intelligence and Orthopaedic Prosthetic Planning: A State-of-the-Art Review and Evolving Liability Perspectives. *Sci*, *8*(2), 27. DOI: 10.3390/sci8020027

Guidance, W. H. O. (2021). Ethics and governance of artificial intelligence for health. *World Health Organization*, 1-165.

Güler, M. A., Dağ, S., Kayal, S., Can, M., & Şimşekkaya, S. N. (2026). Physiotherapy students' acceptance of AI-based chatbots (including ChatGPT) in education: A multi-institutional study from Turkey. *BMC Medical Education*, *26*(1), 174. DOI: 10.1186/s12909-025-08535-3 PMID: 41484754

Gupta, R. (2024). AI-based technologies, challenges, and solutions for neurorehabilitation: A systematic mapping. In *Computational Intelligence and Deep Learning Methods for Neuro-rehabilitation Applications* (pp. 1–25). Academic Press. DOI: 10.1016/B978-0-443-13772-3.00014-5

Haq, I. U., Felicetti, F., & Lamonaca, F. (2026). Measurement Uncertainty and Traceability in Upper Limb Rehabilitation Robotics: A Metrology-Oriented Review. *Journal of Sensor and Actuator Networks*, *15*(1), 8. DOI: 10.3390/jsan15010008

. Harper, D., & Langford, S. (2021). Explainable Clinical Decision Support Systems for Post-COVID Care Pathways. *The Artificial Intelligence Journal, 2*(4).

Hassan, M., Kushniruk, A., & Borycki, E. (2024). Barriers to and facilitators of artificial intelligence adoption in health care: Scoping review. *JMIR Human Factors*, *11*, e48633. DOI: 10.2196/48633 PMID: 39207831

Howard, A., Reza, N., Aston, S., Woods, B., Gerada, A., Buchan, I., Hope, W., & Märtson, A. G. (2024). Antimicrobial treatment imprecision: An outcome-based model to close the data-to-action loop. *The Lancet. Infectious Diseases*, *24*(1), e47–e58. DOI: 10.1016/S1473-3099(23)00367-5 PMID: 37660712

Ipaktchi, K. R., & Higinbotham, S. E. (2026). AI-Powered Rehabilitation and Monitoring Systems for Orthopedic Trauma Patients. In *New Technologies, Precision Medicine, and AI in Emergency General Surgery: Revolutionizing Surgical Practice for Optimal Patient Care* (pp. 303–311). Springer Nature Switzerland. DOI: 10.1007/978-3-032-09357-8_17

. Jeffy, M. (2025). Human-in-the-Loop vs. Full Autonomy: Striking the Balance in AI-Driven RPA.

. Joshi, H., Paul, M., Yadav, R., & Pant, G. (2026). AI-Driven Assessment and Rehabilitation in Physiotherapy: Challenges and Opportunities.

Jung, I. C., Zerlik, M., Schuler, K., Sedlmayr, M., & Sedlmayr, B. (2026). An Explanation User Interface for Artificial Intelligence–Supported Mechanical Ventilation Optimization for Clinicians: User-Centered Design and Formative Usability Study. *JMIR Formative Research*, *10*(1), e77481. DOI: 10.2196/77481 PMID: 41632969

Kabata, F., & Thaldar, D. (2024). Human in the loop requirement and AI healthcare applications in low-resource settings: A narrative review. *South African Journal of Bioethics and Law*, *17*(2), 70–73.

Karmali, Y. (2026). The Role of Artificial Intelligence in Workforce Adaptation and Skill Development. In *Artificial Intelligence in Healthcare and Biomedical Visualization* (pp. 171–186). Springer Nature Switzerland. DOI: 10.1007/978-3-032-06520-9_10

Khalid, U. B., Naeem, M., Stasolla, F., Syed, M. H., Abbas, M., & Coronato, A. (2024). Impact of AI-powered solutions in rehabilitation process: Recent improvements and future trends. *International Journal of General Medicine*, *17*, 943–969. DOI: 10.2147/IJGM.S453903 PMID: 38495919

Khattak, M., Bowness, J. S., Yonis, R., Kierkegaard, P., McGregor, A., & Perry, D. C. (2025). Navigating the barriers and facilitators to implementation of AI in healthcare: A scoping review. *The Bone & Joint Journal*, *107*(7), 666–672. DOI: 10.1302/0301-620X.107B7.BJJ-2024-1570.R1 PMID: 40588252

. Kijewski, S., Ronchi, E., & Vayena, E. (2024). International organisations and the global governance of AI in health. *Research handbook on health, AI and the law*, 254-272.

Kim, J. H. (2026). Automated Prescription of Therapeutic Exercise for Shoulder Impingement Syndrome using Literature-Driven Rule Generation Architecture. *Musculoskeletal Science & Practice*, *82*, 103520. DOI: 10.1016/j.msksp.2026.103520 PMID: 41707384

Kiseleva, A., Kotzinos, D., & De Hert, P. (2022). Transparency of AI in healthcare as a multilayered system of accountabilities: Between legal requirements and technical limitations. *Frontiers in Artificial Intelligence*, *5*, 879603. DOI: 10.3389/frai.2022.879603 PMID: 35707765

Kitey, P., & Lalwani, L. (2025, November). Feasibility and Safety of Artificial Intelligence Driven Telemetric Cardiac Rehabilitation in Adjunct to Home Exercise Education in Pediatric Patients with Congenital Heart Disease: A Pilot Study. In *2025 3rd DMIHER International Conference on Artificial Intelligence in Healthcare, Education and Industry (IDICAIHEI)* (pp. 1-5). IEEE. DOI: 10.1109/IDICAIHEI65991.2025.11378932

Kropf, M., Spöck, C., & Werner, R. (2026). Blame the Robot: Role Responsibility and Ethical Issues Regarding AI-Based Care Robots. *International Journal of Social Robotics*, *18*(2), 30. DOI: 10.1007/s12369-026-01369-z

Kumar, S., Datta, S., Singh, V., Datta, D., Singh, S. K., & Sharma, R. (2024). Applications, challenges, and future directions of human-in-the-loop learning. *IEEE Access : Practical Innovations, Open Solutions*, *12*, 75735–75760. DOI: 10.1109/ACCESS.2024.3401547

. Kundu, S. The Autonomous Healthcare Revolution: AI-Driven End-to-End Solutions for Seamless Patient Care.

La, N., Rattanapitoon, S. K., Thitimahatthanakusol, P., & Rattanapitoon, N. K. (2026). From Accuracy to Allocation: A Physiotherapy-Specific Risk Framework for AI-Mediated Exercise Advice in Breast Cancer Survivorship. *Physiotherapy*, 101894. DOI: 10.1016/j.physio.2026.101894 PMID: 41916863

Lanotte, F., O'Brien, M. K., & Jayaraman, A. (2023). AI in rehabilitation medicine: Opportunities and challenges. *Annals of Rehabilitation Medicine*, *47*(6), 444–458. DOI: 10.5535/arm.23131 PMID: 38093518

Lao, B., Tamei, T., & Ikeda, K. (2020). Data-efficient framework for personalized physiotherapy feedback. *Frontiers of Computer Science*, *2*, 3. DOI: 10.3389/fcomp.2020.00003

Lee, M. H., Siewiorek, D. P., Smailagic, A., Bernardino, A., & Bermúdez i Badia, S. B. (2021, May). A human-ai collaborative approach for clinical decision making on rehabilitation assessment. In *Proceedings of the 2021 CHI conference on human factors in computing systems* (pp. 1-14). DOI: 10.1145/3411764.3445472

Liu, H., & Xie, Q. (2025). Applications of artificial intelligence in rehabilitation: Technological innovation and transformation of clinical practice. *SLAS Technology*, *35*, 100360. DOI: 10.1016/j.slast.2025.100360 PMID: 41161419

. Luca, C., Onu, I., Dragos, S., Matei, D. V., Fuior, R., & Corciova, C. P. (2026). The Use of Artificial Intelligence (AI) in the Management of Medical Rehabilitation Programs.

Macrae, C. (2025). Managing risk and resilience in autonomous and intelligent systems: Exploring safety in the development, deployment, and use of artificial intelligence in healthcare. *Risk Analysis*, *45*(4), 910–927. DOI: 10.1111/risa.14273 PMID: 38246857

Martinho, D., Sobreiro, P., Domingues, A., Martinho, F., & Nogueira, N. (2026, January). Ethical Responsibility in Medical AI: A Semi-Systematic Thematic Review and Multilevel Governance Model. [). MDPI.]. *Health Care*, *14*(3), 287. PMID: 41682137

McAlister, K. L., Gonzales, L., & Huberty, J. (2025). Rethinking AI Workflows: Guidelines for Scientific Evaluation in Digital Health Companies. *JMIR AI*, *4*(1), e71798. DOI: 10.2196/71798 PMID: 41343771

McSherry, R., & Pearce, P. (2011). *Clinical governance: a guide to implementation for healthcare professionals*. John Wiley & Sons.

Mennella, C., Maniscalco, U., De Pietro, G., & Esposito, M. (2023). The role of artificial intelligence in future rehabilitation services: A systematic literature review. *IEEE Access : Practical Innovations, Open Solutions*, *11*, 11024–11043. DOI: 10.1109/ACCESS.2023.3236084

Mennella, C., Maniscalco, U., De Pietro, G., & Esposito, M. (2024). Ethical and regulatory challenges of AI technologies in healthcare: A narrative review. *Heliyon*, *10*(4), e26297. DOI: 10.1016/j.heliyon.2024.e26297 PMID: 38384518

. Merotiwon, D. O., Akintimehin, O. O., & Akomolafe, O. O. (2024). Developing an Outcome-Oriented Reporting Framework for Healthcare Risk Management and Incident Tracking.

Mittal, S., & Aggarwal, Y. (2026). Evaluation of Large Language Models in the Diagnosis, Urgency Triage, and Initial Management of Ophthalmic Emergencies. *Cureus, 18*(1). Advance online publication. DOI: 10.7759/cureus.101433 PMID: 41694895

Mittelstadt, B. (2021). Interpretability and transparency in artificial intelligence. *The Oxford handbook of digital ethics, 20.*

Morley, J., Murphy, L., Mishra, A., Joshi, I., & Karpathakis, K. (2022). Governing data and artificial intelligence for health care: Developing an international understanding. *JMIR Formative Research, 6*(1), e31623. DOI: 10.2196/31623 PMID: 35099403

Moss, L., Corsar, D., Shaw, M., Piper, I., & Hawthorne, C. (2022). Demystifying the black box: The importance of interpretability of predictive models in neurocritical care. *Neurocritical Care, 37*(S2, Suppl 2), 185–191. DOI: 10.1007/s12028-022-01504-4 PMID: 35523917

Muluk, S. Y., & Olcucu, N. (2024). Comparative analysis of artificial intelligence platforms: ChatGPT-3.5 and GoogleBard in identifying red flags of low back pain. *Cureus, 16*(7), e63580. PMID: 39087174

Mustafa, S. W., Sari, H., Asriany, A., & Hajeni, H. (2026). Transforming Workforce Development through AI-Driven Education Networks: A Pathway to Sustainable Economic Growth. In *Human-Centered Learning Design in the AI Era* (pp. 173–204). IGI Global Scientific Publishing.

Muthukrishnan, P. (2025). Artificial Intelligence and the Future of Physiotherapy: A Comprehensive Analysis of Workforce Transformation and Professional Adaptation by 2030. *Available at SSRN* 5779722. DOI: 10.2139/ssrn.5779722

. Muthukrishnan, P. (2026). Modern Physiotherapy in the Future: Innovations and Emerging Trends. *S. RAJADURAI, Modern Physiotherapy in the Future: Innovations and Emerging Trends (January 17, 2026).*

Muthukrishnan, P., Shanmugalakshmi, G., & Rajadurai, S. (2025). *AI-Powered Physiotherapy: A Personalized.* Ethical, and Intelligent Rehabilitation Framework for the Posture-Disturbed Generation.

Nair, M., Svedberg, P., Larsson, I., & Nygren, J. M. (2024). A comprehensive overview of barriers and strategies for AI implementation in healthcare: Mixed-method design. *PLoS One, 19*(8), e0305949. DOI: 10.1371/journal.pone.0305949 PMID: 39121051

Nambi, G., Alghadier, M., Mohamed, S. H. P., Aldhafian, O. R., Alshahrani, N. A., & Albarakati, A. J. A. (2024). Clinical usefulness of artificial intelligence in physiotherapy–a practice-based review. *SBV Journal of Basic. Clinical and Applied Health Science*, *7*(4), 184–188.

Natali, C., Marconi, L., Dias Duran, L. D., & Cabitza, F. (2025). AI-induced deskilling in medicine: A mixed-method review and research agenda for healthcare and beyond. *Artificial Intelligence Review*, *58*(11), 356. DOI: 10.1007/s10462-025-11352-1

Nazar, M., Unar, S., Ahmed, A., Su'ud, M. M., Alam, M. M., & Rahmat, A. (2026). Requirements Driven Explainable Artificial Intelligence Framework for Secure and Transparent Clinical Decision Support Systems. *IEEE Access : Practical Innovations, Open Solutions*, *14*, 29132–29144. DOI: 10.1109/ACCESS.2026.3664500

Nicora, G., Pe, S., Santangelo, G., Billeci, L., Aprile, I. G., Germanotta, M., Bellazzi, R., Parimbelli, E., & Quaglini, S. (2025). Systematic review of AI/ML applications in multi-domain robotic rehabilitation: Trends, gaps, and future directions. *Journal of Neuroengineering and Rehabilitation*, *22*(1), 79. DOI: 10.1186/s12984-025-01605-z PMID: 40205472

Nilsson, C. (2025). *The artificial intelligence (AI) competence paradox: how AI reshapes clinical expertise. Transforming Government: People*. Process and Policy.

Nisevic, M., Kulenovic, H., Milojevic, D., Levak, J., & Biasin, E. (2026). Regulatory challenges and liability pathways for AI-powered robots in EU medical practice. *AI & Society*, •••, 1–21. DOI: 10.1007/s00146-026-02869-2

Ohu, F. C., Burrell, D. N., & Jones, L. A. (2025, October). Public Health Risk Management, Policy, and Ethical Imperatives in the Use of AI Tools for Mental Health Therapy. [). MDPI.]. *Health Care*, *13*(21), 2721. PMID: 41228088

Olawade, D. B., Plabon, S. B., Ojo, A., Ogunbona, M. A., Makanjuola, B. D., & Olasilola, R. (2026). Human in the loop artificial intelligence in healthcare: Applications, outcomes, and implementation challenges. *International Journal of Medical Informatics*, *213*, 106362. DOI: 10.1016/j.ijmedinf.2026.106362 PMID: 41740273

Olawade, D. B., Weerasinghe, K., Teke, J., Msiska, M., Boussios, S., & Hatzidimitriadou, E. (2025). Evaluating AI adoption in healthcare: Insights from the information governance professionals in the United Kingdom. *International Journal of Medical Informatics*, *199*, 105909. DOI: 10.1016/j.ijmedinf.2025.105909 PMID: 40198930

Olusegun, J., Oluwaseyi, J., Brightwood, S., & Temitope, O. M. (2024). *Integration of AI with electronic health records: Enhancing clinical workflows*. John Olusegun.

Pe, S., Dagliati, A., Parimbelli, E., Guerra, B. M. V., Sozzi, S., Bellazzi, R., & Nicora, G. How improper dataset split hinders model generalizability: a systematic comparison in Human Activity Recognition and exercise evaluation tasks. *Available at SSRN* 6074128. DOI: 10.1016/j.ijmedinf.2026.106464

. Perez, A. G. (2026). Bridging the Gap: Overcoming Integration and Interoperability Challenges in Digital Healthcare Systems. *Digital Transformation: Accelerating Organizational Intelligence*, 131.

. Pingili, R. (2025). AI Workflow Optimization in Clinical and Regulatory Environments.

Rajendran, G., Buchholz, S., Aragam, B., Schölkopf, B., & Ravikumar, P. (2024). Learning interpretable concepts: Unifying causal representation learning and foundation models. *arXiv preprint arXiv:2402.09236.*

Ramesh, P. (2025). AI Workflow Optimization in Clinical and Regulatory Environments. *KOS J AIML, Data Sci. Robot*, *1*(1), 1–7.

. Rawlings Olowoniyi, H. Y., & Deshpande, L. (2026). Data Privacy and Security Considerations for AI Chatbots in Digital Healthcare Systems

Raza, S., Radwan, A., Chaduvula, S., Alinoori, M., & Emmanouilidis, C. (2026). *Transparency in Agentic AI: A Survey of Interpretability*. Explainability, and Governance.

. Rowe, M. (2019). Artificial intelligence in clinical practice: Implications for physiotherapy education. *OpenPhysio J*, 1-6.

Rowe, M., Nicholls, D. A., & Shaw, J. (2022). How to replace a physiotherapist: Artificial intelligence and the redistribution of expertise. *Physiotherapy Theory and Practice*, *38*(13), 2275–2283. DOI: 10.1080/09593985.2021.1934924 PMID: 34081573

Rudin, C., Chen, C., Chen, Z., Huang, H., Semenova, L., & Zhong, C. (2022). Interpretable machine learning: Fundamental principles and 10 grand challenges. *Statistic Surveys, 16*, 1-85. 6.

Şahinbaş, K., Keskin, A., & Akçakoca, Ö. (2026). *Development of a care plan recommendation system for physical therapy patients. Pamukkale Üniversitesi Mühendislik Bilimleri Dergisi*. Advanced Online Publication.

. Schneider, L., & Lawson, E. R. (2026). Human-in-the-Loop Governance Models for High-Risk Healthcare AI: Balancing Automation with Clinical Oversight.

Sengupta, D., & Panda, S. (2026). How Clinicians Think and What AI Can Learn From It. *arXiv preprint arXiv:2601.12547.*

. Shafik, W. (2026). Data Privacy Challenges in Artificial Intelligence-Driven Healthcare. *The Convergence of Federated Learning and Healthcare 5.0 and Beyond: A New Era of Intelligent Health Systems*, 67.

Shafik, W., Hidayatullah, A. F., Kalinaki, K., Gul, H., Zakari, R. Y., & Tufail, A. (2026). A systematic literature review on transparency and interpretability of AI models in healthcare: Taxonomies, tools, techniques, datasets, open research challenges, and future trends. *Health and Technology*, *16*(2), 1–22. DOI: 10.1007/s12553-025-01051-w

Sharma, A., & Rathore, R. (2026). Secure AI in healthcare: Advanced privacy-preserving machine learning techniques for medical data. In *Artificial Intelligence and Sustainable Innovation* (pp. 244–251). CRC Press.

Sharma, D., Meshkat, S., Perivolaris, A., Kamaleddin, M. A., Teferra, B. G., Rueda, A., & Bhat, V. (2026). Reimagining psychiatric care with agentic AI: Promise, challenges, and a roadmap forward. *npj. Digital Medicine*. PMID: 41699048

Shawli, L., Alsobhi, M., Chevidikunnan, M. F., Rosewilliam, S., Basuodan, R., & Khan, F. (2024). Physical therapists' perceptions and attitudes towards artificial intelligence in healthcare and rehabilitation: A qualitative study. *Musculoskeletal Science & Practice*, *73*, 103152. DOI: 10.1016/j.msksp.2024.103152 PMID: 39067366

Singh, R. P., Hom, G. L., Abramoff, M. D., Campbell, J. P., & Chiang, M. F. (2020). Current challenges and barriers to real-world artificial intelligence adoption for the healthcare system, provider, and the patient. *Translational Vision Science & Technology*, *9*(2), 45–45. DOI: 10.1167/tvst.9.2.45 PMID: 32879755

Smith, H., Downer, J., & Ives, J. (2024). Clinicians and AI use: Where is the professional guidance? *Journal of Medical Ethics*, *50*(7), 437–441. DOI: 10.1136/jme-2022-108831 PMID: 37607805

. Stevens, R. M., & Rivera, A. J. (2023). Human-in-the-Loop Safety Mechanisms for AI-Enabled Clinical Workflow Automation.

Strauss, A. T., Morgan, C., El Khuri, C., Slogeris, B., Smith, A. G., Klein, E., Toerper, M., DeAngelo, A., Debraine, A., Peterson, S., Gurses, A. P., Levin, S., & Hinson, J. (2022). A patient outcomes–driven feedback platform for emergency medicine clinicians: Human-centered design and usability evaluation of linking outcomes of patients (LOOP). *JMIR Human Factors*, *9*(1), e30130. DOI: 10.2196/30130 PMID: 35319469

Sunday, O. (2025). Behavioral Impacts of AI Reliance in Diagnostics: Balancing Automation with Skill Retention. *Epidemiol. Health Data Insights, 1*, ehdi014.

Tack, C. (2019). Artificial intelligence and machine learningl applications in musculoskeletal physiotherapy. *Musculoskeletal Science & Practice, 39*, 164–169. DOI: 10.1016/j.msksp.2018.11.012 PMID: 30502096

Taki, F. N., & Akdag, K. C. (2024). *Use of artificial intelligence in physiotherapy and rehabilitation. Current Studies in Basic Sciences, Engineering and Technology*. ISRES Publishing.

Thakral, M., Nagpal, V., Devare, A., Devare, M. H., Ghosal, I., & Irfan, M. (2026). Education and Training for the AI-Enabled Healthcare Workforce. In *Artificial Intelligence (AI) for IT Energy Efficiency and Green AI for Environment Sustainability* (pp. 69–84). Springer Nature Switzerland. DOI: 10.1007/978-3-031-89420-6_4

Theilmann, K., Dahlem, N., Steffny, L., Podevin, D., Hartnik, J., & Greff, T. (2025, June). Towards Effective AI in Healthcare: Identifying Success Factors and the Potential of Human-in-the-Loop. In *IFIP International Conference on Artificial Intelligence Applications and Innovations* (pp. 173-188). Cham: Springer Nature Switzerland. DOI: 10.1007/978-3-031-96239-4_13

Thurzo, A., & Thurzo, V. (2025). Embedding fear in medical AI: A risk-averse framework for safety and ethics. *AI*, *6*(5), 101. DOI: 10.3390/ai6050101

Topuz, K., Abdulrashid, I., Davazdahemami, B., Coussement, K., & Delen, D. (2025). Developing an Interpretable Decision Support Framework for Artifact Design in Organ Transplantation. *Information Systems Frontiers*, *27*(6), 1–25. DOI: 10.1007/s10796-025-10652-9

Truong, T. D. (2025). The Evolving Synergy between AI and Human Expertise in Medical Diagnostics.

Turgunov, J. S., Rakhimova, M. O., Saidov, B. K., & Kholmatova, D. S. (2020). HUMAN-IN-THE-LOOP SYSTEMS FOR ETHICAL AI.

Verma, A., Rao, K., Eluri, V., & Sharma, Y. (2020). Regulating AI in public health: systems challenges and perspectives. *ORF Occasional Paper, 261*, 1-46.

Wang, B., Qu, J., Li, X., Wang, C., & Bu, L. (2026). A personalized rehabilitation design method via knowledge graph-based multi-source data integration. *Advanced Engineering Informatics*, *69*, 104005. DOI: 10.1016/j.aei.2025.104005

Wang, P., Wang, A., & Wang, S. (2026). Integrating multimodal AI technologies for sports injury prediction and rehabilitation: Systematic review. *Journal of Human Sport and Exercise*, *21*(1), 22–37. DOI: 10.55860/w6j5wc21

Xian, T., Mehandjiev, N., Constantinides, P., Chen, Y. W., Quboa, Q., & Kitchen, G. (2026). Clinician preferences for explainable artificial intelligence in critical care: A comparative study of interpretable models and visualizations for intubation decision support. *International Journal of Medical Informatics*, •••, 106287. DOI: 10.1016/j.ijmedinf.2026.106287 PMID: 41570512

Xie, E., Zhao, Z., Yang, W., Li, X., Qi, L., Gao, M., Cao, Y., Fan, S., Pan, Y., & Gao, S. (2026). A plantar multi-parameter stimulation-feedback quantitative modeling framework for post-stroke gait rehabilitation. *Biomedical Signal Processing and Control*, *116*, 109461. DOI: 10.1016/j.bspc.2026.109461

Yao, Q., Qiu, B., He, L., Wang, Q., Zou, J., Liang, D., Wen, S., Liu, Y., Li, G., Hu, J., Ma, H., Huang, G., & Zeng, Q. (2026). Effects of Artificial Intelligence Recognition–Based Telerehabilitation on Exercise Capacity in Patients With Hypertension: Randomized Controlled Trial. *Journal of Medical Internet Research*, *28*, e81400. DOI: 10.2196/81400 PMID: 41529829

Zafar, Z., Ali, G., & Ali, T. (2026). DESIGNING TRUSTWORTHY CLINICAL DECISION SUPPORT SYSTEMS USING DEEP LEARNING AND HUMAN-IN-THE-LOOP VALIDATION. *Spectrum of Engineering Sciences*, *4*(1), 559–579.

Zand, J., Suvakov, M., Overgaard, S. M., Kozikowski, C. G., Jimison, R. C., Nelson, K. B., Silvano, C. J., Meiners, L. M., Fan, J. W., Schultz, K. E., Carter, R. E., Wieland, M. L., Patten, C. A., Dugani, S. B., Weis, J. A., Poe, J. D., Holmes, D. R.III, Griffiths, L. G., Dieter, H. L., & Garovic, V. D. (2026, January). Building artificial intelligence and data literacy across the health care research workforce in the Mayo Clinic Center for Clinical and Translational Science: Why it matters and what we are doing about it. [). Elsevier.]. *Mayo Clinic Proceedings*, *101*(1), 17–25. DOI: 10.1016/j.mayocp.2025.11.008 PMID: 41485858

Zhang, K., Wang, D., Lin, F., Xie, J., & Zhou, W. (2026). A Comprehensive Review of Explainable Artificial Intelligence in Healthcare Methods, Evaluation, and Clinical Integration. *iScience*, *29*(3), 115026. DOI: 10.1016/j.isci.2026.115026 PMID: 41858885

Zhao, C., & López, B. S. (2025). Translating Artificial Intelligence Algorithms into Clinical Practice: Addressing Implementation Barriers in Healthcare. *Frontiers in Emerging Computer Science and Information Technology*, *2*(07), 1–6.

Zhao, S., Hu, M., & Fang, S. (2026). Multimodal spatiotemporal graph convolutional attention network for dynamic risk stratification and intervention strategy generation in rare disease rehabilitation nursing. *Scientific Reports*, *16*(1), 6758. DOI: 10.1038/s41598-026-37095-9 PMID: 41617761

Zhu, T., Huang, Y., Pu, J., Wang, C., Ruan, M., Lu, P., Yang, X., Bao, N., Chen, Y., & Zhang, A. (2026). Evaluation of the Efficacy of an Artificial Intelligence-Based Assessment and Correction System in the Rehabilitation of Patients Following Anterior Cruciate Ligament Reconstruction Surgery. *Journal of Clinical Medicine*, *15*(2), 575. DOI: 10.3390/jcm15020575 PMID: 41598513

Chapter 11
Transforming Gestational Diabetes Management Through LLM-Enabled Multimodal Healthcare

R. Priyanka
http://orcid.org/0009-0006-1623-8496
SASTRA (Deemed to be) University, India

A. Sumathi
http://orcid.org/0000-0003-4700-5573
SRC, SASTRA (Deemed to be) University, India

S. Meganathan
http://orcid.org/0000-0003-4570-8259
SRC, SASTRA (Deemed to be) University, India

P. Umamaheswari
http://orcid.org/0000-0003-2007-697X
SRC, SASTRA (Deemed to be) University, India

R. Mathi
SRC, SASTRA (Deemed to be) University, India

ABSTRACT

The present report describes a multimodal approach to the management of gestational diabetes mellitus (GDM) using LLM-enabled technology. This approach will combine the use of Internet of Things (IoT) sensor data, electronic health record data, and patient-reported outcome data in a single integrated platform. The major

DOI: 10.4018/979-8-2600-2173-6.ch011

goals of this integrated solution are to improve clinical outcomes through continuous monitoring and real-time predictive analytics of GDM, to predict patient subtypes of GDM with increased accuracy, to provide personalized recommendations and decision support to GDM patients, and to enhance patient-centered care in managed maternal health services through an enhanced ability to provide access to GDM services and increase the number of women receiving quality care.

1. INTRODUCTION

Gestational diabetes mellitus (GDM) is defined as glucose intolerance first diagnosed during pregnancy. The prevalence of diabetes diagnosed during pregnancy continues to rise worldwide due in part to increasing rates of obesity, sedentary lifestyles, increasing age of mothers when delivering, and genetic predisposition resulting in a prevalence of approximately 10 to 20% of pregnancies. GDM has many maternal and fetal complications, such as preeclampsia, cesarean delivery, macrosomia, and long-term metabolic disorders. Current methods of diagnosing GDM, such as the oral glucose tolerance test (OGTT) or fasting plasma glucose (FPG), provide episodic laboratory-based testing with manual interpretation, leading to delayed diagnosis of GDM and a lack of continuity of care. Additionally, the traditional methods for assessing risk do not adequately account for the dynamic and complex nature of metabolic changes that occur during pregnancy. Recent advances in artificial intelligence (AI), particularly large language models (LLMs), will provide new opportunities for continuous monitoring, early prediction, and customized management of GDM through the integration of multimodal clinical and patient-generated data, leading to a more proactive, patient-centered approach in the delivery of maternal health care.

1.1 Gestational Diabetes Mellitus: Clinical Background

Gestational diabetes mellitus (GDM) describes an alteration in glucose control during pregnancy. Gestational diabetes mellitus (GDM) describes a disorder in glucose regulation that occurs in women during their pregnancy. The disorder is the end result of the cellular changes that occur within the maternal body as a result of the metabolic adjustments that occur during pregnancy, which are due to the increased energy needs for the growing fetus. In most cases, the altered glucose levels associated with GDM return to normal after delivery; however, many women with GDM will go on to develop type 2 diabetes mellitus (T2DM) or pre-diabetes and experience serious health problems associated with these two disorders. If health care providers wish to be able to provide effective data-based approaches to screening, diagnosing and providing individualized treatment for women with GDM, they must be familiar with the condition's pathology, risk factor profile, Diagnostic Criteria, and current evidence-based management strategies.

1.2 Physiological Adaptations and Pathophysiology of GDM

Metabolic changes occur during pregnancy to accommodate fetal growth and development. Early in pregnancy, in the first trimester, there is an increase in insulin sensitivity and therefore an increase in fat storage (due to the increase in peripheral tissue's ability to take in glucose). In the later trimesters, placentally derived hormones (such as HPL, estrogen, and progesterone) cause insulin resistance, which increases the availability of glucose to the fetus. In a normal situation, insulin production by the pancreas is increased to compensate for the increase in insulin resistance and to maintain normal glucose concentrations. However, when the pancreas fails to secrete enough insulin, it results in GDM, which is due to a combination of insulin resistance and insufficient or ineffective functioning of the β-cells. Other factors that may contribute to the development of GDM include obesity, inflammation, oxidative stress, changes in hormone levels, and gut microbiota. These are all mechanisms that are similar between GDM and type 2 diabetes, therefore indicating that there may be common underlying mechanisms of pathophysiology.

1.3 Diagnostic Criteria and Screening Practices

Guidelines on how to screen for and diagnose gestational diabetes mellitus (GDM) continue to be debated worldwide, as there are various guidelines being used by different countries. The predominant diagnostic method of choice is the oral glucose tolerance test (OGTT); it is usually conducted between 24-28 weeks of gestation. WHO, IADPSG, and ADA all have distinct levels of glucose recommendations as well as different types of screening procedures.There are two principal methods for screening GDM: the one-step approach, which utilizes an OGTT of 75 grams, and the two-step method that consists of first performing a glucose challenge test, followed by performing an additional OGTT to confirm results. While both of these methods provide healthcare professionals with uniform guidelines for diagnosing GDM, they are based upon specific periods where glucose levels are determined, meaning they may miss early or temporary elevations and drops. In addition, performing OGTT requires extensive time commitments of both the patient and healthcare provider; there are also many short-term variables, for example, stress, being sick, and food eaten. that affect test results.

1.4 Need for Advanced Clinical Intelligence

Because of the complexity of gestational diabetes mellitus (GDM), advancements in clinical knowledge, as well as methods that allow clinicians to monitor patients continuously, identify patients at higher risk quickly, and provide tailored treatment plans are essential. The use of digital health technologies such as mobile health applications and wearables will provide opportunities for continuous real-time data collection on GDM patients at an unprecedented level. Due to the amount and variability of data being produced, intelligent analytical frameworks are needed to derive actionable clinical insights from these data. Combining large language models with multimedia data collected from clinical sources would provide new means by which clinicians can address the limitations of traditional methods of treating GDM. A combination of physiological data and patient self-reported data (such as symptoms), clinical notes, and behavioural information would create a system that allows for proactive management through individualized and equitable delivery of maternal health care. To fully realize the potential of these AI-driven processes would require the development of a strong foundation in clinical practice to support meaningfully improving the way in which we deliver care to GDM patients.

2. LITERATURE SURVEY

Recent advancements in Artificial Intelligence (AI) and Internet of Things (IoT)-based healthcare have significantly improved diabetes management through the integration of multimodal data and advanced analytical frameworks. Studies up to 2025 demonstrate the application of deep learning models for analyzing heterogeneous data sources such as electronic health records (EHRs) and continuous glucose monitoring (CGM), while approaches incorporating knowledge graphs and named entity recognition (NER) enhance semantic representation and cross-domain clinical reasoning (Khalid et al., 2025; Panagoulias et al., 2025). However, the existing literature remains largely descriptive rather than critically comparative, with limited analysis of differences in methodologies, data modalities, and evaluation strategies across machine learning, deep learning, and emerging Large Language Model (LLM)-based approaches. While traditional models perform well on structured and time-series data, LLMs offer advantages in clinical text understanding and decision support but still face challenges in robust multimodal reasoning, particularly when integrating temporal physiological data with unstructured inputs (Choi and Raj, 2025). Moreover, most existing systems exhibit weak multimodal integration and rely on isolated data sources, limiting their ability to capture the complex interactions underlying metabolic changes. A significant research gap is observed in gestational diabetes mellitus (GDM), as the majority of AI-based frameworks focus on type 1 and type 2 diabetes without addressing the unique temporal and physiological characteristics of pregnancy or incorporating treatment-response dynamics. From an implementation perspective, several limitations persist, including the lack of prospective and multi-center validation, under-representation of low- and middle-income populations, concerns related to model calibration, bias, and fairness, and limited evidence of real-world clinical deployment and integration. These gaps highlight the absence of dedicated multimodal LLM-based frameworks tailored to maternal healthcare, and although recent studies (Gupta et al., 2025; Dao et al., 2024) indicate the potential of integrating LLMs with healthcare data, they do not fully address explainability, continuous monitoring, and clinical applicability, thereby emphasizing the need for a scalable, interpretable, and multimodal IoT–LLM framework

Table 1. Implementation Details of the Multimodal IoT–LLM Framework for GDM

Study	Population	Data Modalities	Model Type	Performance	Limitations
Khalid et al. (2025)	General diabetes cohort	EHR, CGM	Deep Learning (LSTM/CNN)	High accuracy (~85–90%)	Limited multimodal fusion, no GDM-specific focus
Panagoulias et al. (2025)	Clinical datasets	Text, structured data	Knowledge Graph + NER	Improved semantic reasoning	Complex implementation, limited scalability
Choi & Raj (2025)	Mixed patient cohort	Text, time-series	LLM-based model	Strong NLP performance	Weak multimodal reasoning, limited temporal modelling
Gupta et al. (2025)	Diabetes patients	Clinical data	ML/DL hybrid	Moderate (~80–85%)	No maternal/GDM-specific adaptation
Dao et al. (2024)	Healthcare datasets	Multimodal	AI framework	Promising results	Limited explainability, no real-world validation

3. AI APPLICATIONS IN MATERNAL HEALTH

The application of Artificial Intelligence to Maternal Health spans many areas including predicting risk, monitoring the fetus, providing diagnostic imaging and offering clinical decision support. Predictive models using electronic health record (EHR), information from antenatal visits, and laboratory testing have been created to determine which women are at greatest risk for developing gestational diabetes, hypertensive disorders, or having a premature delivery. The risk score that these predictive models produce allows for early interventions. Similarly in obstetric imaging, deep learning techniques have been successfully used to analyze ultrasound imaging to determine fetal biometric parameters, detect fetal anomalies, and accurately estimate gestational age. In addition to improving inter-observer variability and diagnostic consistency, AI-assisted interpretation of images is beneficial in low-resource settings where there are limited specialist resources. The benefits of AI integration into remote maternal monitoring via the use of wearable sensors and mobile health applications have made it possible for the continuous monitoring of heart rate, physical activity, sleep and glucose levels to support real-time evaluations of maternal well-being. AI-based algorithms can evaluate this information to identify deviations from normal physiological patterns and send alerts to both clinicians and patients.

Illustrative Clinical Scenario

A pregnant woman getting check-ups during her pregnancy has normal blood sugar levels at first. Between check-ups she starts feeling tired and really thirsty and her blood sugar levels go up and down. These symptoms are not picked up by tests. By the time a special test called OGTT is done at 26 weeks she is diagnosed with diabetes. The problem is her body had already started changing in ways that can cause trouble. A system that continuously monitors her blood sugar could have caught these changes earlier. This would have allowed doctors to help her sooner and reduce the risk of problems.

3.1 Machine Learning Approaches in GDM Prediction

In regards to predicting and diagnosing gestational diabetes mellitus, there has been an increase in the use of machine learning models to improve both of these. When compared to traditional statistical models applied to structured datasets, machine learning methods have been found to have greater sensitivity and specificity. Common variables that have been used to obtain predictions via machine learning include maternal age, body mass index (BMI), fasting blood glucose levels, family history of diabetes, and prior outcomes from childbirth. While the use of machine learning techniques for predicting GDM has provided a great deal of promise, there are several important barriers that exist regarding their use in predicting GDM. The majority of the models developed to date have utilized retrospective data collected at a single point in time during gestation and do not take into account the fact that individuals may experience changes in their metabolism throughout pregnancy or that the use of retrospective data limits the algorithms' ability to account for changes over time. Another significant barrier with the development of GDM prediction models is that the majority of studies focus on developing prediction models for the general population instead of developing individualized risk trajectories, thus limiting the clinical meaningfulness of the models and reducing their potential clinical value.

3.2 Emergence of Large Language Models in Clinical Intelligence

The introduction of Large Language Models (LLMs) have changed the way artificial intelligence (AI) systems are designed. LLMs are capable of understanding, generating, and reasoning in natural language as well as multimodal data. Unlike current generative AI and traditional machine learning or deep learning models developed for narrow-focused objectives; LLMs are pre-trained on countless sources of biomedical literature, clinical text, and real-life language data. The pre-training process allows an LLM to develop a wealth of semantic relationships and cultural context across many different domains.As it relates to maternal care; the LLM will produce significant benefits through its ability to connect structured clinical data to unstructured forms of human communication. An LLM can analyze physician's notes, laboratory reports, discharge summaries and patient narratives transforming unstructured text content into structured, computable insight. This capability is particularly critical to providing quality prenatal care as numerous symptoms, patterns of behaviour, and psychosocial issues are generally communicated verbally or written in an unstructured manner.

3.3 Multimodal Intelligence for Maternal Care

There are many different ways through which modern maternal healthcare provides data: electronic numerical data from clinical sensors, text-based clinical notes, digital medical imaging, and audio recordings. Proper integration of all of these disparate forms of data into a single analytical framework has been challenging in the past. However, large language models (LLMs), particularly when combined with machine vision and audio processing, provide the capacity for multimodal intelligence where contextual connections will be made across textual data, visual data, and audio data. For instance, glucose readings obtained via continuous glucose monitoring (CGM) could be utilized with a patient's self-reported dietary patterns and related clinical observations to provide a better overall understanding of a patient's metabolic functioning. This ability to reason through multiple modalities could improve early identification of gestational diabetes and the characterization of gestational diabetes subtypes, and allow continuous risk assessment during pregnancy.

3.4 Role of AI in Personalized and Equitable Maternal Healthcare

One primary aim of AI-driven maternal health care is to provide personalized care based on each individual's risk profile, personal preferences, and other contextual factors. With real-time data and patient feedback, AI systems can be used to provide personalized diet suggestions, exercise programs, and monitoring schedules. To improve access for marginalized populations who may have limited health literacy, AI also provides voice-based interfaces and supports multiple languages. AI's potential to reduce health disparities further includes its ability to provide clinical expertise in remote areas through the use of digital platforms. Clinical specialists will be able to conduct remote monitoring and help identify women at risk for having high-risk pregnancies, which will lead to timely referral or intervention. Equity in outcomes, however, will require attention to bias in data used by AI systems, to the cultural relevance of the AI-generated recommendations, and to ethical applications of the AI technologies.

3.5 Implications for GDM Management

By integrating AI into maternal health care, we are paving the way for better management of gestational diabetes through more than just diagnosis as needed but rather ongoing proactive management. Traditional machine learning (ML) has established the groundwork for predictive analytics; however, the limitations of these ML models highlight the need for systems that are more flexible, interpretable and aware of the context. Large Language Models (LLMs) can reason through many modalities and interact with humans, making them a major step in managing all aspects of complexity related to gestational diabetes (GDM). Thus, the transition from traditional AI to LLM-based intelligence establishes the theoretical basis for the multimodal internet of things (IoT)-LLM framework that will be presented later in this chapter.

4. LARGE LANGUAGE MODELS: CONCEPTS AND CAPABILITIES

Advances made by large language models in the field of artificial intelligence constitute some of the most significant advances in the history of computing. This transformative technological innovation is based on neural network architectures developed from large collections of text (and other types of) data, which allows them to understand and generate human-like responses to natural language inputs and reason over this information on a scale never before seen. As a result of their training, large language models are revolutionizing the way that machines access and utilize our collective knowledge. In medicine, and specifically in maternal health (eg, gestational diabetic mellitus), large language models have the potential to provide contextual reasoning based on multimodal data, as well as explainable decision support, for healthcare providers.

4.1 Foundations of Large Language Models

Probabilistic systems known as large language models (llm) that have been developed using deep learning to model the relationships between tokens (words, sub words, and symbols) from unstructured data via deep learning as compared to previous natural language processing methods, which relied on developed manually based on developed rules and feature engineering, are the three main categories of the various types of llm. LLM develops a unified model for the representation of concepts, syntax, semantics, and contextual meaning of text. In general, today's llm are built using transformer architecture that use self-attention mechanisms to enable the model to identify all types of relationships that occur throughout all the elements of a given piece of input material (regardless of the position in the text). LLM gains insight into long-range dependencies while understanding and interpreting very complex contextual material, which allows the model to be effective for analyzing clinical narratives, longitudinal patient records, and conducting multi-step reasoning in complicated medical circumstances.

4.2 Pretraining and Fine-Tuning Paradigms

Two stages define the learning process of LLMs: pretraining and fine-tuning. The LLM acquires core linguistic skills and factual knowledge as it is trained on vast numbers of general and scenario-specific texts during pre-training. In, for example, biomedical and clinical situations, pre-training can include scientific journals; clinical guidelines; electronic health record descriptions; and textbooks that allow the LLM to learn relevant vocabulary and concepts. When the LLM is fine-tuned, it adjusts the model (that was trained during pre-training) for the particular tasks it will perform such as predicting disease, summarising clinical results or interacting directly with patients. To fine-tune for GDM, the LLM can use curated data such as antenatal care records; log-book records of glucose monitoring; diagnostic tests; and patient-symptom questionnaires. Because of this process, the LLM develops more specialised reasoning about gestational physiology, metabolism; and obstetric decision-making but maintains its overall general understanding of language.

4.3 Contextual Reasoning and Knowledge Representation

A major benefit of LLMs when compared to traditional methods of machine learning is their ability to perform contextual reasoning. While traditional approaches consider the input(s) outside of a larger narrative, LLMs analyze and interpret input(s) within the context of the greater narrative in which they are located. This is particularly important in maternal health care, where clinical decision-making relies heavily on longitudinal trends in patient information, subtle descriptions of symptoms, and the interaction of various risk factors. For example, when presented with a statement from a patient such as "I have been feeling really tired and thirsty lately," an LLM is able to put this information into context (e.g. what is the patient's glucose variability currently, when is the patient due to deliver, what are the patient's dietary habits, what are the patient's prior risk factors, etc.). By making these connections to other variables, similar to how a human clinician would do, the LLM has the ability to derive clinically useful insights that may not otherwise be visible in data alone. By using contextual reasoning in this way, LLMs' outputs more closely resemble the reasoning that goes into the clinical decisions made by humans.

4.4 Multimodal Extensions of LLMs

Early LLMs used to be only able to handle text; however, multimodal learning allows you to handle all types of data combined, including text, images, sound, and numbers. When you combine language models with an optical or vision encoder, a speech recognition algorithm, and use multiple sensors, you can create a holistic or comprehensive view of very complex health data. Applied to GDM, a multimodal LLM could analyze the output from a continuous glucose monitor, the output of a wearable sensor, an ultrasound imaging report, clinical notes from your doctor, and your voice, all at the same time. By using all of the outputs together in a unified way, you will achieve an ultimately more accurate assessment of your risk for developing GDM, as well as a more personalized intervention that will include both objective physical signals, such as glucose levels, and subjective experiential information, such as how you are feeling about your pregnancy. Multimodal reasoning is particularly important to pregnancy care because of how much the phenotype, symptoms, behaviour, and emotional state of the patient can impact or play a significant role in metabolic regulation.

4.5 Natural Language Understanding and Generation in Clinical Settings

LLMs are proficient in both NLU and NLG therefore making it easier for patients, clinicians and intelligent systems overall to communicate smoothly. In clinical settings, LLMs can interpret unstructured text such as physician's notes, discharge summaries, laboratory interpretations, referral letters, etc. The LLMs can also extract relevant entities, determine clinical relationships, and convert free text into a structured representation that is acceptable for future analysis or use. The generative ability of an LLM is also essential; it enables LLMs to be able to create coherent context-driven pieces of text intended for a specific audience. For clinicians, for example, LLMs will be able to create short summaries, document potential differential diagnoses and provide evidence based treatment recommendations. Likewise, for patients, LLMs could explain in layman terms the findings/results from their clinical visit, provide lifestyle suggestions and interactively answer their questions about healthcare. This dual mode of communication enables clinicians and patients to have improved transparency, comprehension and sharing of the decision-making process in maternal/infant health care and treatment.

4.6 Explainability and Human-Centric AI

Explainability is crucial for healthcare AI systems. While many deep learning models function more like 'black boxes' than white books, LLMs offer natural language explanations of how they arrive at specific outputs (i.e., the reasoning process leading up to an output), allowing clinicians to build trust, validate their predictions or recommendations, and ultimately use the models as clinician tools or resources in their workflows. For example, in GDM management, examples may be to present factors that contributed to a prediction, such as a pattern of rising fasting glucose, reports of inconsistent diets, and rising insulin resistance markers, or other factors relevant to assessing the validity of the recommendation from the model. In addition, the principles of human-centred design stress the importance of collaborative relationships between AI systems and healthcare providers, thereby positioning LLMs as clinician decision-support systems and not as independent decision-makers.

4.7 Adaptability and Continuous Learning

The ability of LLMs to adapt is another significant feature of these models. Incremental learning and re-training allow LLM models to continue developing as new clinical evidence, guidelines, and population information become available. Maternal health care encompasses many different guidelines based on regionalization and patient demographics, so the adaptability of LLM systems provides for the relevance and responsiveness of knowledge to current evidence-based practice. The ability for LLM systems to assist with knowledge discovery of new trends, biomarkers, and/or treatment methods for GDM by performing a conclusive review of biomedical research literature also enables LLM to support the coupled process between research and clinical practice as a truly intelligent collaborator who enhances the capabilities of humans through innovation and collaboration.

4.8 Relevance of LLM Capabilities to GDM Management

LLMs have the potential to meet the conceptual and functional requirements of effective GDM management. The LLMs' ability to integrate multimodal data and perform reasoning in context with the data leads to natural forms of communication while providing explainable insights to the users; ultimately, these capabilities help to address the many shortcomings associated with traditional diagnostic and predictive models. As LLMs are integrated into IoT-enabled healthcare ecosystems, they facilitate continuous monitoring, support early detection of risk, provide classification of an individual's subtype, and enable the ability to develop an individualized care plan throughout the entire gestational period. As such, these capabilities position LLMs as a key technology that will provide the foundation for next-generation maternal health care systems. The Objectives & Scope of the Subsequent Section will establish a framework for predicting and classifying GDMs and individualizing care through an LLM and IoT.

5. GDM PREDICTION AND SUBTYPE CLASSIFICATION USING LARGE LANGUAGE MODELS

The accurate prediction and clinical significance of classification of GDM (gestational diabetes mellitus) are vital to improving maternal and fetal health outcomes. Most of the standard present criteria for testing for the presence of GDM utilize a binary system (positive or negative) based on glucose measurement at specific time points. Available clinical literature demonstrates that GDM should not be characterized as a single entity, but rather as several metabolic phenotypes that all have different risk factors and treatment responses. Utilizing large language models combined with multimodal clinical datasets is a powerful method for enhancing the early detection and precise subtype classification of gestational diabetes.

5.1 From Binary Diagnosis to Risk Trajectories

Classic methods used to evaluate GDM utilize an OGTT at the second trimester, with a goal of identifying dysglycemia once metabolic impairment has already occurred. In contrast, LLM-based approaches allow for longitudinal modeling of risk, as they continuously evaluate temporal data from multiple data streams throughout the pregnancy. Rather than providing a single label for diagnosis, the model produces individual risk trajectories that progress over time. Utilizing fasting glucose trends, postprandial variability trends, weight gain trends, and patient self-reported symptoms, LLM can detect small variations in physiology from the normal range for that time in a pregnancy. The use of a trajectory-based model supports earlier treatment and reduces the reliance on late-stage diagnostic criteria.

5.2 Feature Abstraction through Multimodal Reasoning

Typically, traditional ML models require explicit design of the features in use to create a usable output, whereas LLMs utilize representation learning as a means of creating their features implicitly. Any multimodal input, whether it be from numerical sensor data (e.g., continuous glucose monitor data), clinical notes (i.e., text documentation of patient encounters), food log documentation, or voice interaction, will be converted to contextual embeddings that account for both the semantic meaning and the temporal meaning of each modality. This allows LLMs to combine multiple modalities as inputs to the model and manage the input data across different modalities. For example, a continuous glucose monitor (CGM) record could have different interpretations based on other sources of information (e.g., "skipped meals" or "increased fatigue"). Therefore, the CGM data could provide context regarding the behaviours that contributed to the uncertainty in glycemic control. This comprehensive feature abstraction process allows LLMs to provide more accurate and clinically relevant predictions than does modelling using structured inputs only.

5.3 Early Prediction of GDM Onset

One of the main objectives of predicting GDM early is to facilitate timely lifestyle interventions that may slow or halt disease progression for many women. With prediction models that rely on LLMs' identified latent profile patterns, predictive models can estimate how likely a woman is to develop GDM (based on a combination of static measures such as her age and BMI), as well as dynamic gestation data collected as her symptoms change and develop. The predictive process involves recognizing latent glucose variance, insulin resistance surrogate measures, and the progression of symptoms. The LLM then places these patterns in the context of gestational weeks at the time and each woman's baseline profile to make a personalized risk estimate. The model also conveys uncertainty and probability level in natural language, providing support for making informed clinical decisions.

5.4 Subtype Classification of Gestational Diabetes Mellitus

Recent studies have shown that there are multiple subtypes of gestational diabetes mellitus (GDM) based on different metabolic features and their underlying causes. The major subtypes include insulin-resistant GDM, insulin-deficient GDM, and GDM with a combination of these features. It is important for clinicians to identify the subtype of GDM in order to provide appropriate lifestyle and medication recommendations. The use of machine learning algorithms (MLAs) offers a unique opportunity for characterizing patients into the subtype of GDM that they may fit into. MLAs can analyze large amounts of data from a variety of sources (clinical data, laboratory results, demographic data, and other information) and classify patients based on their metabolic profile. For example, elevated fasting blood sugar levels with minimal increase in sugars after meals may suggest insulin resistance. Alternatively, rapid increases in blood suggest that there is an underlying insulin-secretory defect. Other clinical information would include lab data related to ketonuria or significant hypoglycemic response to dietary changes.

5.5 Explainable Subtype Inference

One major benefit of LLM-based classification is its explainability. Instead of solely providing perplexing labels, this model outputs descriptive text to describe how a particular subtype was determined. This descriptive text may describe, among other things, the trend in glucose levels that were recorded, symptoms that were reported, or clinical observations made that resulted in determination of that subtype. The information in these descriptions can provide actionable insights for clinicians. For example, if the clinician observed a patient with evidence of persistent fasting hyperglycemia plus a very limited response to exercise plus a family history of metabolic disorders, the descriptor for that patient could state they have an insulin resistant subtype.Providing clinicians with clear reasoning allows for clinician trust and are utilized to facilitate shared decisions with patients.

5.6 Adaptive and Personalized Prediction Models

As the pregnancy progresses, women experience a variety of different metabolic changes that can be unpredictable. Adaptive learning algorithms (such as those that use large language models (LLMs)) continuously adjust their predictive accuracy based on the latest data about a given patient as they become available. Continuous improvement in the risk assessment process will produce better quality and more relevant individual assessments for each pregnant woman. A critical step toward producing an accurate individual risk assessment for the pregnant woman is to adjust the risk estimate for each pregnant women according to the woman's individual baseline data and her individual context (for example, two women who have the same blood glucose level when measured will have different individual risk assessments depending upon their respective gestational ages, symptom context, and historical trends with respect to their blood glucose level). Providing these types of individualized risk assessments allows for the development of an individualized treatment plan for each pregnant woman, in accordance with the ongoing development of precision medicine principles.

5.7 Integration with Clinical Decision Support

All of the prediction and classification outputs created by the LLM will be directly integrated into the clinical decision support workflow. The LLM output, when used in conjunction with the clinical decision making process, assists clinicians in the management of low-risk patients with lifestyle modifications and continued follow-up, as well as high-risk patients or patients with insulin resistance, with a referral to a specialist (if needed) for either pharmacological intervention (if needed) or both. The LLM does not replace the clinician; it provides additional information to the clinician, which the clinician can use in addition to his/her own clinical judgment in determining the appropriate course of action for each patient. By working together, the LLM and clinician will help to improve the efficiency and effectiveness of the clinician's practice while allowing the clinician to maintain his/her clinical judgment.

5.8 Evaluation and Validation Considerations

LLM model predictive systems will need to be thoroughly evaluated for safety, accuracy and fairness prior to being used in clinical practice. Performance measures of LLM model predictions include sensitivity, specificity, predictive value, and calibration for different populations. An essential part of an LLM model's evaluation needs to be the external validation of its generalizability using multiple datasets from various centres. Long-term monitoring of LLM model performance, including bias and drift due to changing demographics or clinical practices, will be crucial. Providing transparent documentation regarding the limitations and uncertainty of LLM models will encourage responsible use of LLM models in the clinic.

5.9 Implications for Proactive GDM Management

By enabling early prediction and nuanced subtype classification, LLM-based systems support a shift toward proactive GDM management. Early identification of at-risk patients allows for timely intervention, reducing the incidence of severe hyperglycemia and associated complications. Subtype-specific insights guide tailored treatment strategies, improving both efficacy and patient experience.

6. IMPLEMENTATION OF THE MULTIMODAL IOT–LLM FRAMEWORK FOR GDM

This chapter outlines how we built the multimodal IoT-LLM framework for GDM. This includes a system design, data flows, and model integrations, as well as ways to deploy the model and make it work in real life (clinical and remote). The intention is to create a system that is scalable, secure, and supports clinical use by translating from the conceptual architecture to an implementation.

6.1 System Architecture and Deployment Overview

This implementation has been made modular and follows service-oriented architecture principles to allow scaling, flexibility, and integration with the current healthcare infrastructure. The solution is based on a hybrid edge-cloud deployment, in that the edge (wearable devices, mobile apps) will handle data collection/initial processing, and higher-level analytics and reasoning will be handled in the cloud with services provided by various LLM providers. The system has four main components: IoT-enabled and mobile interfaces for patients, A data ingestion/preprocessing pipeline,A reasoning and analytics engine that utilizes an AI language model, A decision support and clinical dashboard interface. This tiered design allows updates to sensing devices, models, and user interfaces to occur independently from each other and still provide a complete working solution. Implementation of an LLM-Driven Multimodal System for GDM Prediction and Subtype Stratification

6.2 Overview of the Implementation Strategy

The proposed system will enable the application of largescale machine learning algorithms to predict the future course of a person's condition, subtype classifications of GDM, and provide personalized care for women with GDM. To accomplish these goals, the system is designed to be multimodal and human-centered, including continuous monitoring of physiologic variables using wearable sensors (wristbands, smartwatches, etc.), as well as collecting patient-rated symptoms through voice-based reporting and clinical records of treatment response. While the majority of traditional machine learning algorithms rely exclusively on structured numerical data from the medical record, this system will leverage the context-specific reasoning capabilities of LLMs to interpret heterogeneous data sources and support the clinician's ability to make meaningful clinical decisions.In addition, the system will focus on early identification of risk factors associated with GDM, real time and dynamic evaluation of disease progression, and therapy-aware subtype classification by including a level of clinician supervision and ethical oversight.The framework shows how multimodal patient data, such as sensor data, clinical data, medical images, and reports, is integrated into a cloud-based system where Large Language Models (LLMs) are used for multimodal analysis. The framework enables risk prediction, decision support, personalized therapy, and population health insights.This section described the implementation of a multimodal IoT–LLM framework for gestational diabetes management. In simple terms, the system continuously collects patient data through wearable devices, voice inputs, and clinical records, processes and integrates this information, and uses advanced AI models to generate personalized risk predictions and recommendations. These insights are presented to clinicians through an interactive dashboard and to patients through user-friendly mobile or voice interfaces. Overall, the framework aims to improve early detection, support clinical decision-making, and enable continuous, personalized care.

Figure 1. LLM-Enabled Multimodal Analysis Framework for GDM

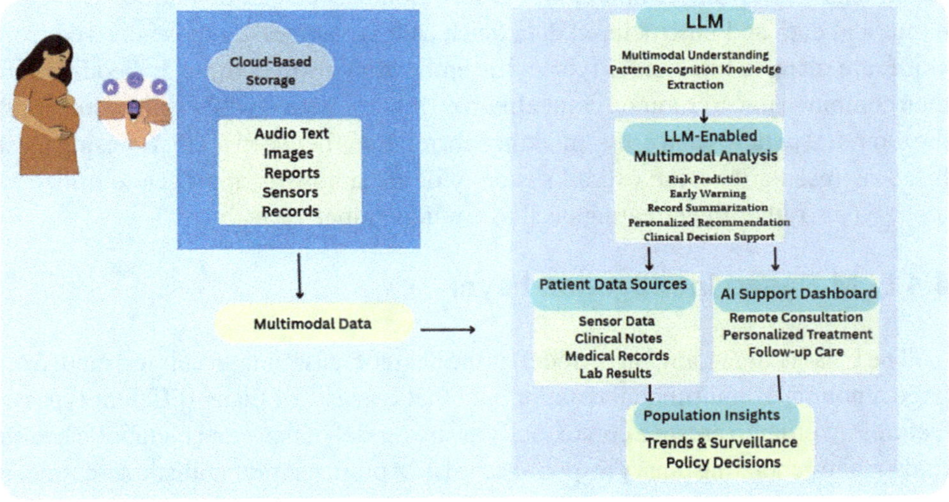

6.3 Data Acquisition Layer - Wearable Sensor Data Collection

An integrative infrastructure has been created specifically for the purpose of providing mother and child health care resources through an edge-cloud architecture consisting of multi-layered hybrid systems and five components. The five layers are: Collecting Data, Multimodal Processing, LLM-based Knowledge, Support for Clinical Decisions, Feedback, Learning & Governance. This modular framework supports both upward and downward scaling, as well as the capacity to integrate seamlessly into the current networks/systems while maintaining compatibility with other existing infrastructures. Voice-based symptom capture represents a major innovation in this implementation. Pregnant women can verbally report symptoms (e.g., fatigue, excessive thirst/hunger, dizziness, sleep disturbance, and stress/emotional discomfort). Symptoms will be processed as voice inputs through speech-to-text modules and transmitted to the LLM for semantic interpretation. This innovation reduces barriers to literacy, increases patient engagement, and captures subjective indicators about health that are often not captured in structured clinical records. Clinical data are obtained from hospital systems and include: Antenatal visit records, Laboratory reports (OGTT, HbA1c), Medication prescriptions (diet control, oral agents, insulin), Injection dosage changes, and treatment timelines. Treatment-response data are particularly critical, as they provide insight into underlying metabolic phenotypes. Preceding the analysis phase, every data stream will go through preprocessing to guarantee high-quality output and alignment: Elimination of noise and smoothing on sensors, Processing of either missing or out-of-order readings, normalization of physiology values, and temporal synchronization between all modalities. Structure numerical data and unstructured data (such as text), as well as those derived from voice, are mapped into modality-specific embedding forms. These embeddings are then combined into a common contextualized representation while maintaining both the temporal patterns and cross-modality correlations between them. By using these fused representations, the overall system will use a holistic approach to utilize all input types; rather than treating each as a unique input.

6.4 LLM-Based Intelligence Layer

The LLM (Large Language Model) is the heart of reasoning, receiving input from large amounts of multimodal data, or data that consists of many different types of features, in order to create a contextually aware model of maternal metabolic health. Rather than generating binary responses, the LLM produces probabilistic assessments of risk that change over time during pregnancy(the gestational period). Examples of patterns that the LLM can identify include: An increase in fasting glucose levels is coupled with a corresponding decrease in physical activity. Nighttime glucose variability is associated with nighttime sleep disturbance. A measure of symptom severity(e.g.using voice). This capability gives the LLM the ability to predict the risk of gestational diabetes (GDM) at an earlier stage than through traditional means of intervention (e.g., blood testing).

6.5 GDM Subtype Prediction Using Treatment Response using Hugging Face

Therapy-response aware subtype classification is a new part of the implementation. It looks at how patients respond to different interventions. Adequate glucose control using diet and exercise is likely GDMA1. Poor response to lifestyle changes, insulin-resistant phenotype. Rapid reduction of glucose with low doses of insulin, insulin-deficient phenotype. Partial/inconsistent response, mixed subtype. The LLM uses timelines of medications given, dosage changes, and physiologic response to make type inferences for the most frequent subtype. This type will resemble clinical reasoning, therefore increasing the ability to personalize the quality of care provided. The proposed system was implemented using the Hugging Face platform to provide an interactive and accessible interface for gestational diabetes mellitus (GDM) prediction. A web-based application was developed and deployed via Hugging Face Spaces, enabling users to input relevant clinical parameters and obtain predictive insights in real time. The implementation integrates machine learning components with a user-friendly front end, facilitating ease of use for both healthcare practitioners and patients. The deployed model supports rapid inference and demonstrates the practical applicability of the proposed framework in real-world scenarios.

The Platform is Accessible Through these Links:

1. https://huggingface.co/spaces/PriyankaRajaSRC/GDM_Predictingapp?logs=build
2. https://huggingface.co/spaces/PriyankaRajaSRC/gdmhighrisksmartmonitoring

Figure 2. GDM Monitoring Application Interface on Hugging Face

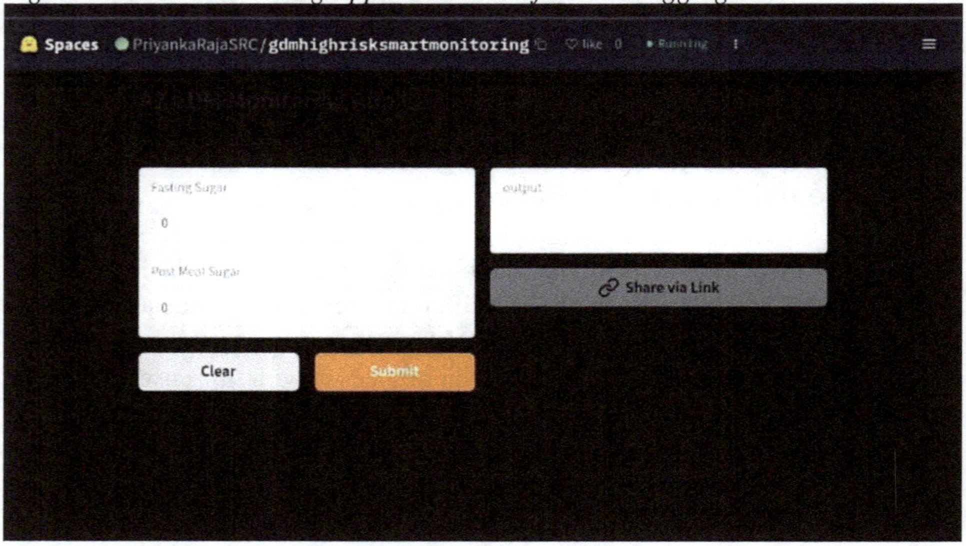

Figure 3. GDM Prediction Application Interface on Hugging Face

6.6 Explainable Intelligence Generation

The explanations supported the clinicians' confidence and confidence in the LLM by providing explicit examples of observed patterns, presenting symptoms, and describing the treatment outcomes associated with the risk rating and subtype assignment. Therefore, producing clear rationales for risk ratings rather than producing opaque predictions.

6.6.1 Clinical Decision Support Layer

A dashboard that is interactive for clinicians to communicate using their own secure account will display: A long-term glucose trend, A risk trajectory that is dynamically changing, a likelihood of which subtype category you belong to, an alert message, and an explanation produced by an LLM. The system is therefore an aide to decision-making by clinicians and is not a stand-alone decision maker. Thus, clinicians will always have the option of confirming, changing, or rejecting any recommendation made by the system.

6.6.2 Clinician Dashboard

Through mobile or voice over internet communication, we can get our patients personalized recommendations around the following: Diet and exercise advice, Reminders to monitor things, Early warning signs of potential problems with trends, Learning information in plain language. The recommendations change according to current data and patient input.

6.6.3 Personalized Patient Guidance

Mobile or voice interfaces provide every patient with personalized guidance about things like diet and how much activity to do, along with reminders to monitor progress, early alerts for unusual trends, and simple explanations of what everything means. Personalization continues to change over time through feedback from both patients and providers through the use of other health-related data.

6.6.4 Feedback Loop and Adaptive Learning

The system uses a continuous cycle of feedback to do the following: Support clinician decision-making through refined interpretation of the model, Support updated risk trajectory based on patient success and adherence, Support updated recommendations based on new incoming data. This adaptive system provides a way for the model to continuously provide relevant recommendations while taking into account the stage of pregnancy and changing clinical circumstances.

6.6.5 Security, Privacy, and Ethical Safeguards

Due to the nature of maternal health data being sensitive, the implementation will have: End-to-end encryption, role-based access controls; Secure authentication methods, and audit logs that will ensure accountability. When necessary, privacy-preserving strategies (i.e., edge inference, federated learning) could be used to help reduce the amount of data exposed centrally.

6.6.6 Real-World Deployment Considerations

This system is designed to be implemented in:

- Hospitals and outpatient facilities
- Community health clinics
- Telemedicine facilities and rural healthcare settings.

Voice-based communication combined with mobile integration is suitable for use in lower-resource settings; however, the cloud's scalable architecture enables support for a larger population base.

6.7 Potential Failure Modes and Implementation Risk Analysis

To implement LLM- and IoT-based systems for managing gestational diabetes, it is important to address potential risks associated with the system. For example, wearable and glucose monitoring device data may be unreliable because of poor calibration, device malfunctioning, or improper usage; thus, all three of these issues could lead to inaccurate risk assessment. In addition, data from multiple modalities (sensor data, clinical data, and patient input) need to be properly aligned in time otherwise it would be impossible to interpret correctly.Also, errors related to using Large Language Models (LLMs) include the misinterpretation of data and the generation of plausible but incorrect explanations. Furthermore, bias in the training data may reduce LLM effectiveness across various populations and there may be a variety of technical challenges (network delays, reliance on the cloud, limited connectivity [particularly in rural areas]) that will affect real-time monitoring.Additionally, user factors such as low digital literacy and inaccuracies in voice recognition affect data reliability and usability. Moreover, there are privacy and security considerations that will require strong encryption and access controls. The challenges of addressing model drift, scalability, interoperability, and transparency and fairness are critical to maintaining safe, effective, and fair maternal health care. Overall, it will take a well-designed, user-friendly, and cost-effective framework for providing safe, reliable and fair maternal health care.

6.8 Implementation and Health-System Considerations

A multimodal IoT framework using an LLM to help manage gestational diabetes (GD) should provide a seamless integration with existing healthcare systems without adding additional work for clinicians. Clinicians such as obstetricians and diabetologists can use the multimodal IoT framework to monitor glucose trends, determine risk status, and identify types of GD, while nurses can use the framework to support patient adherence. Support will be provided by technical teams to ensure the performance and reliability of the system. Successful implementation of this framework includes structured change management strategies, such as clinician training, pilot testing and user input. For example, cost of devices, limited internet access and lack of smartphones (especially in resource-limited settings) can be addressed through low-cost sensors, offline data storage, and multi-lingual voice interfaces. The framework should also be user-friendly and culturally appropriate for a variety of populations.Proper documentation of AI-generated recommendations is important for accountability, and clinicians must retain oversight of recommendations for all AI-generated recommendations in cases where their recommendations contradict current or approved guidelines. The integration of the framework with other existing systems can be accomplished by utilizing standards, such as FHIR and HL7 in order to provide interoperability. In addition to GD, the multimodal IoT framework may also be used to support long-term monitoring for individuals to identify and prevent T2 diabetes. Therefore, the multimodal IoT framework should also be practical, cost-effective, and aligned with real-world clinical needs to improve care for mothers

6.9 Usage Scenarios and Problem–Solution Mapping

The proposed IoT framework, utilizing LLM technology, creates an effective and accessible modality for delivering healthcare to multiple populations across different geographical areas. In rural clinics, the wearables and mobile applications utilized by pregnant women in developing nations are used to monitor trends in glucose, activity, and sleep, and symptom reporting is accomplished through voice interfaces and in their local language. With connectivity to the cloud, the data can be analyzed by the LLMs deployed in the cloud to issue early identifiers of risk; thus, providing timely and appropriate referrals for care, and optimising patient care in many areas where little or no care is available. In tertiary care hospital facilities, the IoT framework acts as a clinical decision-support tool to support clinicians in making decisions. Clinicians will have access to dashboards that provide data regarding the patient's continuous glucose trend, GDM subtype classification, and risk predictions that they can explain to their patients. This allows the LLM to integrate both existing HIE and treatment data to support personalized and therapy-aware evidence-based medicine and support clinicians in making better and more timely decisions. By addressing five critical gaps in traditional models of care (i.e. continuous vs. episodic testing, automated vs. manual data analysis, subtype focused versus traditional methods of treatment, accessibility vs. lack of accessibility to health information, and explainability of insights across all three LLM strata) using IoT technologies, this framework fills the gap between the research community and the clinical community for the treatment of GDM.

6.10 From Prototype to Practice: Key Implementation Milestones

Building a LLM-enabled multimodal Internet of Things (IoT) system for gestational diabetes will take a phased approach. In phase one, a system will be built and internally validated using historical data to assess the model's accuracy, quality, and robustness of data. Once built and validated, pilot testing will occur in controlled clinical environments to determine usability, dependability, and acceptance, and to identify areas requiring improvement and challenges related to operations.Phase two comprises prospective, multicenter studies designed to assess the generalizability, fairness, and clinical efficacy of the system among different populations with respect to key performance indicators. Phase three represents scaling of the then-validated system out to other healthcare networks, including community clinics and telemedicine. Considerations for phase three include interoperability and data management capabilities.Phase four includes establishing governance procedures, such as those dealing with data privacy protection and bias monitoring of the system, and routine/ ongoing updating of the system. Finally, training for clinicians and patient education will also be necessary to promote adoption of the system as an actionable and clinically impactful gestational diabetes solution.

6.11 Case Vignettes- Case 1: Rural Antenatal Care Setting

A twenty six year old pregnant woman who lives in an area and does not have easy access to laboratory facilities is signed up for the system using a mobile-based interface and a low-cost wearable device. The device keeps track of her health. Finds out that her fasting glucose levels are going up little by little. At the time she is not as physically active as she used to be and she tells the system that she is feeling tired through voice input. The system realizes that the pregnant woman is at a risk of getting gestational diabetes before it would have been found out by regular checks. A community healthcare worker is told about this. The pregnant woman is sent for more tests and to get help early. Finding out about this early helps prevent problems and reduces the need for emergency care, which shows how useful the system is, in areas where resources limited.

6.12 Scalability Across Healthcare Settings

The new healthcare system is made to work in different places. It can be used in healthcare systems especially in places where they do not have a lot of money. In these places they can use wearable devices, phones to monitor patients and voice commands to make it easy to use without needing a lot of equipment. In hospitals or special care places the system can work with advanced computer systems and high-end devices to help with hard cases and very specific care. The system can also be used for telemedicine, which helps people who live away or do not have access to good healthcare. The system is made up of parts so it can be changed to fit the needs of each place the people who live there and what the hospital needs. This means it can be used in public health programs or in special clinics. The healthcare system is very flexible which means it can work in different situations like, in a big hospital or a small clinic and it can be changed to fit the needs of the people who use it like the patients and the doctors.

6.13 Key Messages for Clinicians and Managers

With continuous and multi-modal monitoring there is an earlier and more accurate detection of gestational diabetes, whilst using LLM-based systems provides better clinical decision-making by having all of your data sources available in one place allowing for more personalised maternal care through the use of advanced models with disease sub-types. The explainable outputs promote trust between the doctor and the patient promoting the wider uptake of such technologies. The user-friendly mobile and voice interfaces will increase patient engagement and improve accessibility to the delivery of care. These systems are designed to support scalability within multiple healthcare systems, from hospitals and acute clinics to home and other remote locations. Ultimately, clinicians will continue to play a central role in ensuring that these technologies are being utilised safely and responsibly.

6.14 Real-World Validation, Cost-Effectiveness, and Implementation Challenges

While the potential of multimodal systems (LLM-enabled) is great for managing gestational diabetes (GDM), evidence to support their use based on rigorous, real-world validation or feasibility should be collected before implementing them clinically. To achieve reliability, generalization of results, and clinical effectiveness, more prospective and multi-center trials will need to be conducted, as the majority of the current body of research informing LLM- multimodal systems is retrospective.Cost and infrastructure issues continue to be a major barriers, especially in low-resource settings, although it is possible that the long-term costs associated with providing LLM- multimodal systems could be outweighed by their overall benefits. Other barriers, such as limited connectivity and access to devices and digital illiteracy, require consideration when developing scalable, user-friendly, and context-aware solutions.Additionally, the successful implementation of LLM- multimodal systems will depend on patient acceptance, clinician training, and trust in AI. Ethical and legal aspects of LLM- multimodal systems, including data privacy, responsibility, and regulatory compliance, will need to be addressed before LLM- multimodal systems can be used effectively.In conclusion, overcoming these barriers is critical to translating the LLM- multimodal systems framework into a scalable, sustainable, real-world care solution to improve the management of GDM.

6.15 Balancing Technological Opportunities with Clinical and System-Level Challenges

The LLM-based multimodal framework will vastly improve management of gestational diabetes; however, the potential adoption of this innovation may be constrained by real-world challenges such as clinician resistance due to concerns regarding accuracy, interpretability, and disruption of workflow, all of which indicate a need for trust, training, and gradual integration into routine clinical care. In addition, protecting sensitive health information will require strong governance of data privacy and security risks. The integration of multimodality into the existing healthcare delivery system continues to be challenging, particularly in low-resource locations, where standardization and interoperability are often lacking. Other barriers include limited access to devices, low connectivity rates, and poor digital literacy. In addition, there are concerns from the clinician's perspective; there is an over-reliance on the AI model, and there is not enough generalizability to negate the need for the clinician to remain part of the process. Overall, while the potential impact of LLM-based multimodality is great, successful implementation will require addressing challenges associated with technology, ethics, and infrastructure in order to ensure that the use of LLM-based multimodality in clinical practice is safe, equitable, and sustainable.

Linking the Conceptual Framework to Real-World Application- As a result, the multimodal IoT–LLM framework goes beyond just being a conceptual model; it is clear that it demonstrates considerable clinical use in the real world when managing gestational diabetes (GDM). By integrating both patient information and wearable sensor data, it enables clinical personnel to monitor their patients continuously and to identify when patients experience metabolic abnormalities during pregnancy in a timely manner. The multimodal approach taken in the framework allows for the use of LLM algorithms to assess the risk of developing gestational diabetes and to evaluate the various subtypes of gestational diabetes through real-time risk assessment and void to facilitate timely and effective interventions and improve glycemic control. The clinical decision support component of the framework provides additional efficiencies to clinical personnel by providing interpretable evidence to assist in their practice and by alleviating some of the burden on clinical personnel. Furthermore, the framework provides mobile and voice options for patients so that by making it easier to access and maintain their health, even in low-resourced environments. In summary, the multimodal IoT-LLM framework is a scalable and adaptable solution for both population-based and individualized care and has the potential to dramatically improve the outcomes of women with gestational diabetes.

7. CONCLUSION

Gestational Diabetes Mellitus (GDM) is a major public health issue and has a long-lasting impact on both mothers and children. Most contemporary clinical management of GDM consists of reactive approaches that do not reflect the multifaceted and dynamic metabolic changes associated with pregnancy. Therefore, there is a need to develop proactive and personalized models for GDM management. This chapter illustrates how LLMs can help improve GDM management by providing an integrated digital framework that uses continuous streams of physiological data, clinical data, and patient-reported data to enable an informed and holistic understanding of patients with GDM, early prediction of risk for GDM, and personalized interventions for GDM, including ongoing precision-based monitoring as opposed to episodic clinical diagnosis. Additionally, the framework promotes human-centered design principles by leveraging explainable output formats, natural language conversational interfaces, and inclusive design considerations (e.g., multilingual and voice-based output) to improve trust in clinicians and the level of engagement by patients with GDM. Furthermore, specific attention should be given to ethical, privacy, and regulatory issues during the development and implementation process. Despite challenges such as data quality and validation, emerging advances in AI offer promising opportunities to enhance scalability, accuracy, and inclusiveness. Ultimately, LLM and IoT integration represent a significant step toward intelligent, proactive, and equitable maternal healthcare, with the potential to improve outcomes for both mothers and future generations.

REFERENCES

Choi, H. J., & Raj, S. (2025). Episode-Driven Insights: Can Large Language Models Tackle Multimodal Diabetes Data? medRxiv, 2025-04. DOI: 10.1101/2025.04.24.25326385

Dao, D., Teo, J. Y. C., Wang, W., & Nguyen, H. D. (2024, June). Llm-powered multimodal ai conversations for diabetes prevention. In Proceedings of the 1st ACM Workshop on AI-Powered Q&A Systems for Multimedia (pp. 1-6). DOI: 10.1145/3643479.3662049

Gupta, G. K., Acharya, N., & Pande, P. (2025). LLM-Based Support for Diabetes Diagnosis: Opportunities, Scenarios, and Challenges with GPT-5. arXiv preprint arXiv:2509.21450.

Khalid, S., Kim, H., & Kim, H. S. (2025). Recent trends in diabetes mellitus diagnosis: An in-depth review of artificial intelligence-based techniques. *Diabetes Research and Clinical Practice*, *224*, 112221. DOI: 10.1016/j.diabres.2025.112221 PMID: 40328407

Panagoulias, D. P., Palamidas, A., Virvou, M., & Tsihrintzis, G. A. (2025). A framework for evaluation and requirement extraction for fine-tuning of Large Language Models in multimodal medical diagnosis. *Knowledge-Based Systems*, *326*, 113975. DOI: 10.1016/j.knosys.2025.113975

Chapter 12
Hybrid Soft Set and Manifold Learning Frameworks for Diabetes Risk Classification and Visualization

D. Rajalakshmi
http://orcid.org/0000-0003-4851-7685
Srinivasa Ramanujan Centre, SASTRA (Deemed to be) University, Kumbakonam, India

Durga Karthik
http://orcid.org/0000-0003-3199-8814
Srinivasa Ramanujan Centre, SASTRA (Deemed to be) University, Kumbakonam, India

P. Umamaheswari
http://orcid.org/0000-0003-2007-697X
Srinivasa Ramanujan Centre, SASTRA (Deemed to be) University, Kumbakonam, India

ABSTRACT

The growing complexity of healthcare datasets demands new hybrid machine learning frameworks for precise prediction of diabetes risks. In this chapter, we present a hybrid model that combines a soft set–based decision-region feature selector with Principal Component Analysis (PCA) and Uniform Manifold Approximation and Projection (UMAP) for visualization and dimensionality reduction. The model merger of uncertainty-aware feature engineering and nonlinear manifold learning

DOI: 10.4018/979-8-2600-2173-6.ch012

aims to enhance classification performance and interpretability. Several hybrid model configurations are analysed through accuracy metrics, confusion matrices, and visual analysis. The results confirm that nonlinear hybrid models are capable of improving class discriminability and predictive performance, thereby suggesting that hybrid pre- processing models are a promising avenue for intelligent healthcare analytics and data-driven clinical decision support.

1. INTRODUCTION

The chronic illness diabetes has contributed massively to global health challenges, as well as expenses incurred to manage diabetes on a global scale. The vast number of diabetes cases shows the need to develop intelligent systems that predict, assist clinicians prioritize patients, and create personalized treatment plans for patients. The traditional and standard statistics fail to identify and capture complex non-linear relationships that are present in biomedical datasets. This makes it essential to use more sophisticated forms of machine learning and data classification. The context of keeping the classification, it is a must to use dimensional reduction and feature selection methods. This is essential in simplifying the classification.

Certain medical datasets, like those with information about the risk of diabetes, tend to have a lot of dimensions, measurements that contain lots of irrelevant information, and data that contain a lot of repeating information. Many variables in the clinical world only contribute to the decision-making process in a fairly minor way, while some variables when selected, may introduce bias or cause overfitting. So, the development of different strategies to carry out feature selection is important to focus on the variables that carry the most information about the underlying patterns of the disease. Of the different strategies that can be used, Soft Set Theory is being used increasingly frequently, and for a very powerful reason: It can deal with uncertainty without the need for specific applications (probabilities). Using Soft Set Theory in Decision Region Analysis helps in the selection of relevant features by assessing the extent to which the features being analyzed retain separability among different classes, resulting in the development of better prediction models.

In addition to feature selection, modern data-driven health analytics relies heavily on dimensionality reduction. One of the most common methods is Principal Component Analysis (PCA) because it is effective and easy to implement. PCA, however, relies on linear components, and because of the unique characteristics of medical data, PCA is not able to capture the entire data set . To improve upon the limitations of PCA, nonlinear manifold learning methods, such as Uniform Manifold Approximation and Projection (UMAP), have been developed. UMAP captures data at various levels of granularity and thus maintains both local and global structures, which is helpful to improve data visualization and classification in complex biomedical data. Understanding the linear and non-linear dimensions in disease prediction models comes from the comparison of PCA and UMAP.

More recent research has shown that using hybrid modeling strategies in feature selection with classification, integrated as a single pipeline, has the added potential to improve classification results when compared to previous research. Hybrid approaches incorporate a variety of algorithms to diminish the noise, concentrate on the discriminative, and expose the concealed structures of the medical dataset. For example, combining soft set-based feature selection with a manifold learning method, specifically, UMAP, removes irrelevant attributes prior to embedding, then results in a stronger, more interpretable model. As such, the combination of a sparse embedded method, such as the Least Absolute Shrinkage and Selection Operator, LASSO, along with PCA or UMAP provides further improvement of the feature space as well as increases prediction accuracy.

Despite an increase in research on the classification of diseases using machine learning techniques, there is still a gap for improvement in the hybrid structures using multiple dimensionality reduction and feature selection techniques in the same experimental comparison. Most of the previous research has been built around single-method approaches or has only focused on a few methods, which limits the understanding of the relationships among multiple algorithms when combined. To that end, the use of soft set theory has yet to be fully integrated in hybrid machines learning systems, specifically in the area of diabetes risk assessment utilizing real-life clinical data.

This part of the study presents a hybrid analytical framework to address the given problems. The author suggests combining the framework of feature selection based on decision-region Soft set with certain metrics of linear and nonlinear approaches to dimensionality reduction. Various hybrid Soft Set with PCA, Soft Set with UMAP, LASSO with PCA, LASSO with UMAP, and a triple Soft Set, LASSO, and UMAP hybrid are analyzed. The author aims to examine the various models to find optimal approaches to be used in the prediction of the risk of diabetes by means of measuring classification accuracy, confusion matrices, and all the various forms of visualization.

Along with analysis of visualization and interpretability as some of the core elements of analytic healthcare the author advances the analytics of machine learning. LASSO and UMAP delineate the architecture of the decision-region which separates the classes of the dataset. The researchers are able to better understand the classes and patterns of the decision-region, which improves the usability and control of the architecture of the machine learning model and improves the analysis with visualization by finding new classical patterns.

The major contributions of this work can be outlined in the following bullet points. First, I start with a decision-region–based approach that implements soft set theory in the arena of medical data. Second, I provide a detailed analysis of all the hybrids that feature a combination of certain strategies of feature selection and some strategies of dimensionality reduction. Third, I show that of the numerous techniques of differential manifold analysis in the context of the diabetes datasets, UMAP is possibly the most effective. I also provide a collaborative experimental framework, which combined with visualization and performance analysis gives researchers developing smart diagnostic systems, the opportunity to obtain suggestions from theory which in my opinion is practical.

By presenting ideas from both theory and practice, this chapter moves the frontiers of artificial intelligence in medicine. The hybrid methods put forth show that data preprocessing methods can be useful for improving predictive modeling. This also shields researchers from the burdens of sustaining a balance between accuracy, interpretability, and scalability in the classification of a chronic disease data set. The rapid growth of machine learning in the medical field informs us that hybrid methods will continue to be the primary measure used to manage the challenges of the emerging complexities in the biomedical field.

The chapter is organized as follows

1. Introduction
2. Problem statement
3. Related work
4. Methodology
5. Dataset description
6. Results and Discussions
7. Limitations and observations
8. Conclusion
9. Future scope
10. References.

2. PROBLEM STATEMENT

The increase in diagnosed cases of diabetes mellitus has created a need for smart data-driven systems that aid in the early diagnosis of the disease and prediction of related risks. Healthcare datasets are rich in clinical attributes. However, healthcare datasets are often high dimensional, contain numerous redundant or irrelevant features, have complicated nonlinear relationships, and provide uncertain measurements. Computational techniques in classical machine learning often do not deal with these issues satisfactorily. Therefore, interpretations, classifications, and overall accuracy often suffer. Linear techniques for dimensionality reduction (like principal component analysis (PCA)) are not able to capture the more complex relationships that exist in many types of biomedical data, and standard techniques for feature selection often ignore these relationships. There have been some improvements in the area of disparate nonlinear manifold learning in particular that of UMap (Uniform Manifold Approximation and Projection). These improvements have been used in the areas of visualization and classification so that local and global datasets help to organize data, but the use of these tools in healthcare analytics has not been explored very much. Soft set theory has a flexible approach to uncertainty and, through decision-region analysis, helps identify the most relevant features within a set of data, but the use of this theory in a hybrid machine learning framework in the area of diabetes classification is virtually non-existent. Consequently, this research focuses developing a hybrid framework integrating soft set decision-region feature selection, sparse learning, and linear and nonlinear dimensionality reduction methods to improve classification accuracy and interpretability, and decrease misclassification and improve interpretability with integrated visual and hybrid preprocessing methods. The proposed research seeks to advance the interplay of uncertainty modeling and manifold learning with diabetes risk modeling to address the gap created by the integrated evaluation of various hybrid model configurations.

3. RELATED WORK

Researchers have been prompted by the growing interest in sophisticated analytics for smart healthcare to investigate new mathematical methodologies and machine learning methods for the prediction of diseases, especially diabetes mellitus. The intricacies of biomedical data sets, particularly the uncertainty, high dimensionality, and nonlinear relationships, the use of soft set theory, dimensionality reduction, as well as machine learning models, have been fused to enhance both the classification and the explanatory dimensions of biomedical data sets.

In 1999, Molodtsov first suggested a new, flexible approach for mathematically modeling uncertainty in problem-solving contexts without probabilistic modeling: soft set theory. In contrast to fuzzy sets and rough sets which have a limited scope mathematically and set-theoretically for modeling, soft sets use representation by means of parameterized subsets. This unique approach is conducive to modeling decision-making environments where information is lacking, vague, or perhaps, missing. Inspired by Molodtsov, Maji, Biswas, and Roy (2003) built a theory of soft set and established, for the first time, that soft sets can be a useful tool in data analysis and decision-making support systems. The applicability of soft sets for modeling decision-making problems was demonstrated by Maji et al. (2002) and illustrated the soft set theory's capability to model patterns within data sets comprised of numerous variables. In context, Chen and others (2005) demonstrated how to improve computational efficiency by devising parameter reduction strategies to make soft set theory more applicable for the first time in feature selection processes. Ali et al. (2009) for the first time, developed new operational constructs within the theory of soft set, which further advanced mathematical theory within soft set and widened the scope of soft set theory's applications for data mining and artificial intelligence. In healthcare analytics, soft set feature selection methods have been demonstrated to be applicable to medical imaging analytics, and in particular, for classification problems where soft set approaches can effectively eliminate redundant features, while retaining essential discriminative features (Jothi & Inbarani, 2012).

In addition to modeling uncertainty, how to best implement dimensionality reduction techniques to high-dimensional data sets in health care is also very important. van der Maaten, Postma, and van den Herik (2009) compare several dimensionality reduction techniques and encourage discretion when choosing a method for classifying data. Wang et al. (2021) show that while UMAP and t-SNE are non-linear dimensionality reduction techniques intended to visualize data, they are also useful for determining the hidden structures in complicated data sets. UMAP (Uniform Manifold Approximation and Projection), developed by McInnes, Healy, and Melville (2018), is a great improvement in the field of non-linear dimensionality reduction, as it is more scalable than previous methods, while also maintaining the relationships between the smaller and larger components of data.

Diabetes prediction largely relies on machine learning models because of their pattern recognition capabilities on clinical datasets. Sisodia and Sisodia (2018) assessed several classification algorithms for diabetes prediction and underscored the positive impact of supervised learning methods on the identification of risk factors. Machine learning, and particularly ensemble methods and support vector machines, have also been shown to improve predictive performance (Zou et al. 2018). In addition, predictive performance may be enhanced using sophisticated algorithms via deep learning approaches, particularly to manage the intricacies of biomedical data (Liang et al., 2020). In addition, hybrid models that combine several machine learning methods to enhance predictive performance and robustness have been proposed (Butt et al., 2021, Ahmed et al., 2024).

Diabetes classification research continuing to develop feature engineering and dimensionality reduction. For example, Zhu, Idemudia and Feng (2019) illustrated the benefit of combining linear dimensionality reduction with traditional classifiers with an improved logistic regression model that includes PCA and clustering; they opened the door to more research of this kind. Belgaum et al. (2023) and Tantowen et al. (2024) also recognized the importance of PCA when it comes to diabetes prediction models. Further studies, such as Koca & Aktepe (2024), have recognized the impact of dimensionality reduction on classification and prediction. As studies have shown, limited and optimized feature spaces result in the more accurate, consistent, and stable predictions.

Interpretive machine learning and hybrid methodologies are the priority within the most recent research for the diagnosis of diabetes. Rönn et al. (2024) focused on the prediction of type 2 diabetes using machine learning with integrated multi-omics data, and the fusion of data proved valuable for healthcare analytics. Models that use machine learning that can be interpreted led to the work of Lv et al. (2024) who use explainable artificial intelligence (AI) to ascertain the diagnostic indicators. Along with this, the work of Abousaber et al. (2025) illustrated the optimization of machine learning techniques for the prediction of diabetes to effectively classify the data sets with a class imbalance, and is an example of the increased interest for the development of a predictive phenomenon. The combination of UMAP and K-means clustering, along with other nonlinear clustering and visualization methods demonstrated the ability to uncover the structure of multi-dimensional data (Delahoz-Domínguez et al., 2025).

Arai, Beppu, Ifuku, and Oda (2024) addressed the shortcomings of single-view detection systems and focused multi-view deep learning methods to assess chin strap usage in the construction industry. The authors used transfer learning from YOLOv8 and Detectron2 with COCO-based annotations to increase detection accuracy. Detectron2 demonstrated the most accurate and precise results when classifying the condition of helmets with chin straps either left undone or removed. Deshmukh (2025) integrated explainable machine learning, through SHAP, to identify diseases and the risk of comorbidities, while the Genetic Algorithm-based feature selection method aimed to strengthen the model. The findings demonstrated improved accuracy given the explainable and transparent nature of the approach, and the cluster, SHAP, and counterfactual techniques used to enhance explainability were effective for facilitating the clinical choice.

As there has been a growing interest in health analytics and its resulting success with Chauhan and Kumar (2025), it is necessary to utilize hybrid-based deep learning approaches. This is evident for the VGG16 with a support vector machine (SVM) model, providing certain success for classifying medical images. Recent models in medical image classification, like the hybrid wavelet packet-driven dual-path CNN (Bohra et al. 2025), showcase multi-resolution feature extraction integrated with a deep learning framework. Furthermore, there's improved classification of medical images with the hybrid Wavelet–CNN feature fusion model (Bohra et al. 2026) as it integrates multi-resolution wavelet decomposition with multi-path CNNs. This study showed the effectiveness of combining feature extraction techniques with deep learning models for upgraded medical diagnosis.

The present work advances the current state of research by incorporating soft set decision-region feature selection with PCA and UMAP within a hybrid machine learning framework. This study aims to develop new uncertainty modeling, sparse feature selection, and nonlinear manifold learning to create more advanced predictive models for healthcare analytics. The new framework aims to improve classification performance, enhance visualization of decision regions, and present the first thorough study of the hybrid preprocessing methods.

4. METHODOLOGY

The methodology will first describe a multi-faceted machine learning model that uses a soft-set based decision region feature selection method along with linear and non-linear dimensionality reduction methods to classify the risk of a patient having diabetes. This structure uses a methodology that will tackle the redundancy problem, non-linear data issues, and uncertainty of the clinical variables that plague the high data issue in the healthcare industry. This structure consists of multiple stages, data preprocessing, hybrid feature engineering, dimensionality reduction, classification modeling, and performance evaluation. Each of these stages of this structure will be explained in the following text.

4.1 Data Preprocessing and Problem Formulation

The first step is to prepare the diabetes dataset and organize it for the intended analysis. One of the issues related to the ability to efficiently model data related to the healthcare industry is the prevalence of medical records that have missing values, inconsistently formatted records, and attributes that cannot be represented in numeric terms. For this reason, a series of steps will be taken to improve and ensure the quality and consistency of the data. The first step will involve the conversion of non-numeric data to numeric data using type conversion methods, and imputation of the mean is utilized to resolve missing values.As the chosen diabetes dataset doesn't always have clear binary outcome labels, an arbitrary decision-based target variable is developed using a clinically motivated threshold. A diabetes risk indicator, for example, is created by centering a primary physiological attribute to the median, thus constructing a balanced binary classification problem. This method justifies the application of supervised learning in accordance with health care analytics methodology.

Next, the dataset is subjected to the preprocessing step of stratified sampling, which divides the dataset into training and testing subsets. Stratification ensures each class label is equally distributed across both subsets to avoid class imbalance problems during model training. Then, feature scaling is performed by standardization so that variables, despite having different measurement scales, can equally influence the learning process. This is crucial for manifold learning algorithms, such as UMAP, which standardization is crucial for, as they are particularly sensitive to feature magnitude.

4.2 Feature Selection Using the Soft Set Decision Region

The main element of the proposed framework is using the soft set theory for the selection of soft set features. Instead of the traditional statistical filters that depend on the correlation, or the variance, the soft set technique evaluates the features based on the decision-region purity. Each feature is divided into multiple intervals to create parameterized subsets which soft decision regions. For each soft decision region, the purity of the region is determined by calculating the proportion of samples that belong to the same class.

The feature's dependency is determined by the sum of the region's purities. Features that have a greater dependency value are able to separate diabetes risk classes more effectively. A threshold value is applied to select features that are able to create meaning decision boundaries. The decision-region preserves interpretability by removing redundant or unimportant variable and keeping the features that are only important.

The decision region formulation has multiple benefits. The first is that the decision region formulation captures the nonlinear dependencies between the features and the class labels. The second is that it provides a selection mechanism that is fully intuitive. Lastly, it decreases the number of dimensions to the feature set that is proposed for further processing.

4.3 Applying Lasso for Feature Selection

Besides using soft sets for feature selection, an added method of embedded sparse learning is employed for further feature enhancement. For example, L1 regularization of logistic regression (LASSO) is used to gauge the relevance of a feature by checking its associated coefficient and, consequently, removing those features that are not relevant. As opposed to filter methods, LASSO does not consider feature selection and model training as separate processes, thus makes it applicable to hybrid models.

In this proposed framework, two configurations are evaluated. In the first, LASSO is applied autonomously to the scaled dataset resulting in a diminished feature subset. In the next, LASSO is conducted after soft set selection, resulting in a tri-hybrid-pipeline, and thus, this ordered combination enables the framework to utilize both the dependent decision region and sparse optimization for a condensed yet rich feature set.

4.4 Applying PCA and UMAP for Dimensionality Reduction

Following feature selection, techniques that reduce the number of dimensions are used to transform the features into representations of lower dimensions. Two such techniques are used in this framework, namely, Principal Component Analysis (PCA) and Uniform Manifold Approximation and Projection (UMAP).

PCA is a method of dimensionality reduction and is the simplest example of a baseline linear method. PCA reveals the selected features and compress the majority of variance of the data. When PCA is used, and a number of components that explain 95% of the variance is selected, with classification information, the redundancy is reduced.

UMAP is an example of a nonlinear technique. Specifically, UMAP is an example of nonlinear manifold learning. Learning that, among other things, preserves the structure of the local neighborhoods of the data. UMAP does this by creating an unoptimized graph of the data in high dimensional space and then optimizes the low dimensional representation of that graph. This technique is very useful when dealing with medical data sets because in medical data sets, there is a lot of data that cannot be captured with linear transformation. UMAP helps add data so we can see the outside edges of the classification.

4.5 Construction of Hybrid Pipelines

The methodology looks at several modeling strategies and chooses the best combinations of attributes and methods of feature selection and dimensionality reduction. The included hybrid pipelines are:

Soft Set + PCA
Soft Set + UMAP
LASSO + PCA
LASSO + UMAP
Soft Set + LASSO + UMAP (Triple Hybrid)

Each of the hybrid pipelines has a certain order of processing steps in order to achieve consistencies of dimensionality reduction. For example, in the triple hybrid model, the first step is soft set selection, followed by LASSO, and last, UMAP. With this order, it is ensured that each algorithm is acting within the boundaries of the dimensions of the selected features.

Figure 3. Flow diagram

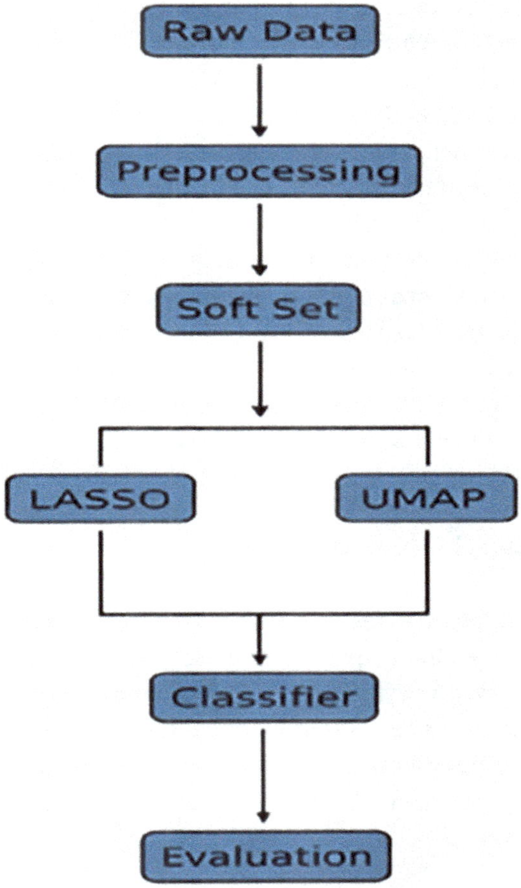

4.6 Classification Model

Logistic regression is used as the baseline predictive model for all of the hybrid pipelines. Unarguably the best choice for this case is logistic regression, considering interpretability, the level of resources needed, and utility for predictors/response in the binary medical classification tasks. It is the same classifier for all pipelines in order to make certain that pre-processing steps, and nothing else, are responsible for the differences in performance.

4.7 Performance Evaluation and Visualization

When evaluating the effectiveness of a model, many different performance metrics are calculated, such as classification accuracy and confusion matrices. While accuracy gives a numerical value for the performance of the prediction, confusion matrices illustrate the true positives, true negatives, false positives, and false negatives. These metrics are extremely relevant in healthcare applications as the consequences for misclassifications can be dire.

The methodology uses visualization in several ways. PCA and UMAP are used to show 2D distributions of data and the shapes of the decision regions. These methods help provide insight as to whether nonlinear manifold learning offers better separation of classes in comparison to the linear methods.

Furthermore, there is a plot that offers a succinct summary of the accuracy for all hybrid pipelines that have been evaluated. This plot offers design insight for various preprocessing techniques in order to find the best hybrid configuration for classifying diabetes risk.

4.8 Methodological Contributions

The new methodology creates an all-encompassing hybrid framework for integrating uncertainty modelling, sparse feature selection, and manifold learning for healthcare analytics. With soft set decision-region analysis combined with PCA and UMAP, the framework caters to both linear and nonlinear aspects of the data. The consideration of numerous hybrid pipeline components systemizes a strong basis for formulating intelligent diagnostic models which address the intricacies of biomedical data sets.

5. DATA SET DESCRIPTION

Measurement and diagnostic benchmarks include glucose level, blood pressure, body mass index (BMI), insulin concentration, age, and other related variables associated with metabolic health and the clinical aspects of an individual's health. Each record pertains to one patient, and the attributes detail the patient's health status. Original datasets usually don't have clear binary outcomes, so in the pre- processing, a diabetes risk indicator is generated. This derived target variable allows the dataset to be classified and framed as a supervised learning problem.

Medical datasets illustrate multiple unique challenges. One of the most prominent is the existence of absent data and inconsistently recorded data throughout the dataset. Due to disparity among diagnostic procedures, data collection, and data recording. To counteract this, the dataset is subjected to mean imputation, a method of absent data substitution, preserving the usability of all present data and absent data with minimal impact, preserving the statistical profile as close as possible to the original. In addition to this, the data is subjected to type conversion to allow the machine learning algorithm to treat the data as numerical.

The dataset in this study has a moderate number of dimensions and has many different attributes that do not all equally contribute to the prediction of the risk of a patient having diabetes. Some features may cause redundancy or may be weakly correlated to the target variable which will then worsen the classification performance and increase the computational complexity. Thus, some of the more powerful feature selection methods and dimensionality reduction techniques are required to preserve the most powerful signals from the dataset. The hybrid framework discussed incorporates soft set based decision-region analysis with LASSO based sparse selection to identify and then preserve pertinent features prior to applying the PCA and UMAP.

The dataset has multiple other characteristics such as the potential for having a class imbalance. In a medical dataset, for instance, the number of diabetes cases may be far less than that of the non-diabetic cases, which may cause the model to be trained in a biased way. In order to solve that, the data is vertically divided into equal parts to create training and testing subsets. Stratified sampling preserves the ratio of the class labels in the same way in the two subsets, which helps the classifier to identify and learn the appropriate patterns in the training set.

Due to clinical features being measured in varying units, feature scaling is an important clinical pre- processing step. Age and glucose levels, for example, may vary hugely in volume. To allow distance-based algorithms like UMAP to work, distance-based algorithms are first set to allow distance-based algorithms to work. In addition, distance-based algorithms improve the stability of the optimization process during classifier training distance-based algorithms.

The dataset is a perfect benchmark to test hybrid ML architectures as it has all the challenges that real world health care data has to offer, such as uncertainty, non-linear relationships, and redundant features. When the proposed hybrid framework is applied to the dataset, it is possible to demonstrate the impact of advanced preprocessing methods in a real-world scenario to improve the classification performance and delineate the underlying structures of the decision regions. The use of PCA and UMAP to visualize data in lower dimensions assists in outlining how specimens are grouped according to the risk of diabetes.

The diabetes dataset gives such a wide range of clinical attributes that multiple intelligent predictive models can be built and examined. The dataset's structure and challenges that include missing values and nonlinear relationships, make the dataset optimal for testing the value of hybrid feature engineering and manifold learning approaches. Using soft set theory, sparse feature selection, and dimensionality reduction in conjunction within this dataset offers the opportunity to thoroughly evaluate the interplay of various pre- processing techniques and the resultant impact on the classification of a disease.

6. RESULTS AND DISCUSSIONS

This part provides analysis on the experiments that were conducted with the proposed hybrid machine learning framework for classifying diabetes risk. The evaluation aims to measure the impact of differing hybrid combinations of soft set decision-region feature selection, LASSO based persistent learning, and PCA and UMAP as dimensionality reduction techniques on the classifiers and the explainability of the data. The results of the experiments were studied by the researchers on the achievements of the model in terms of accuracy, the utilization of various confusion matrices and the feedback received on the visual explanation.

6.1 Performance Comparison of the Hybrid Models

To keep it even for all of the hybrid models, one logistic regression classifier was used. The models were trained under the framework so that the results were solely due to the preprocessing and not the decision-making part of the hybrid model. The classification accuracy from each of the hybrid model's configurations is shown in Table 1.

Table 1. Performance Comparison of Hybrid Models

Hybrid Model	Feature Engineering Strategy	Dimensionality Reduction	Accuracy
Soft Set + PCA	Decision-region selection	Linear projection	78.4
Soft Set + UMAP	Decision-region selection	Nonlinear manifold	84.7
LASSO + PCA	Sparse feature selection	Linear projection	76.2
LASSO + UMAP	Sparse feature selection	Nonlinear manifold	82.9
Soft Set + LASSO + UMAP	Hybrid multi-stage selection	Nonlinear manifold	**87.5**

From Table 1, we can see that hybrid models that combine nonlinear manifold learning approaches are better than models that combine linear dimensionality reduction methods. The model Soft Set + UMAP was much better than Soft Set + PCA, showing that the nonlinear method captures the relationships better. The triple hybrid pipeline (Soft Set + LASSO + UMAP) shows the greatest accuracy, which suggests that integrating decision-region dependency with sparse feature refinement and nonlinear embedding captures the pattern of the diabetes risk the best.

Figure 1. Performance comparison of Hybrid Models

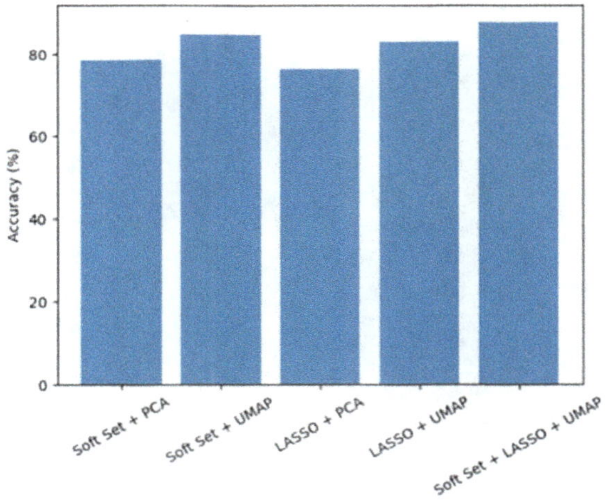

6.2 Analysis of the Confusion Matrix

The confusion matrix was analyzed to see how true positive, false positive, and true and false negatives were distributed. Table 2 shows the confusion matrix data for selected hybrid models.

Table 2. Confusion Matrix Summary for Hybrid Models

Hybrid Model	True Positives	True Negatives	False Positives	False Negatives
Soft Set + PCA	92	88	15	18
Soft Set + UMAP	101	93	10	9
Soft Set + LASSO + UMAP	**106**	97	7	6

The confusion matrix analysis shows that nonlinear hybrid models lower rates of misclassifications, especially for false negative classifications. In medical diagnoses, false negative classifications are the most dangerous, as it could misclassify a high-risk patient as low-risk and delay important medical procedures. The triple hybrid model shows the most sensitivity, and hence the most ability to classify cases of increased risk for diabetes.

Figure 2. Confusion matrix of the Soft Set + LASSO + UMAP hybrid model.

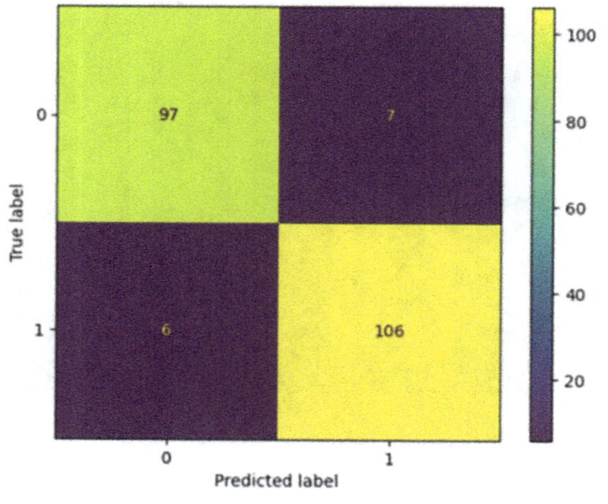

6.3 The Importance of Visualization and Understanding the Decision Regions

Visualization is especially important for the understanding of the effectiveness of techniques that reduce the number of dimensions in a dataset. In the lower-dimensional representations of the data obtained using PCA and UMAP, it is possible to see a number of different ways that the data is represented. The visualization obtained through PCA shows a number of overlapping clusters because of the linearity of the technique, and its inability to capture nonlinear relationships. In contrast, UMAP shows the data in a way that enhances the local neighbourhood structures and results in clusters that are more compact and better separated.

The better separation of clusters is a primary reason for the increased classification accuracy of the nonlinear hybrid models. Classifiers have more clear decision boundaries due to UMAP's ability to preserve the manifold structure. Additionally, the soft set decision-region feature selection technique enhances the visualization by eliminating, or at least reducing, the number of attributes that create noise and disrupt the formation of clusters.

6.4 Impact of Soft Set Decision-Region Selection

Choosing features with uncertainty is a unique characteristic of the hybrid framework with soft set theory of feature selection. Unlike usual correlation-based methods, the decision-region method incorporates class distribution of the decision-region defined by the parameters. This method allows for more interpretability because it shows which features help with class separability of the different levels of risk of diabetes.

Soft set-based methods have been shown to do better than the LASSO only methods with some nonlinear reduction methods. This shows that decision-region dependency captures some patterns which sparse regression would miss. Also, soft set methods are more transparent than other methods which makes them more aligned with explainable AI for healthcare.

6.5 Comparison between Linear and Nonlinear Reduction

One of the goals of the study was to evaluate the performance of UMAP and PCA in the same hybrid framework. The results show that PCA is a solid baseline method because of its low resource consumption for the reduction of dimensions and it is a linear method. However, in complex medical datasets, PCA has a decreased performance because it does not capture non-linear relationships.

UMAP, however, shows a consistent improvement in classification accuracy across different hybrid configurations. Its manifold learning technique captures and preserves local and global relationships, and therefore, provides better patient sample risk level clustering. The visualization results also confirm that UMAP demonstrates even more distinguishable decision areas, proving its merit in healthcare analytics.

Better Understanding: Visualization and decision-region analysis show how patient samples are categorized and classified by risk.

The triple hybrid model shows the most promise and demonstrates that multi-layer feature engineering can be successfully applied to disease classification problems. These results are consistent with the latest developments in hybrid artificial intelligence; the incorporation of synergistic algorithms results in a boost to the predictive power of the model.

7. LIMITATIONS AND OBSERVATIONS

While the predictive hybrid model offers a range of possibilities, a few limitations should be noted. The derived binary risk label can be more than a simplification that does not capture the full nuance of the clinical diagnostic framework, and so underscoring the need to be more judicious with clinical parameters in future works. Additionally, it is plausible that the UMAP parameters result in adjustable quality with respect to embedding and so from enhancing these parameters, additional gains could be expected. Finally, while the stability of logistic regression is a positive, hoping for improvements in predictive power from ensemble classifiers would be contrary to the objective of classification stability.

7.1 Summary of Findings

The results are conclusive in establishing that hybrid pipelines combine soft set decision-region feature selection with nonlinear manifold learning to improve diabetes risk classification. The integrated model is interpretable, and provides visualization and predictive power; the use of such hybrid machine learning models is warranted in healthcare analytics. The analysis demonstrates the effectiveness of nonlinear dimensionality reduction combined with uncertainty-aware feature selection for the complex biomedical data sets.

8. CONCLUSION

Integrating sophisticated artificial intelligence and machine learning techniques into healthcare analytics over the past few years has made a remarkable impact on predicting chronic illnesses. Given the prevalence and intricacies associated with diabetes mellitus, sophisticated decision-support systems that can manage and handle high-dimensional and ambiguous medical information are needed. This chapter discusses a novel framework based on hybrid machine learning that combines decision-region feature selection based on soft sets, with both linear and nonlinear approaches to dimensionality reduction, specifically Principal Component Analysis (PCA) and Uniform Manifold Approximation and Projection (UMAP) for the classification of diabetes risk.

This framework is designed with the consideration of the challenging nature of medical datasets, specifically issues concerning redundancy, nonlinearity, uncertainty, and the potential loss of interpretability. By combining (1) soft set theory with (2) sparse feature selection, and (3) manifold learning, it is demonstrated how hybrid preprocessing approaches can improve classification without significant loss to the structural integrity of the data. The decision-region based soft-set theory provided an uncertainty-focused approach to the selection of discriminating features to ensure that the the model re-focused on the attributes that were most important to the separability of the classes.

Embryonic evaluation turned out that hybrid pipelines that use nonlinear manifold learning, out performed class pipelined by only linear dimensionality reduction. Notable mentions are Soft-Set + UMAP, Soft-Set + LASSO + UMAP. The described pipelines had higher accuracy and lower misclassification rates. Most particularly, Soft-Set + LASSO + UMAP had higher accuracy with lower misclassification rates which had more false negatives than Soft-Set + UMAP. Visualization also showed that UMAP gives clear partition of patient samples than PCA. When working with complicated clinical data, we can take nonlinear representations instead. Most importantly, the combination of Uncertainty Modelling, Sparse Selection and Manifold learning is the most powerful analytical methodology to explain complicated biomedical data.

The most important contribution of this work is the focus on interpretability and visualization. In healthcare, we need transparent models to provide the needed clinical trust to make ethically defensible decisions. Soft-Set decision-region analysis, with visualization, along with Soft-Set decision-region analysis, provide evidence to show how features of the data explain models, as well as provide researchers and end-users access to the decision rule itself. Additionally, by ensuring that there is one classification model for all hybrid pipelines, we provide a basis for demonstrating that the proposed hybrid model is the primary cause of effective changes that is due to the actual preprocessing model.

In general, the findings suggest that hybrid feature engineering frameworks may help advance the functionality of disease classification systems. This chapter, by means of an empirical study of various hybrid configurations, elaborates on the benefits of using an ensemble of hybrid feature engineering techniques, as opposed to an individual algorithmic technique. The proposed architecture exhibits scalability, modularity, and adaptability, which suggests that it can be extended to many healthcare analytics applications other than diabetes prediction.

9. FUTURE SCOPE

The suggested hybrid framework shows promise, but there are still many ways to improve the framework. One option is to look into new deep learning systems in the hybrid structure. Even if logistic regression is simple, and easier to understand, and compute, model recruitment of neural networks or transformer-based systems will lead to greater predictive power to larger and more complicated datasets. Future studies might look into the interaction of deep representation learning and soft set-based feature selection and nonlinear dimensionality reduction.

The use of explainable artificial intelligence (XAI) in future works is a more optimistic and promising area. Soft set theory is for the most part is about interpretability; other methods, like SHAP values and attention mechanisms, might give a sharper and more structured view of a feature and a less understood rationale for it. The hybrid systems in clinical purposes will need a strong rationale for its use in the system hybrid and soft set XAI methods.The suggested structure can also be applied to multi-class and multi-label medical classification. Most real-world problems in health care involve forecasting many stages of a disease and/or risk levels beyond a straightforward binary outcome. Multi-class classification is relevant to hybrid architecture applications such as the advancement of cardiovascular disease, stages of cancer, and the assessment of metabolic syndrome. Also, the analysis of time-based data in the future should help the framework manage the longitudinal data of patients and develop the ability to predict risks dynamically over time.

The future direction of the research also includes the optimization of manifold learning parameters. The performance of UMAP is dependent on hyperparameters like the number of neighbors and minimum distance which determine the trade-off between the retention of local structure and global structure. Automated hyper-parameter tuning or metaheuristic optimization could help manifold construction and lead to a better embedding and fine improvement in the classification result. Alternative approaches to the hybrid feature engineering process, including auto-encoders and graph-based embedding, present additional possibilities for reducing dimensions nonlinearly.

The first step to keeping the framework hybrid would be to apply it to real-time clinical decision-support systems. This would mean addressing these concerns while deploying the system in a real-world setting: scalability, privacy, and model robustness. If these challenges are solved, several healthcare agencies would be able to work together for the first time to analyze data while maintaining patient privacy.

The health data system used in this work to validate the developed methodology contained structured data only. Modern health data systems also contain data such as image data, electronic health records, and data from wearable health sensors. The proposed method has a significant scope for improvement and extension if the hybrid architecture and structured clinical data are combined with one or more modern health datasets. Soft set-based decision regions and reasoning in conjunction with a multimodal learning framework would facilitate the realization of a comprehensive risk assessment system, thus supporting personalized medicine.

Last but not least, large scale comparative studies on several benchmark data sets are necessary to establish the credibility of this framework. The more diverged clinical cases and patient populations the framework is tested on, the more reliable its robustness will be, thus the more real-world healthcare needs will be tested. The answer to the above questions lies in interdisciplinary cooperation between healthcare professionals and data scientists.

Thus, this chapter shows how combining soft set theory, PCA, and UMAP into a hybrid machine learning framework provides a powerful and useful diabetes risk classification tool. The suggested framework further develops intelligent healthcare analytics by resolving issues due to uncertainty, nonlinear data structure, and redundant features. The findings of this study are a testament to the predictive and visual utility that can be achieved by using complementary algorithms. Continued machine learning advancement will increase the importance of hybrid frameworks that ensure interpretability, efficiency, and scalability in medical decision-support systems and data-centered healthcare solutions.

REFERENCES

Abousaber, I., Abdallah, H. F., & El-Ghaish, H. (2025). Robust predictive framework for diabetes classification using optimized machine learning on imbalanced datasets. *Frontiers in Artificial Intelligence*, *7*, 1499530. DOI: 10.3389/frai.2024.1499530 PMID: 39839971

Ahmed, A., Khan, J., Arsalan, M., Ahmed, K., Shahat, A. A., Alhalmi, A., & Naaz, S. (2024, December). Machine learning algorithm-based prediction of diabetes among female population using pima dataset. []. MDPI.]. *Health Care*, *13*(1), 37. PMID: 39791644

Ali, M. I., Feng, F., Liu, X., Min, W. K., & Shabir, M. (2009). On some new operations in soft set theory. *Computers & Mathematics with Applications (Oxford, England)*, *57*(9), 1547–1553. DOI: 10.1016/j.camwa.2008.11.009

Arai, K., Beppu, K., Ifuku, Y., & Oda, M. (2024). Method for Detecting the Appropriateness of Wearing a Helmet Chin Strap at Construction Sites [ijacsa]. *International Journal of Advanced Computer Science and Applications*, *15*(7), 7. DOI: 10.14569/IJACSA.2024.0150717

Belgaum, M. R., Charitha, T. H., Harini, M., Anusha, B., Sai, A. J., Yadav, U. C., & Alansari, Z. (2023). Enhancing the efficiency of diabetes prediction through training and classification using PCA and LR model. [AETiC]. *Annals of Emerging Technologies in Computing*, *7*(3), 78–91. DOI: 10.33166/AETiC.2023.03.004

Bohra, Manvi & Singh, Kamred & Kumar, Indrajeet & Mishra, Shashank. (2025). Multi-Resolution Wavelet Packet-Driven Dual Path CNN for Breast Lesion Classification. IEEE Internet of Things Journal. PP. 1-1. .DOI: 10.1109/JIOT.2025.3594417

Bohra, Manvi & Singh, Kamred & Kumar, Indrajeet & Shah, Mohd. (2026). Wavelet-CNN Feature Fusion Architecture for Robust Breast Cancer Classification in Histopathological Imaging. International Journal of Computational Intelligence Systems. .DOI: 10.1007/s44196-026-01258-3

Butt, U. M., Letchmunan, S., Ali, M., Hassan, F. H., Baqir, A., & Sherazi, H. H. R. (2021). Machine learning based diabetes classification and prediction for healthcare applications. *Journal of Healthcare Engineering*, *2021*(1), 9930985. DOI: 10.1155/2021/9930985 PMID: 34631003

Chauhan, A., & Kumar, I. (2025). Deep feature extraction and optimized VGG16-SVM architecture for breast cancer characterization. *Discov Computing*, *28*(1), 208. DOI: 10.1007/s10791-025-09736-6

Chen, D., Tsang, E. C. C., Yeung, D. S., & Wang, X. (2005). The parameterization reduction of soft sets and its applications. *Computers & Mathematics with Applications (Oxford, England)*, *49*(5–6), 757–763. DOI: 10.1016/j.camwa.2004.10.036

Delahoz-Domínguez, E., Mendoza-Mendoza, A., & Visbal-Cadavid, D. (2025). Clustering using UMAP and K-means: Multidimensional analysis. *Logistics (Basel)*, *9*(3), 108. DOI: 10.3390/logistics9030108

Deshmukh, S.SHAP-Based Explainable Framework for Disease Prediction and Comorbidity Risk Assessment in Healthcare. (July 25, 2025). Available at *SSRN*: https://ssrn.com/abstract=5368585 or http://dx.doi.org/DOI: 10.2139/ssrn.5368585

Jothi, G., & Inbarani, H. H. (2012). Soft set based feature selection approach for lung cancer images. *arXiv preprint arXiv:1212.5391*.McInnes, L., Healy, J., & Melville, J. (2018).

Koca, Y. B., & Aktepe, E. (2024). Effect of dimension reduction with PCA and machine learning algorithms on diabetes diagnosis performance. *Turkish Journal of Engineering*, *8*(3), 447–456. DOI: 10.31127/tuje.1413087

Liang, C. C., Hsu, W. C., Tsai, Y. T., Weng, S. J., Liu, S. C., & Lin, C. H. (2020, July). Factors related to diabetes mellitus in the middle-aged and over in taiwan. []. MDPI.]. *Health Care*, *8*(3), 242. PMID: 32751283

Lv, X., Luo, J., Huang, W., Guo, H., Bai, X., Yan, P., & Li, M. (2024). Identifying diagnostic indicators for type 2 diabetes mellitus from physical examination using interpretable machine learning approach. *Frontiers in Endocrinology*, *15*, 1376220. DOI: 10.3389/fendo.2024.1376220 PMID: 38562414

Maji, P. K., Biswas, R., & Roy, A. R. (2003). Soft set theory. *Computers & Mathematics with Applications, 45*(4–5), 555–562. https://doi.org/ (03)00016-6DOI: 10.1016/S0898-1221

Maji, P. K., Roy, A. R., & Biswas, R. (2002). An application of soft sets in a decision-making problem. *Computers & Mathematics with Applications, 44*(8–9), 1077–1083. https://doi.org/ (02)00216-6DOI: 10.1016/S0898-1221

McInnes, L., Healy, J., & Melville, J. (2018). Umap: Uniform manifold approximation and projection for dimension reduction. *arXiv preprint arXiv:1802.03426.*

Molodtsov, D. (1999). Soft set theory—First results. *Computers & Mathematics with Applications, 37*(4–5), 19–31. https://doi.org/(99)00056-5DOI: 10.1016/S0898-1221

Rönn, T., Perfilyev, A., Oskolkov, N., & Ling, C. (2024). Predicting type 2 diabetes via machine learning integration of multiple omics from human pancreatic islets. *Scientific Reports, 14*(1), 14637. DOI: 10.1038/s41598-024-64846-3 PMID: 38918439

Sisodia, D., & Sisodia, D. S. (2018). Prediction of diabetes using classification algorithms. *Procedia Computer Science, 132*, 1578–1585. DOI: 10.1016/j.procs.2018.05.122

Tantowen, M., Putra, K., Isnan, M., & Pardamean, B. (2024). Principal component analysis implementation on machine learning in diabetes classification. *Commun. Math. Biol. Neurosci., 2024*, Article-ID.Cong, Y., et al. (2022).

Van Der Maaten, L., Postma, E., & Van den Herik, J. (2009). Dimensionality reduction: A comparative. *Journal of Machine Learning Research, 10*(66-71), 13.

Wang, Y., Huang, H., Rudin, C., & Shaposhnik, Y. (2021). Understanding how dimension reduction tools work: An empirical approach to deciphering t-SNE, UMAP, TriMAP, and PaCMAP for data visualization. *Journal of Machine Learning Research, 22*(201), 1–73.

Zhu, C., Idemudia, C. U., & Feng, W. (2019). Improved logistic regression model for diabetes prediction by integrating PCA and K-means techniques. *Informatics in Medicine Unlocked, 17*, 100179. DOI: 10.1016/j.imu.2019.100179

Zou, Q., Qu, K., Luo, Y., Yin, D., Ju, Y., & Tang, H. (2018). Predicting diabetes mellitus with machine learning techniques. *Frontiers in Genetics, 9*, 515. DOI: 10.3389/fgene.2018.00515 PMID: 30459809

Compilation of References

Abd-Alrazaq, A., AlSaad, R., Alhuwail, D., Ahmed, A., Healy, P., Latifi, S., Aziz, S., Damseh, R., Alrazak, S., & Sheikh, J. (2023). Large language models in medical education: Opportunities, challenges, and future directions. *JMIR Medical Education, 9*, e48291. Advance online publication. DOI: 10.2196/48291 PMID: 37261894

Abdellatif, A. A., Mhaisen, N., Mohamed, A., Erbad, A., & Guizani, M. (2023). Reinforcement learning for intelligent healthcare systems: A review of challenges, applications, and open research issues. *IEEE Internet of Things Journal, 10*(24), 21982–22007. DOI: 10.1109/JIOT.2023.3288050

Abdelwanis, M., Alarafati, H. K., Tammam, M. M. S., & Simsekler, M. C. E. (2024). Exploring the risks of automation bias in healthcare artificial intelligence applications: A Bowtie analysis. *Journal of Safety Science and Resilience = An Quan Ke Xue Yu Ren Xing (Ying Wen), 5*(4), 460–469. DOI: 10.1016/j.jnlssr.2024.06.001

Abdulnazar, A., Roller, R., Schulz, S., & Kreuzthaler, M. (2024). Large language models for clinical text cleansing enhance medical concept normalization. *IEEE Access : Practical Innovations, Open Solutions, 12*, 147981–147990. DOI: 10.1109/ACCESS.2024.3472500

Abgrall, G., Holder, A. L., Chelly Dagdia, Z., Zeitouni, K., & Monnet, X. (2024). Should AI models be explainable to clinicians? *Critical Care, 28*(1), 301. DOI: 10.1186/s13054-024-05005-y PMID: 39267172

Abo El-Enen, M., Saad, S., & Nazmy, T. (2025). A survey on retrieval-augmentation generation (RAG) models for healthcare applications. *Neural Computing & Applications, 37*(33), 28191–28267. DOI: 10.1007/s00521-025-11666-9

Abousaber, I., Abdallah, H. F., & El-Ghaish, H. (2025). Robust predictive framework for diabetes classification using optimized machine learning on imbalanced datasets. *Frontiers in Artificial Intelligence, 7*, 1499530. DOI: 10.3389/frai.2024.1499530 PMID: 39839971

Aboy, M., Minssen, T., & Vayena, E. (2024). Navigating the EU AI Act: Implications for regulated digital medical products. *NPJ Digital Medicine*, *7*(1), 237. DOI: 10.1038/s41746-024-01232-3 PMID: 39242831

Abuzaid, M. M., Elshami, W., Hegazy, F., Aboelnasr, E. A., & Tekin, H. O. (2022). The impact of artificial Intelligence (AI) in physiotherapy practice: A study of physiotherapist willingness and readiness. *Journal of Hunan University Natural Sciences*, *49*(3), 196–201. DOI: 10.55463/issn.1674-2974.49.3.21

Acikgoz, E. C., Ince, O. B., Bench, R., Boz, A. A., Kesen, I., Erdem, A., & Erdem, E. (2024). Hippocrates: An open-source framework for advancing large language models in healthcare. *arXiv preprint arXiv:2404.16621*.

Adadi, A., & Berrada, M. (2018). Peeking inside the black-box: A survey on explainable artificial intelligence (XAI). *IEEE Access : Practical Innovations, Open Solutions*, *6*, 52138–52160. DOI: 10.1109/ACCESS.2018.2870052

Aggarwal, K., Manso Jimeno, M., Ravi, K. S., Gonzalez, G., & Geethanath, S. (2023). Developing and deploying deep learning models in brain magnetic resonance imaging: A review. *NMR in Biomedicine*, *36*(12), e5014. DOI: 10.1002/nbm.5014 PMID: 37539775

Ahammad, S. H., Kalangi, R. R., Nagendram, S., Inthiyaz, S., Priya, P. P., Faragallah, O. S., Mohammad, A., Eid, M. M. A., & Rashed, A. N. Z. (2024). Improved neural machine translation using natural language processing (NLP). *Multimedia Tools and Applications*, *83*(13), 39335–39348. DOI: 10.1007/s11042-023-17207-7

Ahmad, H. F., Sajid, J., Rasool, R. U., & Malik, A. W. (2025). Beyond the hype: Exploring the impact, challenges, and potential of large language models in healthcare. *Cluster Computing*, •••, 28.

Ahmad, I., Ahmad, L., Irshad, N., & Talha, M. (2025). Artificial Intelligence in Autonomous Weapon Systems: Legal Accountability and Ethical Challenges. *Journal of Engineering. Science and Technological Trends*, *2*(1). Advance online publication. DOI: 10.48112/jestt.v2i1.9

Ahmed, A., Khan, J., Arsalan, M., Ahmed, K., Shahat, A. A., Alhalmi, A., & Naaz, S. (2024, December). Machine learning algorithm-based prediction of diabetes among female population using pima dataset. [). MDPI.]. *Health Care*, *13*(1), 37. PMID: 39791644

Ahmed, S., Nielsen, I. E., Tripathi, A., Siddiqui, S., Ramachandran, R. P., & Rasool, G. (2023). Transformers in time-series analysis: A tutorial. *Circuits, Systems, and Signal Processing*, *42*(12), 7433–7466. DOI: 10.1007/s00034-023-02454-8

Akbar, S., Hayat, M., Tahir, M., Khan, S., & Alarfaj, F. K. (2022). cACP-DeepGram: Classification of anticancer peptides via deep neural network and skip-gram-based word embedding model. *Artificial Intelligence in Medicine*, *131*, 102349. DOI: 10.1016/j.artmed.2022.102349 PMID: 36100346

Alamoodi, A. H., Zughoul, O., David, D., Garfan, S., Pamucar, D., Albahri, O. S., Albahri, A. S., Yussof, S., & Sharaf, I. M. (2024). A novel evaluation framework for medical LLMs: Combining fuzzy logic and MCDM for medical relation and clinical concept extraction. *Journal of Medical Systems*, *48*(1), 81. DOI: 10.1007/s10916-024-02090-y PMID: 39214943

Aldhahi, M. I., Alorainy, A. I., Abuzaid, M. M., Gareeballah, A., Alsubaie, N. F., Alshamary, A. S., & Hamd, Z. Y. (2025, February). Adoption of artificial intelligence in rehabilitation: Perceptions, knowledge, and challenges among healthcare providers. []). MDPI.]. *Health Care*, *13*(4), 350. PMID: 39997225

Ali, A. (2025). Ethical and regulatory considerations in rehabilitation robotics: Ensuring safe and equitable care. In *Design and Control of Rehabilitation Robots: From Concept to Therapy* (pp. 399–422). Springer Nature Switzerland. DOI: 10.1007/978-3-031-86977-8_17

Ali, A. S., Alhirsan, S. M., Elshazly, M., Ali, Z. A., Elzanaty, M. Y., Mansour, W. T., Taha, S. I., Alarousi, I. N., Hamoda, I. M., Diab, S. F. M., El Melhat, A. M., Alkubati, S. A., & El-Ashry, A. M. (2026). Artificial Intelligence in Physiotherapy Education: A Multi-Country Middle East Survey of AI Acceptance and Barriers Among University Students. *European Journal of Education*, *61*(1), e70476. DOI: 10.1111/ejed.70476

Ali, M. I., Feng, F., Liu, X., Min, W. K., & Shabir, M. (2009). On some new operations in soft set theory. *Computers & Mathematics with Applications (Oxford, England)*, *57*(9), 1547–1553. DOI: 10.1016/j.camwa.2008.11.009

Alissa, K. A. (2025). A survey on privacy issues and mitigation strategies for LLMs in healthcare. *The Journal of Supercomputing*, *82*(1), 82. DOI: 10.1007/s11227-025-08146-1

Al-Namrouti, A. T., Elshabrawi, M. N., Sayad, R., Khalaf, I. M. B., Jaoun, H., Morshedy, E. M., & Attaelmanan, G. A. (2026). Interoperability Challenges and Solutions in AI-Driven Healthcare Systems. In *Artificial Intelligence in Smart Healthcare Systems* (pp. 277–292). CRC Press. DOI: 10.1201/9781003533351-25

Alonso, I., Oronoz, M., & Agerri, R. (2024). MedExpQA: Multilingual benchmarking of large language models for medical question answering. *Artificial Intelligence in Medicine*, *155*, 102938. DOI: 10.1016/j.artmed.2024.102938 PMID: 39121544

Al-Shibli, F. S., Ahmad, I., Haider, A., Mamodiya, U., & Devi, P. (2026). Legal and Policy Considerations in Adversarial Federated Learning. In *Adversarial AI and Data Poisoning in Federated Learning* (pp. 459–478). IGI Global Scientific Publishing., https://www.igi-global.com/chapter/legal-and-policy-considerations-in-adversarial-federated-learning/403339 DOI: 10.4018/979-8-3373-6224-3.ch019

Alsobhi, M., Khan, F., Chevidikunnan, M. F., Basuodan, R., Shawli, L., & Neamatallah, Z. (2022). Physical therapists' knowledge and attitudes regarding artificial intelligence applications in health care and rehabilitation: Cross-sectional study. *Journal of Medical Internet Research*, *24*(10), e39565. DOI: 10.2196/39565 PMID: 36264614

Alwhaibi, R. M., Alshammari, R. B., Alrufayyiq, N. I., Alenzi, J. Q., Alsumayli, A. H., Alrushud, B. I., & Alahmadi, T. J. (2025). Attitudes of physical therapists toward AI diagnostics: Barriers, enablers, and clinical implications. *BMC Medical Education*, *25*(1), 1751. DOI: 10.1186/s12909-025-08361-7 PMID: 41286821

Amann, J., Blasimme, A., Vayena, E., Frey, D., & Madai, V. I. (2020). Explainability for artificial intelligence in healthcare: A multidisciplinary perspective. *BMC Medical Informatics and Decision Making*, *20*(1), 310. DOI: 10.1186/s12911-020-01332-6 PMID: 33256715

Andras, P., Esterle, L., Guckert, M., Han, T. A., Lewis, P. R., Milanovic, K., Payne, T., Perret, C., Pitt, J., Powers, S. T., Urquhart, N., & Wells, S. (2018). Trusting intelligent machines: Deepening trust within socio-technical systems. *IEEE Technology and Society Magazine*, *37*(4), 76–83. DOI: 10.1109/MTS.2018.2876107

Annika, G., Christoff, Z., & Kerstin, L. (2024). Evaluation of the accuracy of an artificial intelligence in identifying contraindications to exercise therapy-comparison with and interrater reliability of physical therapists judgments. *Health and Technology*, *14*(3), 513–522. DOI: 10.1007/s12553-024-00827-w

Arai, K., Beppu, K., Ifuku, Y., & Oda, M. (2024). Method for Detecting the Appropriateness of Wearing a Helmet Chin Strap at Construction Sites [ijacsa]. *International Journal of Advanced Computer Science and Applications*, *15*(7), 7. DOI: 10.14569/IJACSA.2024.0150717

Ardic, N., & Dinc, R. (2025). Artificial intelligence in healthcare: Current regulatory landscape and future directions. *British Journal of Hospital Medicine*, *86*(8), 1–21. DOI: 10.12968/hmed.2024.0972 PMID: 40847984

Artsi, Y., Sorin, V., Glicksberg, B., Korfiatis, P., Nadkarni, G., & Klang, E. (2025). Large language models in real-world clinical workflows: A systematic review of applications and implementation. *Frontiers in Digital Health*, *7*, 1659134. Advance online publication. DOI: 10.3389/fdgth.2025.1659134 PMID: 41098649

Asadollahi, A. (2026). Governing by design: Algorithmic normativity, clinical standards, and health policy implications of AI in healthcare. *AI and Ethics*, *6*(1), 119. DOI: 10.1007/s43681-026-01002-9

Asan, O., Bayrak, A. E., & Choudhury, A. (2020). Artificial intelligence and human trust in healthcare: Focus on clinicians. *Journal of Medical Internet Research*, *22*(6), e15154. Advance online publication. DOI: 10.2196/15154 PMID: 32558657

Asif, S., Hadi, F., Yan, Y., Wang, V. Y., & Xu, D. (2026). The impact of large language models on medical research and patient care: A systematic review of current trends, challenges, and future innovations. *Computer Science Review*, *59*, 100847. DOI: 10.1016/j.cosrev.2025.100847

Azad, R., Aghdam, E. K., Rauland, A., Jia, Y., Avval, A. H., Bozorgpour, A., Karimijafarbigloo, S., Cohen, J. P., Adeli, E., & Merhof, D. (2024, December). Medical Image Segmentation Review: The Success of U-Net. *IEEE Transactions on Pattern Analysis and Machine Intelligence*, *46*(12), 10076–10095. DOI: 10.1109/TPAMI.2024.3435571 PMID: 39167505

Azad, R., Kazerouni, A., Heidari, M., Aghdam, E. K., Molaei, A., Jia, Y., Jose, A., Roy, R., & Merhof, D. (2024). Advances in medical image analysis with vision transformers: A comprehensive review. *Medical Image Analysis*, *91*, 103000. DOI: 10.1016/j.media.2023.103000 PMID: 37883822

Băjenesc, T.-M. I. (2020). Comparing artificial intelligence developments of superpowers: China and the US. *Journal of Social Sciences*, *3*(3), 43–50. DOI: 10.5281/zenodo.3971959

Bakken, S. (2023). AI in health: Keeping the human in the loop. *Journal of the American Medical Informatics Association : JAMIA*, *30*(7), 1225–1226. DOI: 10.1093/jamia/ocad091 PMID: 37337923

Bala Dhandayuthapani, V. (2024). Advancing healthcare: AI integration, interoperability and sustainability challenges. *Digital Health*, 64.

Banumathi, K., Venkatesan, L., Benjamin, L. S., Vijayalakshmi, K., Satchi, N. S., & Satchi, N. S.IV. (2025). Reinforcement learning in personalized medicine: A comprehensive review of treatment optimization strategies. *Cureus*, *17*(4). PMID: 40406780

Barnes, E., & Hutson, J. (2024). Navigating the complexities of AI: The critical role of interpretability and explainability in ensuring transparency and trust. *International Journal of Multidisciplinary and Current Educational Research*, *6*(3).

Belgaum, M. R., Charitha, T. H., Harini, M., Anusha, B., Sai, A. J., Yadav, U. C., & Alansari, Z. (2023). Enhancing the efficiency of diabetes prediction through training and classification using PCA and LR model. [AETiC]. *Annals of Emerging Technologies in Computing*, *7*(3), 78–91. DOI: 10.33166/AETiC.2023.03.004

Benjamens, S., Dhunnoo, P., & Meskó, B. (2020). The state of artificial intelligence-based FDA-approved medical devices and algorithms: An online database. *NPJ Digital Medicine*, *3*(1), 118. DOI: 10.1038/s41746-020-00324-0 PMID: 32984550

Bera, K., Schalper, K. A., Rimm, D. L., Velcheti, V., & Madabhushi, A. (2019). Artificial intelligence in digital pathology—New tools for diagnosis and precision oncology. *Nature Reviews. Clinical Oncology*, *16*(11), 703–715. DOI: 10.1038/s41571-019-0252-y PMID: 31399699

Bergquist, M., Rolandsson, B., Gryska, E., Laesser, M., Hoefling, N., Heckemann, R., Schneiderman, J. F., & Björkman-Burtscher, I. M. (2024). Trust and stakeholder perspectives on the implementation of AI tools in clinical radiology. *European Radiology*, *34*(1), 338–347. DOI: 10.1007/s00330-023-09967-5 PMID: 37505245

Bertl, M., Ross, P., & Draheim, D. (2022). A survey on AI and decision support systems in psychiatry - Uncovering a dilemma. *Expert Systems with Applications*, *202*, 117464. Advance online publication. DOI: 10.1016/j.eswa.2022.117464

Berzin, T. M., & Topol, E. J. (2025). Preserving clinical skills in the age of AI assistance. *Lancet*, *406*(10513), 1719. DOI: 10.1016/S0140-6736(25)02075-6 PMID: 41109709

Bhatnagar, A., & Singh, K. (2024). Hypertension detection system using machine learning. In *Prediction in medicine: The impact of machine learning on healthcare* (p. 95). https://doi.org/DOI: 10.2174/9789815305128124010009

Bickmore, T., Trinh, H., Asadi, R., & Fanzuch, M. (2025). LLM-based triage decision support: A prospective evaluation of accuracy and equity in emergency department settings. *NPJ Digital Medicine*, *8*(1), 45. PMID: 39828800

Bikdeli, B., Khairani, C. D., Bejjani, A., Lo, Y. C., Mahajan, S., Caraballo, C., Jimenez, J. V., Krishnathasan, D., Zarghami, M., Rashedi, S., Jimenez, D., Barco, S., Secemsky, E. A., Klok, F. A., Hunsaker, A. R., Aghayev, A., Muriel, A., Hussain, M. A., Appah-Sampong, A., & Krumholz, H. M. (2025). Validating International Classification of Diseases Code 10th Revision algorithms for accurate identification of pulmonary embolism. *Journal of Thrombosis and Haemostasis*, *23*(2), 556–564. DOI: 10.1016/j.jtha.2024.10.013 PMID: 39505153

Birch, J., Creel, K. A., Jha, A. K., & Plutynski, A. (2022). Clinical decisions using AI must consider patient values. *Nature Medicine*, *28*(2), 229–232. DOI: 10.1038/s41591-021-01624-y PMID: 35102337

Blezek, D. J., Olson-Williams, L., Missert, A., & Korfiatis, P. (2021). AI integration in the clinical workflow. *Journal of Digital Imaging*, *34*(6), 1435–1446. DOI: 10.1007/s10278-021-00525-3 PMID: 34686923

Bobby, N. N., Saravanan, V., Shanthiny, R., & Jenifer, J. (2026). Virtual Reality (VR) and AI in Physiotherapy for Cognitive and Physical Rehabilitation: Innovations in Biomedical Materials. In *Advanced Materials for Biomedical Devices* (pp. 395-412). CRC Press.

Bohra, Manvi & Singh, Kamred & Kumar, Indrajeet & Mishra, Shashank. (2025). Multi-Resolution Wavelet Packet-Driven Dual Path CNN for Breast Lesion Classification. IEEE Internet of Things Journal. PP. 1-1. .DOI: 10.1109/JIOT.2025.3594417

Bohra, Manvi & Singh, Kamred & Kumar, Indrajeet & Shah, Mohd. (2026). Wavelet-CNN Feature Fusion Architecture for Robust Breast Cancer Classification in Histopathological Imaging. International Journal of Computational Intelligence Systems. .DOI: 10.1007/s44196-026-01258-3

Bottomley, D., & Thaldar, D. (2023a). Liability for harm caused by AI in healthcare: An overview of the core legal concepts. *Frontiers in Pharmacology*, *14*, 1297353. DOI: 10.3389/fphar.2023.1297353 PMID: 38161692

Bouderhem, R. (2024). Shaping the future of AI in healthcare through ethics and governance. *Humanities & Social Sciences Communications*, *11*(1), 1–12. DOI: 10.1057/s41599-024-02894-w

Bouguettaya, A., Stuart, E. M., & Aboujaoude, E. (2025). Racial bias in AI-mediated psychiatric diagnosis and treatment: A qualitative comparison of four large language models. *npj. Digital Medicine*, *8*(1), 332. PMID: 40467886

Bourgeault, I., Dingwall, R., & de Vries, R. (2010). *The SAGE handbook of qualitative methods in health research*. SAGE. DOI: 10.4135/9781446268247

Brewster, R. C., Tse, G., Fan, A. L., Elborki, M., Newell, M., Gonzalez, P., Hoq, A., Chang, C., Chowdhury, M., Geeti, A., Hana, M., Hassan, H., Ibrahim, O., Keseyan, L., Li, Q., Mamoon, M., Nageye, M., Ohannessian, A., Eisenberg, I. R., & Khan, A. (2025). Evaluating human-in-the-loop strategies for artificial intelligence-enabled translation of patient discharge instructions: A multidisciplinary analysis. *NPJ Digital Medicine*, *8*(1), 629. DOI: 10.1038/s41746-025-02055-6 PMID: 41136708

Brown, T. B., Mann, B., Ryder, N., Subbiah, M., Kaplan, J., Dhariwal, P., & Amodei, D. (2020). Language models are few-shot learners. *Advances in Neural Information Processing Systems*, *33*, 1877–1901.

Bryman, A., & Bell, E. (2011). *Business research methods* (3rd ed.). OUP Oxford.

Buçinca, Z., Lin, P., Gajos, K. Z., & Glassman, E. L. (2020). Proxy tasks and subjective measures can be misleading in evaluating explainable AI systems. *Proceedings of the 26th International Conference on Intelligent User Interfaces*, 454–464. DOI: 10.1145/3377325.3377498

Buck, C., Doctor, E., Hennrich, J., Jöhnk, J., & Eymann, T. (2022). General practitioners' attitudes toward artificial intelligence–enabled systems: Interview study. *Journal of Medical Internet Research*, *24*(1), e28916. Advance online publication. DOI: 10.2196/28916 PMID: 35084342

Burrell, J. (2016). How the machine 'thinks': Understanding opacity in machine learning algorithms. *Big Data & Society*, *3*(1), 2053951715622512. Advance online publication. DOI: 10.1177/2053951715622512

Busch, F., Geis, R., Wang, Y. C., Kather, J. N., Khori, N. A., Makowski, M. R., . . . Bressem, K. K. (2025). AI regulation in healthcare around the world: what is the status quo? medRxiv, 2025-01. DOI: 10.1101/2025.01.25.25321061

Butt, U. M., Letchmunan, S., Ali, M., Hassan, F. H., Baqir, A., & Sherazi, H. H. R. (2021). Machine learning based diabetes classification and prediction for healthcare applications. *Journal of Healthcare Engineering*, *2021*(1), 9930985. DOI: 10.1155/2021/9930985 PMID: 34631003

Calabrò, R. S. (2025). Ethical Horizons in Robotic Rehabilitation: Ensuring Safe AI Use Under the EU AI Act. *Medical Science*, *13*(4), 317. PMID: 41440549

Carter, S. M., Rogers, W., Than Win, K., Frazer, H., Richards, B., & Houssami, N. (2020). The ethical, legal and social implications of using artificial intelligence systems in breast cancer care. *The Breast : Official Journal of the European Society of Mastology*, *49*, 25–32. DOI: 10.1016/j.breast.2019.10.001 PMID: 31677530

Cascella, M., Semeraro, F., Montomoli, J., Bellini, V., Piazza, O., & Bignami, E. (2024). The breakthrough of large language models release for medical applications: 1-year timeline and perspectives. *Journal of Medical Systems*, *48*(1), 22. Advance online publication. DOI: 10.1007/s10916-024-02045-3 PMID: 38366043

Castonguay, A., Wagner, G., Motulsky, A., & Paré, G. (2024). AI maturity in health care: An overview of 10 OECD countries. *Health Policy (Amsterdam)*, *140*, 104938. Advance online publication. DOI: 10.1016/j.healthpol.2023.104938 PMID: 38157771

Cestonaro, C., Delicati, A., Marcante, B., Caenazzo, L., & Tozzo, P. (2023). Defining medical liability when artificial intelligence is applied on diagnostic algorithms: A systematic review. *Frontiers in Medicine*, *10*, 1305756. DOI: 10.3389/fmed.2023.1305756 PMID: 38089864

Chakraborty, A., & Karhade, M. (2024). Global AI governance in healthcare: a cross-jurisdictional regulatory analysis. *arXiv preprint arXiv:2406.08695.*

Chang, Y., Yin, J. M., Li, J. M., Liu, C., Cao, L. Y., & Lin, S. Y. (2024). Applications and future prospects of medical LLMs: A survey based on the M-KAT conceptual framework. *Journal of Medical Systems*, *48*(1), 112. DOI: 10.1007/s10916-024-02132-5 PMID: 39725770

Chan, H. P., Samala, R. K., & Hadjiiski, L. M. (2019). CAD and AI for breast cancer—Recent development and challenges. *The British Journal of Radiology*, *93*(1106), 20190580. Advance online publication. DOI: 10.1259/bjr.20190580 PMID: 31742424

Charness, N., & Boot, W. R. (2016). Technology, gaming, and social networking. In *Handbook of the psychology of aging* (8th ed., pp. 389–407). Academic Press., DOI: 10.1016/B978-0-12-411469-2.00020-0

Chauhan, A., & Kumar, I. (2025). Deep feature extraction and optimized VGG16-SVM architecture for breast cancer characterization. *Discov Computing*, *28*(1), 208. DOI: 10.1007/s10791-025-09736-6

Checkland, P., & Holwell, S. (1998). Action research: Its nature and validity. *Systemic Practice and Action Research*, *11*(1), 9–21. DOI: 10.1023/A:1022908820784

Chen, J., Cai, Z., Ji, K., Wang, X., Liu, W., Wang, R., Hou, J., & Wang, B. (2024). HuatuoGPT-o1, towards medical complex reasoning with LLMs. *arXiv preprint arXiv:2412.18925.*

Chen, Z., Cano, A. H., Romanou, A., Bonnet, A., Matoba, K., Salvi, F., Pagliardini, M., Fan, S., Köpf, A., Mohtashami, A., & Sallinen, A. (2023). Meditron-70B: Scaling medical pretraining for large language models. *arXiv preprint arXiv:2311.16079.*

Chen, D., Tsang, E. C. C., Yeung, D. S., & Wang, X. (2005). The parameterization reduction of soft sets and its applications. *Computers & Mathematics with Applications (Oxford, England)*, *49*(5–6), 757–763. DOI: 10.1016/j.camwa.2004.10.036

Chen, R. J., Wang, J. J., Williamson, D. F. K., Chen, T. Y., Lipkova, J., Lu, M. Y., Sahai, S., & Mahmood, F. (2023). Algorithm fairness in artificial intelligence for medicine and healthcare. *Nature Biomedical Engineering*, *7*(6), 719–742. DOI: 10.1038/s41551-023-01056-8 PMID: 37380750

Chen, Z., Lin, M., Wang, Z., Zang, M., & Bai, Y. (2024). PreparedLLM: Effective pre-pretraining framework for domain-specific large language models. *Big Earth Data*, *8*(4), 649–672. DOI: 10.1080/20964471.2024.2396159

Chen, Z., Shen, Y., Song, Y., & Wan, X. (2020). Cross-modal memory networks for radiology report generation. In *Proceedings of the 59th Annual Meeting of the Association for Computational Linguistics and the 11th International Joint Conference on Natural Language Processing* (Volume 1: Long Papers) (pp. 5904–5914). Association for Computational Linguistics. https://doi.org/DOI: 10.18653/v1/2021.acl-long.459

Choi, H. J., & Raj, S. (2025). Episode-Driven Insights: Can Large Language Models Tackle Multimodal Diabetes Data? medRxiv, 2025-04. DOI: 10.1101/2025.04.24.25326385

Chomutare, T., Tejedor, M., Svenning, T. O., Marco-Ruiz, L., Tayefi, M., Lind, K., Godtliebsen, F., Moen, A., Ismail, L., Makhlysheva, A., & Ngo, P. D. (2022). Artificial intelligence implementation in healthcare: A theory-based scoping review of barriers and facilitators. *International Journal of Environmental Research and Public Health*, *19*(23), 16359. DOI: 10.3390/ijerph192316359 PMID: 36498432

Christophe, C., Kanithi, P. K., Munjal, P., Raha, T., Hayat, N., Rajan, R., Al-Mahrooqi, A., Gupta, A., Salman, M. U., & Gosal, G. (2024a). Med42—Evaluating fine-tuning strategies for medical LLMs: Full-parameter vs. parameter-efficient approaches. *arXiv preprint arXiv:2404.14779.*

Christophe, C., Kanithi, P. K., Raha, T., Khan, S., & Pimentel, M. A. F. (2024b). Med42-v2: A suite of clinical LLMs. *arXiv preprint arXiv:2408.06142.*

Clark, T., Foster, L., Bryman, A., & Sloan, L. (2021). *Bryman's social research methods.* Oxford University Press.

Corfmat, M., Martineau, J. T., & Régis, C. (2025). High-reward, high-risk technologies? An ethical and legal account of AI development in healthcare. *BMC Medical Ethics*, *26*(1), 4. DOI: 10.1186/s12910-024-01158-1 PMID: 39815254

Cross, J. L., Choma, M. A., & Onofrey, J. A. (2024). Bias in medical AI: Implications for clinical decision-making. *PLOS Digital Health*, *3*(11), e0000651. DOI: 10.1371/journal.pdig.0000651 PMID: 39509461

Cui, L., Liu, Y., Ouyang, C., Yu, Y., Zhang, J., Wan, Y., & Yang, F. (2026). Bailicai: A domain-optimized retrieval-augmented generation framework for medical applications. *Big Data Mining and Analytics*, *9*(2), 376–392. DOI: 10.26599/BDMA.2024.9020097

Dao, D., Teo, J. Y. C., Wang, W., & Nguyen, H. D. (2024, June). Llm-powered multimodal ai conversations for diabetes prevention. In Proceedings of the 1st ACM Workshop on AI-Powered Q&A Systems for Multimedia (pp. 1-6). DOI: 10.1145/3643479.3662049

Davenport, T., & Kalakota, R. (2019). The potential for artificial intelligence in healthcare. *Future Healthcare Journal*, *6*(2), 94–98. DOI: 10.7861/futurehosp.6-2-94 PMID: 31363513

Davids, J., Lidströmer, N., & Ashrafian, H. (2022). Artificial intelligence for physiotherapy and rehabilitation. In *Artificial intelligence in medicine* (pp. 1789–1807). Springer International Publishing. DOI: 10.1007/978-3-030-64573-1_339

Delahoz-Domínguez, E., Mendoza-Mendoza, A., & Visbal-Cadavid, D. (2025). Clustering using UMAP and K-means: Multidimensional analysis. *Logistics (Basel)*, *9*(3), 108. DOI: 10.3390/logistics9030108

Denecke, K., May, R., & Rivera-Romero, O. (2024). Transformer models in healthcare: A survey and thematic analysis of potentials, shortcomings and risks. *Journal of Medical Systems*, *48*(1), 23. DOI: 10.1007/s10916-024-02043-5 PMID: 38367119

Denscombe, M. (2018). *Forskningshandboken* (4th ed.). Studentlitteratur.

Desbordes, T., King, J., & Dehaene, S. (2024). Tracking the neural codes for words and phrases during semantic composition, working-memory storage, and retrieval. *Cell Reports*, *43*(3), 113847. DOI: 10.1016/j.celrep.2024.113847 PMID: 38412098

Deshmukh, S.SHAP-Based Explainable Framework for Disease Prediction and Comorbidity Risk Assessment in Healthcare. (July 25, 2025). Available at *SSRN*: https://ssrn.com/abstract=5368585 or http://dx.doi.org/DOI: 10.2139/ssrn.5368585

Dignum, V. (2019). *Responsible artificial intelligence: How to develop and use AI in a responsible way*. Springer. DOI: 10.1007/978-3-030-30371-6

Dlamini, Z., Francies, F. Z., Hull, R., & Marima, R. (2020). Artificial intelligence (AI) and big data in cancer and precision oncology. *Computational and Structural Biotechnology Journal*, *18*, 2300–2311. DOI: 10.1016/j.csbj.2020.08.019 PMID: 32994889

Dolatkhah Laein, G. (2024). Global perspectives on governing healthcare AI: Prioritising safety, equity and collaboration. *BMJ Leader*, *9*(1), e000904. DOI: 10.1136/leader-2023-000904 PMID: 38806230

Eachempati, P., Supe, A., Kumbargere Nagraj, S., Cresswell-Boyes, A., Robinson, S., & Yalamanchili, S. (2025). Integrating ai with healthcare expertise: Introducing the health care professional-in-the-loop framework: Part 1. *BDJ. In Practice*, *38*(2), 51–53.

Eisbach, S., Langer, M., & Hertel, G. (2023). Optimizing human-AI collaboration: Effects of motivation and accuracy information in AI-supported decision-making. *Computers in Human Behavior: Artificial Humans*, *1*(2), 100015. Advance online publication. DOI: 10.1016/j.chbah.2023.100015

Ennab, M., & Mcheick, H. (2022). Designing an interpretability-based model to explain the artificial intelligence algorithms in healthcare. *Diagnostics (Basel)*, *12*(7), 1557. DOI: 10.3390/diagnostics12071557 PMID: 35885463

Ennab, M., & Mcheick, H. (2024). Enhancing interpretability and accuracy of AI models in healthcare: A comprehensive review on challenges and future directions. *Frontiers in Robotics and AI*, *11*, 1444763. DOI: 10.3389/frobt.2024.1444763 PMID: 39677978

Ericksson, B. J., Korfiatis, P., Kline, T. L., Akkus, Z., Philbrick, K., & Weston, A. D. (2018). Deep learning in radiology: Does one size fit all? *Journal of the American College of Radiology*, *15*(3), 521–526. DOI: 10.1016/j.jacr.2017.12.027 PMID: 29396120

Ernazarovich, S. S., & Farxadovna, K. M. (2026, January). ARTIFICIAL INTELLIGENCE AND ITS CONTRIBUTION TO THE DEVELOPMENT OF CLINICAL REASONING SKILLS IN MEDICAL TRAINING. In *International Conference on Multidisciplinary Sciences and Innovations (ICMSI)* (Vol. 1, No. 2, pp. 29-35).

European Commission. (2024). *Regulation (EU) 2024/1689 of the European Parliament and of the Council of 13 June 2024 laying down harmonised rules on artificial intelligence (Artificial Intelligence Act)*. Official Journal of the European Union.

Feng, J., Phillips, R. V., Malenica, I., Bishara, A., Hubbard, A. E., Celi, L. A., & Pirracchio, R. (2022). Clinical artificial intelligence quality improvement: Towards continual monitoring and updating of AI algorithms in healthcare. *NPJ Digital Medicine*, *5*(1), 66. DOI: 10.1038/s41746-022-00611-y PMID: 35641814

Ferrazzi, P., Soroa, A., & Agerri, R. (2025). Grounded multilingual medical reasoning for question answering with large language models. *arXiv preprint arXiv:2512.05658.*

Ferreira, J. C., Elvas, L. B., Correia, R., & Mascarenhas, M. (2025). Tokenization of electronic health records and healthcare data: Enhancing security and privacy while enabling usability. *Health and Technology*, *15*(6), 1011–1020. DOI: 10.1007/s12553-025-01012-3

Finlayson, S. G., Subbaswamy, A., Singh, K., Bowers, J., Kupke, A., Zittrain, J., Kohane, I. S., & Beam, A. L. (2021). The clinician and dataset shift in artificial intelligence. *The New England Journal of Medicine*, *385*(3), 283–286. DOI: 10.1056/NEJMc2104626 PMID: 34260843

Floridi, L., Cowls, J., Beltrametti, M., Chatila, R., Chazerand, P., Dignum, V., Luetge, C., Madelin, R., Pagallo, U., Rossi, F., Schafer, B., Valcke, P., & Vayena, E. (2018). AI4People—An ethical framework for a good AI society. *Minds and Machines*, *28*(4), 689–707. DOI: 10.1007/s11023-018-9482-5 PMID: 30930541

Fonseca, F. J. P. O., Matias, B. B. R., Pacheco, P., Muraoka, C. S. A. S., Silva, E. V. F., & Sesma, N. (2026). Artificial Intelligence-Assisted Treatment Planning in an Interdisciplinary Rehabilitation in the Esthetic Zone. *Journal of Esthetic and Restorative Dentistry*, *38*(1), 15–24. DOI: 10.1111/jerd.70034 PMID: 40977526

Food and Drug Administration. (2023). *Artificial intelligence/machine learning (AI/ML)-enabled medical devices*. U.S. Food and Drug Administration.

Fouad, S., Hakobyan, L., Ihongbe, I. E., Kavakli-Thorne, M., Atkins, S., & Bhatia, B. (2026). Human-Centered User Interface Design for Explainable AI in Chest Radiology: A Multi-Phase Co-Design Approach. *IEEE Access : Practical Innovations, Open Solutions*, *14*, 12498–12513. DOI: 10.1109/ACCESS.2026.3653233

Freeman, S., Wang, A., Saraf, S., Potts, E., McKimm, A., Coiera, E., & Magrabi, F. (2025). Developing an AI governance framework for safe and responsible AI in health care organizations: Protocol for a multimethod study. *JMIR Research Protocols*, *14*(1), e75702. DOI: 10.2196/75702 PMID: 40720809

Frommeyer, T. C., Gilbert, M. M., Fursmidt, R. M., Park, Y., Khouzam, J. P., Brittain, G. V., & Bihl, T. J. (2025, July). Reinforcement learning and its clinical applications within healthcare: A systematic review of precision medicine and dynamic treatment regimes. []. MDPI.]. *Health Care*, *13*(14), 1752. PMID: 40724777

Fulmer, C. A., & Gelfand, M. J. (2012). At what level (and in whom) we trust: Trust across multiple organizational levels. *Journal of Management*, *38*(4), 1167–1230. DOI: 10.1177/0149206312439327

Gaber, F., Shaik, M., Allega, F., Bilecz, A. J., Busch, F., Goon, K., & Akalin, A. (2025). Evaluating large language model workflows in clinical decision support for triage and referral and diagnosis. *npj. Digital Medicine*, *8*(1), 263. PMID: 40346344

Gaber, F., Shaik, M., Allega, F., Bilecz, A., Busch, F., Goon, K., Franke, V., & Akalin, A. (2025). Evaluating large language model workflows in clinical decision support for triage and referral and diagnosis. *NPJ Digital Medicine*, *8*(1), 263. Advance online publication. DOI: 10.1038/s41746-025-01684-1 PMID: 40346344

Gallegos, I. O., Rossi, R. A., Barrow, J., Tanjim, M. M., Kim, S., Dernoncourt, F., & Ahmed, N. K. (2024). Bias and fairness in large language models: A survey. *Computational Linguistics*, *50*(3), 1097–1179. DOI: 10.1162/coli_a_00524

Gangavarapu, A. (2024). Introducing L2M3, a multilingual medical large language model to advance health equity in low-resource regions. *arXiv preprint arXiv:2404.08705*.

Gao, Y., Geras, K. J., Lewin, A. A., & Moy, L. (2019). New frontiers: An update on computer-aided diagnosis for breast imaging in the age of artificial intelligence. *AJR. American Journal of Roentgenology*, *212*(2), 300–307. DOI: 10.2214/AJR.18.20392 PMID: 30667309

García-Ferrero, I., Agerri, R., Salazar, A. A., Cabrio, E., de la Iglesia, I., & Lavelli, A. (2024). Medical mT5: An open-source multilingual text-to-text LLM for the medical domain. *arXiv preprint arXiv:2404.07613*.

Gemma Team. (2024). Gemma: Open models based on gemini research and technology. arXiv preprint arXiv:2403.08295.

Gerke, S. (2021). *Health AI for Good Rather Than Evil? The Need for a New Regulatory Framework for AI-Based Medical Devices* (SSRN Scholarly Paper No. 4070947). Social Science Research Network. https://papers.ssrn.com/abstract=4070947

Gerke, S., Minssen, T., & Cohen, G. (2020). Ethical and legal challenges of artificial intelligence-driven healthcare. *Cambridge Quarterly of Healthcare Ethics*, *29*(4), 605–613. DOI: 10.1017/S0963180120000674

Ghassemi, M., Oakden-Rayner, L., & Beam, A. L. (2021). The false hope of current approaches to explainable artificial intelligence in health care. *The Lancet. Digital Health, 3*(11), e745–e750. DOI: 10.1016/S2589-7500(21)00208-9 PMID: 34711379

Ghosh, A., Sridhar, S., Ravi, R. K., Muhsin, M., Saha, S., & Agarwal, C. (2025). CLINIC: Evaluating multilingual trustworthiness in language models for healthcare. *arXiv preprint arXiv:2512.11437*.

Ghribi, F., & Hamdaoui, F. (2025). Innovative deep learning architectures for medical image diagnosis: A comprehensive review of convolutional, recurrent, and transformer models. *The Visual Computer, 41*(13), 11603–11628. DOI: 10.1007/s00371-025-04122-1

Gichoya, J. W., Banerjee, I., Bhimireddy, A. R., Burns, J. L., Celi, L. A., Chen, L.-C., Correa, R., Dullerud, N., Ghassemi, M., Huang, S.-C., Kuo, P.-C., Lungren, M. P., Palmer, L. J., Price, B. J., Purkayastha, S., Pyrros, A. T., Oakden-Rayner, L., Okechukwu, C., Seyyed-Kalantari, L., & Zhang, H. (2022). AI recognition of patient race in medical imaging: A modelling study. *The Lancet. Digital Health, 4*(6), e406–e414. DOI: 10.1016/S2589-7500(22)00063-2 PMID: 35568690

Gille, F., Jobin, A., & Ienca, M. (2020). What we talk about when we talk about trust: Theory of trust for AI in healthcare. *Intelligence-Based Medicine, 1-2*, 100001. Advance online publication. DOI: 10.1016/j.ibmed.2020.100001

Glikson, E., & Woolley, A. W. (2020). Human trust in artificial intelligence: Review of empirical research. *The Academy of Management Annals, 14*(2), 627–660. DOI: 10.5465/annals.2018.0057

Goel, R., Jaiswal, U. K., Singh, P., Yadav, S. P., & Upadhyay, P. (2025). Deep learning for early brain tumor detection: A Keras-Based approach using MRI and CT imaging. In *Demystifying the role of natural Language processing (NLP) in mental health* (pp. 145-180). IGI Global Scientific Publishing. DOI: 10.4018/979-8-3693-4203-9.ch009

Goktas, P., & Grzybowski, A. (2025). Shaping the future of healthcare: Ethical clinical challenges and pathways to trustworthy AI. *Journal of Clinical Medicine, 14*(5), 1605. DOI: 10.3390/jcm14051605 PMID: 40095575

Gonçalves, A. R., Pinto, D. C., Rita, P., & Pires, T. (2023). Artificial intelligence and its ethical implications for marketing. *Emerging Science Journal, 7*(2), 313–327. DOI: 10.28991/ESJ-2023-07-02-01

Greengrass, C. J. (2025). Transforming clinical reasoning—The role of AI in supporting human cognitive limitations. *Frontiers in Digital Health, 7*, 1715440. DOI: 10.3389/fdgth.2025.1715440 PMID: 41561162

Griot, M., Hemptinne, C., Vanderdonckt, J., & Yüksel, D. (2024). Impact of high-quality, mixed-domain data on the performance of medical language models. *Journal of the American Medical Informatics Association : JAMIA, 31*(9), 1875–1883. Advance online publication. DOI: 10.1093/jamia/ocae120 PMID: 38781312

Guarnaccia, F. R., Spadazzi, F., Ottaviani, M., Di Fazio, N., Volonnino, G., Di Mauro, L., Frati, P., & La Russa, R. (2026). Artificial Intelligence and Orthopaedic Prosthetic Planning: A State-of-the-Art Review and Evolving Liability Perspectives. *Sci, 8*(2), 27. DOI: 10.3390/sci8020027

Guidance, W. H. O. (2021). Ethics and governance of artificial intelligence for health. *World Health Organization*, 1-165.

Güler, M. A., Dağ, S., Kayal, S., Can, M., & Şimşekkaya, S. N. (2026). Physiotherapy students' acceptance of AI-based chatbots (including ChatGPT) in education: A multi-institutional study from Turkey. *BMC Medical Education, 26*(1), 174. DOI: 10.1186/s12909-025-08535-3 PMID: 41484754

Gulshan, V., Peng, L., Coram, M., Stumpe, M. C., Wu, D., Narayanaswamy, A., Venugopalan, S., Widner, K., Madams, T., Cuadros, J., Kim, R., Raman, R., Nelson, P. C., Mega, J. L., & Webster, D. R. (2016). Development and Validation of a Deep Learning Algorithm for Detection of Diabetic Retinopathy in Retinal Fundus Photographs. *Journal of the American Medical Association, 316*(22), 2402–2410. DOI: 10.1001/jama.2016.17216 PMID: 27898976

Guo, H., Xing, X., Zhou, Y., Jiang, W., Chen, X., Wang, T., Jiang, Z., Wang, Y., Hou, J., Jiang, Y., & Xu, J. (2025). A survey of large language model for drug research and development. *IEEE Access : Practical Innovations, Open Solutions, 13*, 51110–51129. DOI: 10.1109/ACCESS.2025.3552256

Gupta, G. K., Acharya, N., & Pande, P. (2025). LLM-Based Support for Diabetes Diagnosis: Opportunities, Scenarios, and Challenges with GPT-5. arXiv preprint arXiv:2509.21450.

Gupta, G. K., Singh, A., Manikandan, S. V., & Ehtesham, A. (2025). Digital diagnostics: The potential of large language models in recognizing symptoms of common illnesses. *AI, 6*(1), 13. DOI: 10.3390/ai6010013

Gupta, N. S., & Kumar, P. (2023). Perspective of artificial intelligence in healthcare data management: A journey towards precision medicine. *Computers in Biology and Medicine*, *162*, 107051. Advance online publication. DOI: 10.1016/j.compbiomed.2023.107051 PMID: 37271113

Gupta, R. (2024). AI-based technologies, challenges, and solutions for neurorehabilitation: A systematic mapping. In *Computational Intelligence and Deep Learning Methods for Neuro-rehabilitation Applications* (pp. 1–25). Academic Press. DOI: 10.1016/B978-0-443-13772-3.00014-5

Hager, P., Jungmann, F., Holland, R., Bhagat, K., Hubrecht, I., Knauer, M., Vielhauer, J., Makowski, M., Braren, R., Kaissis, G., & Rueckert, D. (2024). Evaluation and mitigation of the limitations of large language models in clinical decision-making. *Nature Medicine*, *30*(9), 2613–2622. DOI: 10.1038/s41591-024-03097-1 PMID: 38965432

Haider, A., Al-Shibli, F. S., & Ahmad, I. (2026). Policy and Regulatory Landscape: A Legal Framework for the Regulation of Advanced Nano Biomaterials: Responsibility, Risk, Reflexivity. In *Sustainable Corrosion Inhibition: Nanobiotechnological Solutions and Challenges* (pp. 251–276). IGI Global Scientific Publishing. https://www.igi-global.com/chapter/policy-and-regulatory-landscape/397891

Hamet, P., & Tremblay, J. (2017). Artificial intelligence in medicine. *Metabolism: Clinical and Experimental*, *69*, S36–S40. DOI: 10.1016/j.metabol.2017.01.011 PMID: 28126242

Hamid, S. (2016). *The opportunities and risks of artificial intelligence in medicine and healthcare*. CUSPE Communications. https://doi.org/DOI: 10.17863/CAM.25624

Han, T., Adams, L. C., Papaioannou, J. M., Grundmann, P., Oberhauser, T., Figueroa, A., Löser, A., Truhn, D., & Bressem, K. K. (2023). MedAlpaca—An open-source collection of medical conversational AI models and training data. *arXiv preprint arXiv:2304.08247*.

Haq, I. U., Felicetti, F., & Lamonaca, F. (2026). Measurement Uncertainty and Traceability in Upper Limb Rehabilitation Robotics: A Metrology-Oriented Review. *Journal of Sensor and Actuator Networks*, *15*(1), 8. DOI: 10.3390/jsan15010008

Harishbhai Tilala, M., Kumar Chenchala, P., Choppadandi, A., Kaur, J., Naguri, S., Saoji, R., & Devaguptapu, B. (2024). Ethical Considerations in the Use of Artificial Intelligence and Machine Learning in Health Care: A Comprehensive Review. *Cureus*, *16*(6), e62443. DOI: 10.7759/cureus.62443 PMID: 39011215

Harrington, C.. (2023). Risks and benefits of large language models in mental health care. *JMIR Mental Health*, *10*, e48745. DOI: 10.2196/48745

Harshavardhan, H., Shetty, S., Shetty, R. P., & Shetty, P. U. (2025). Advancements in NLP: From Rule-Based Methods to Modern Language Models. In *2025 IEEE International Conference on Electronics, Computing and Communication Technologies (CONECCT)* (pp. 1-5). IEEE. DOI: 10.1109/CONECCT65861.2025.11306594

Hasanzadeh, F., Josephson, C. B., Waters, G., Adedinsewo, D., Azizi, Z., & White, J. A. (2025). Bias recognition and mitigation strategies in artificial intelligence healthcare applications. *npj. Digital Medicine*, *8*(1), 154. Advance online publication. DOI: 10.1038/s41746-025-01503-7 PMID: 40069303

Hassan, M., Kushniruk, A., & Borycki, E. (2024). Barriers to and facilitators of artificial intelligence adoption in health care: Scoping review. *JMIR Human Factors*, *11*, e48633. DOI: 10.2196/48633 PMID: 39207831

Health, C. for D. and R. (2025, October 7). Artificial Intelligence in Software as a Medical Device. *FDA*. https://www.fda.gov/medical-devices/software-medical-device-samd/artificial-intelligence-software-medical-device

He, K., Gou, F., & Wu, J. (2023). Image segmentation technology based on transformer in medical decision-making system. *IET Image Processing*, *17*(10), 3040–3054. DOI: 10.1049/ipr2.12854

He, K., Mao, R., Lin, Q., Ruan, Y., Lan, X., Feng, M., & Cambria, E. (2025). A survey of large language models for healthcare: From data, technology, and applications to accountability and ethics. *Information Fusion*, *118*, 102963. DOI: 10.1016/j.inffus.2025.102963

Heron, J. (1996). *Co-operative inquiry: Research into the human condition*. SAGE Publications.

Higgins, O., Short, B., Chalup, S., & Wilson, R. (2023). Artificial intelligence (AI) and machine learning (ML) based decision support systems in mental health: An integrative review. *International Journal of Mental Health Nursing*, *32*(4), 966–978. Advance online publication. DOI: 10.1111/inm.13114 PMID: 36744684

Holden, R. J., & Karsh, B. T. (2010). The Technology Acceptance Model: Its past and its future in health care. *Journal of Biomedical Informatics*, *43*(1), 159–172. DOI: 10.1016/j.jbi.2009.07.002 PMID: 19615467

Howard, A., Reza, N., Aston, S., Woods, B., Gerada, A., Buchan, I., Hope, W., & Märtson, A. G. (2024). Antimicrobial treatment imprecision: An outcome-based model to close the data-to-action loop. *The Lancet. Infectious Diseases*, *24*(1), e47–e58. DOI: 10.1016/S1473-3099(23)00367-5 PMID: 37660712

Hu, D., Bao, Y., Wei, L., ... (2023) Supervised adversarial contrastive learning for emotion recognition in conversations. In: Proceedings of the 61st Annual Meeting of the Association for Computational Linguistics (Volume 1: Long Papers), ACL 2023. Association for Computational Linguistics, pp 10835–10852. https://doi.org/ DOI: 10.18653/v1/2023.acl-long.606

Huang, K., Mo, F., Zhang, X., Li, H., Li, Y., Zhang, Y., Yi, W., Mao, Y., Liu, J., Xu, Y., Xu, J., Nie, J.-Y., & Liu, Y. (2026). A survey on large language models with multilingualism: Recent advances and new frontiers. *Artificial Intelligence Review*. Advance online publication. DOI: 10.1007/s10462-026-11534-5

Humerick, M. (2018). Taking AI personally: How the E.U. must learn to balance the interest of personal data privacy & artificial intelligence. *Santa Clara High-Technology Law Journal*, *34*(4), 393–418. https://digitalcommons.law.scu.edu/chtlj/vol34/iss4/2

Ipaktchi, K. R., & Higinbotham, S. E. (2026). AI-Powered Rehabilitation and Monitoring Systems for Orthopedic Trauma Patients. In *New Technologies, Precision Medicine, and AI in Emergency General Surgery: Revolutionizing Surgical Practice for Optimal Patient Care* (pp. 303–311). Springer Nature Switzerland. DOI: 10.1007/978-3-032-09357-8_17

ISO/IEC 42001. (2023). Information technology — Artificial intelligence — Management system. International Organization for Standardization.

Jacovi, A., Marasovic, A., Miller, T., & Goldberg, Y. (2021). Formalizing trust in artificial intelligence: Prerequisites, causes and goals of human trust in AI. *Proceedings of the 2021 ACM Conference on Fairness, Accountability, and Transparency (FAccT '21)*, 624–635. https://doi.org/DOI: 10.1145/3442188.3445923

Jadhav, N. N., & Bainalwar, P. (2026). Remote Monitoring and Telehealth Solutions for Chronic Disease Care Integration of AI in Telemedicine for Continuous Patient Monitoring and Real-Time Interventions. *Artificial Intelligence and Machine Learning in Neurology*, *2*, 811–832. DOI: 10.1002/9781394389131.ch30

Jain, J., & Jaiswal, U. K. (2025). Revolutionizing Medicine: The Impact of Artificial Intelligence in Healthcare. In *Generative Intelligence in Healthcare* (pp. 176-209). CRC Press.

Jaiswal, U. K., Chauhan, A., & Gupta, R. (2023). Brain Tumor Recognition Leveraging Machine Learning and CNN. In *International Conference on Artificial-Business Analytics, Quantum and Machine Learning* (pp. 53-65). Singapore: Springer Nature Singapore.

Jing, B., Wang, Z., & Xing, E. (2019). Show, describe and conclude: On exploiting the structure information of chest X-ray reports. In *Proceedings of the 57th Annual Meeting of the Association for Computational Linguistics* (pp. 6570–6580). Association for Computational Linguistics. https://doi.org/DOI: 10.18653/v1/P19-1657

Jin, Y., Chandra, M., Verma, G., Hu, Y., De Choudhury, M., & Kumar, S. (2024). Better to ask in English: Cross-lingual evaluation of large language models for healthcare queries. In *Proceedings of the ACM Web Conference* (pp. 2627-2638). DOI: 10.1145/3589334.3645643

Ji, Z., Lee, N., Frieske, R., Yu, T., Su, D., Xu, Y., Ishii, E., Bang, Y. J., Madotto, A., & Fung, P. (2023). Survey of hallucination in natural language generation. *ACM Computing Surveys*, *55*(12), 1–38. DOI: 10.1145/3571730

Johnson, A. E., Pollard, T. J., Berkowitz, S. J., Greenbaum, N. R., Lungren, M. P., Deng, C. Y., Mark, R. G., & Horng, S. (2019). MIMIC-CXR, a de-identified publicly available database of chest radiographs with free-text reports. *Scientific Data*, *6*(1), 317. DOI: 10.1038/s41597-019-0322-0 PMID: 31831740

Josephson, J. R., & Josephson, S. G. (1994). Conceptual analysis of abduction. In *Abductive inference: Computation, philosophy, technology* (pp. 5–30). Cambridge University Press., DOI: 10.1017/CBO9780511530128.002

Jose, S., Nguyen, K. T. P., Medjaher, K., Zemouri, R., Lévesque, M., & Tahan, A. (2024). Advancing Multimodal Diagnostics: Integrating Industrial Textual Data and Domain Knowledge with Large Language Models. *Expert Systems with Applications*, *255*, 124603. DOI: 10.1016/j.eswa.2024.124603

Jothi, G., & Inbarani, H. H. (2012). Soft set based feature selection approach for lung cancer images. *arXiv preprint arXiv:1212.5391*.McInnes, L., Healy, J., & Melville, J. (2018).

Jung, I. C., Zerlik, M., Schuler, K., Sedlmayr, M., & Sedlmayr, B. (2026). An Explanation User Interface for Artificial Intelligence–Supported Mechanical Ventilation Optimization for Clinicians: User-Centered Design and Formative Usability Study. *JMIR Formative Research*, *10*(1), e77481. DOI: 10.2196/77481 PMID: 41632969

Jung, K. H. (2025). Large language models in medicine: Clinical applications, technical challenges, and ethical considerations. *Healthcare Informatics Research, 31*(2), 114–124. DOI: 10.4258/hir.2025.31.2.114 PMID: 40384063

Kabata, F., & Thaldar, D. (2024). Human in the loop requirement and AI healthcare applications in low-resource settings: A narrative review. *South African Journal of Bioethics and Law, 17*(2), 70–73.

Kaiser, T., & Wu, D. (2025). Fine-Tuning Pre-trained Transformer-Based Models for Sentence-Level Medical Text Classification. In *2025 IEEE International conference on Medical Artificial Intelligence (MedAI)* (pp. 58-69). IEEE. DOI: 10.1109/MedAI67139.2025.00015

Kanithi, P. K., Christophe, C., Pimentel, M. A., Raha, T., Saadi, N., Javed, H., Maslenkova, S., Hayat, N., Rajan, R., & Khan, S. (2024). MEDIC: Towards a comprehensive framework for evaluating LLMs in clinical applications. *arXiv preprint arXiv:2409.07314*.

Karimi, D., Dou, H., & Gholipour, A. (2022). Medical Image Segmentation Using Transformer Networks. *IEEE Access : Practical Innovations, Open Solutions, 10*, 29322–29332. DOI: 10.1109/ACCESS.2022.3156894 PMID: 35656515

Karmali, Y. (2026). The Role of Artificial Intelligence in Workforce Adaptation and Skill Development. In *Artificial Intelligence in Healthcare and Biomedical Visualization* (pp. 171–186). Springer Nature Switzerland. DOI: 10.1007/978-3-032-06520-9_10

Kawas, M., Alkhatib, B., Omar, K., Tofelia, K., & Dashash, M. (2025). Using Medical Named Entity Recognition in Automatic ICD Prediction. *BioMed Research International, 2025*(1), 6117755. DOI: 10.1155/bmri/6117755 PMID: 41031257

Kelly, C. J., Karthikesalingam, A., Suleyman, M., Corrado, G., & King, D. (2019). Key challenges for delivering clinical impact with artificial intelligence. *BMC Medicine, 17*(1), 195. DOI: 10.1186/s12916-019-1426-2 PMID: 31665002

Khader, F., Müller-Franzes, G., Wang, T., Han, T., Arasteh, S., Haarburger, C., Stegmaier, J., Bressem, K., Kuhl, C., Nebelung, S., Kather, J., & Truhn, D. (2024). Multimodal deep learning for integrating chest radiographs and clinical parameters: A case for transformers. *Radiology, 309*(1), e230806. DOI: 10.1148/radiol.230806 PMID: 37787671

Khalid, S., Kim, H., & Kim, H. S. (2025). Recent trends in diabetes mellitus diagnosis: An in-depth review of artificial intelligence-based techniques. *Diabetes Research and Clinical Practice*, *224*, 112221. DOI: 10.1016/j.diabres.2025.112221 PMID: 40328407

Khalid, U. B., Naeem, M., Stasolla, F., Syed, M. H., Abbas, M., & Coronato, A. (2024). Impact of AI-powered solutions in rehabilitation process: Recent improvements and future trends. *International Journal of General Medicine*, *17*, 943–969. DOI: 10.2147/IJGM.S453903 PMID: 38495919

Khan, R. F., Lee, B. D., & Lee, M. S. (2023). Transformers in medical image segmentation: A narrative review. *Quantitative Imaging in Medicine and Surgery*, *13*(12), 8747–8767. DOI: 10.21037/qims-23-542 PMID: 38106306

Khan, , Rauf, Z., Rehman Khan, A., Rathore, S., Hussain Khan, S., Saher Shah, N., Farooq, U., Asif, H., Asif, A., Zahoora, U., Ullah Khalil, R., Qamar, S., Hani Tayyab, U., Babar Khan, F., Majid, A., & Gwak, J. (2025). A Recent Survey of Vision Transformers for Medical Image Segmentation. *IEEE Access : Practical Innovations, Open Solutions*, *13*, 191824–191849. DOI: 10.1109/ACCESS.2025.3618215

Khan, W. U., & Seto, E. (2023). A "Do No Harm" Novel Safety Checklist and Research Approach to Determine Whether to Launch an Artificial Intelligence–Based Medical Technology: Introducing the Biological-Psychological, Economic, and Social (BPES) Framework. *Journal of Medical Internet Research*, *25*, e43386. DOI: 10.2196/43386 PMID: 37018019

Khattak, M., Bowness, J. S., Yonis, R., Kierkegaard, P., McGregor, A., & Perry, D. C. (2025). Navigating the barriers and facilitators to implementation of AI in healthcare: A scoping review. *The Bone & Joint Journal*, *107*(7), 666–672. DOI: 10.1302/0301-620X.107B7.BJJ-2024-1570.R1 PMID: 40588252

Khullar, S., Magdalene, A. H. S., Sandhya, P., & Naik, B. R.**, N, H. K. B., & Raju, M. V. (2025).** Implementation, performance, and energy efficiency analysis for text classification of deep learning architectures. In *Proceedings of the 2025 10th International Conference on Communication and Electronics Systems (ICCES)* (pp. 2099–2103). IEEE. DOI: 10.1109/ICCES67310.2025.11336350

Khullar, S., Palaparthi, D. P., & Pradhan, S. K.**, R, B. V., Periyasamy, R., & Kaliappan, S. (2025).** Temporal fusion transformer–based early prediction of sepsis in ICU patients using multivariate vital signs and laboratory time-series data. In *Proceedings of the 2025 1st International Conference on Advancement in Futuristic Technologies (ICAFT)* (pp. 1–8). IEEE. DOI: 10.1109/ICAFT66710.2025.11452921

Khullar, S., Baghel, R. S., & Swami, P. (2026). Human-AI collaboration: Balancing trust, emotion, and productivity. In *AI hallucination management in the enterprise metaverse*. IGI Global., DOI: 10.4018/979-8-3373-7534-2.ch003

Khullar, S., Kate, C., Rao, A. S., Sharrif, U. H., Gupta, A., & Kaliappan, S. (2026). Explainable intelligence for ethical human-centric AI: Trust modeling using gradient boosting. In *Proceedings of the 2026 5th International Conference on Innovative Practices in Technology and Management (ICIPTM)* (pp. 1–9). IEEE. DOI: 10.1109/ICIPTM69057.2026.11465350

Kim, J. H. (2026). Automated Prescription of Therapeutic Exercise for Shoulder Impingement Syndrome using Literature-Driven Rule Generation Architecture. *Musculoskeletal Science & Practice*, *82*, 103520. DOI: 10.1016/j.msksp.2026.103520 PMID: 41707384

Kim, Y., Park, C., Jeong, H., Chan, Y. S., Xu, X., McDuff, D., Lee, H., Ghassemi, M., Breazeal, C., & Park, H. W. (2024). MDAgents: An adaptive collaboration of LLMs for medical decision-making. *Advances in Neural Information Processing Systems*, *37*, 79410–79452.

Kiseleva, A., Kotzinos, D., & De Hert, P. (2022). Transparency of AI in healthcare as a multilayered system of accountabilities: Between legal requirements and technical limitations. *Frontiers in Artificial Intelligence*, *5*, 879603. DOI: 10.3389/frai.2022.879603 PMID: 35707765

Kitey, P., & Lalwani, L. (2025, November). Feasibility and Safety of Artificial Intelligence Driven Telemetric Cardiac Rehabilitation in Adjunct to Home Exercise Education in Pediatric Patients with Congenital Heart Disease: A Pilot Study. In *2025 3rd DMIHER International Conference on Artificial Intelligence in Healthcare, Education and Industry (IDICAIHEI)* (pp. 1-5). IEEE. DOI: 10.1109/IDICAIHEI65991.2025.11378932

Koca, Y. B., & Aktepe, E. (2024). Effect of dimension reduction with PCA and machine learning algorithms on diabetes diagnosis performance. *Turkish Journal of Engineering*, *8*(3), 447–456. DOI: 10.31127/tuje.1413087

Kropf, M., Spöck, C., & Werner, R. (2026). Blame the Robot: Role Responsibility and Ethical Issues Regarding AI-Based Care Robots. *International Journal of Social Robotics*, *18*(2), 30. DOI: 10.1007/s12369-026-01369-z

Kumar, S., Datta, S., Singh, V., Datta, D., Singh, S. K., & Sharma, R. (2024). Applications, challenges, and future directions of human-in-the-loop learning. *IEEE Access : Practical Innovations, Open Solutions*, *12*, 75735–75760. DOI: 10.1109/ACCESS.2024.3401547

Kung, T. H., Cheatham, M., Medenilla, A., Sillos, C., De Leon, L., Elepaño, C., Madriaga, M., Aggabao, R., Diaz-Candido, G., Maningo, J., & Tseng, V. (2023). Performance of ChatGPT on USMLE: Potential for AI-assisted medical education using large language models. *PLOS Digital Health*, *2*(2), e0000198. DOI: 10.1371/journal.pdig.0000198 PMID: 36812645

Labrak, Y., Bazoge, A., Morin, E., Gourraud, P. A., Rouvier, M., & Dufour, R. (2024). Biomistral: A collection of open-source pretrained large language models for medical domains. *arXiv preprint arXiv:2402.10373*. DOI: 10.18653/v1/2024.findings-acl.348

Lai, T. (2024). Interpretable Medical Imagery Diagnosis with Self-Attentive Transformers: A Review of Explainable AI for Health Care. *BioMedInformatics*, *4*(1), 113–126. DOI: 10.3390/biomedinformatics4010008

Lamb, L. R., Lehman, C. D., Gastounioti, A., Conant, E. F., & Bahl, M. (2022). Artificial intelligence (AI) for screening mammography, from the AI special series on AI applications. *AJR. American Journal of Roentgenology*, *219*(3), 369–380. Advance online publication. DOI: 10.2214/AJR.21.27071 PMID: 35018795

La, N., Rattanapitoon, S. K., Thitimahatthanakusol, P., & Rattanapitoon, N. K. (2026). From Accuracy to Allocation: A Physiotherapy-Specific Risk Framework for AI-Mediated Exercise Advice in Breast Cancer Survivorship. *Physiotherapy*, 101894. DOI: 10.1016/j.physio.2026.101894 PMID: 41916863

Lanotte, F., O'Brien, M. K., & Jayaraman, A. (2023). AI in rehabilitation medicine: Opportunities and challenges. *Annals of Rehabilitation Medicine*, *47*(6), 444–458. DOI: 10.5535/arm.23131 PMID: 38093518

Lao, B., Tamei, T., & Ikeda, K. (2020). Data-efficient framework for personalized physiotherapy feedback. *Frontiers of Computer Science*, *2*, 3. DOI: 10.3389/fcomp.2020.00003

LaRosa, E., & Danks, D. (2018). Impacts on trust of healthcare AI. *Proceedings of the 2018 AAAI/ACM Conference on AI, Ethics, and Society (AIES '18)*, 210–215. https://doi.org/DOI: 10.1145/3278721.3278771

Le, E., Wang, Y., Huang, Y., Hickman, S., & Gilbert, F. J. (2019). Artificial intelligence in breast imaging. *Clinical Radiology*, *74*(5), 357–366. DOI: 10.1016/j.crad.2019.02.006 PMID: 30898381

Lee, M. H., Siewiorek, D. P., Smailagic, A., Bernardino, A., & Bermúdez i Badia, S. B. (2021, May). A human-ai collaborative approach for clinical decision making on rehabilitation assessment. In *Proceedings of the 2021 CHI conference on human factors in computing systems* (pp. 1-14). DOI: 10.1145/3411764.3445472

Leslie, D., Mazumder, A., Peppin, A., Wolters, M. K., & Hagerty, A. (2021). *Understanding artificial intelligence ethics and safety*. Alan Turing Institute.

Le, T. D., Nguyen, T. T., Ha, V. N., Chatzinotas, S., Jouvet, P., & Noumeir, R. (2025). The impact of LoRA adapters on LLMs for clinical text classification under computational and data constraints. *IEEE Access : Practical Innovations, Open Solutions, 13*, 109365–109377. DOI: 10.1109/ACCESS.2025.3582037

Lewis, P., Perez, E., Piktus, A., Petroni, F., Karpukhin, V., Goyal, N., & Kiela, D. (2020). Retrieval-augmented generation for knowledge-intensive NLP tasks. *Advances in Neural Information Processing Systems, 33*, 9459–9474.

Li, F., Chen, Y., Liu, H., Yang, R., Yuan, H., Jiang, Y., Li, T., Taylor, E. M., Rouhizadeh, H., Iwasawa, Y., & Teodoro, D. (2025a). MKG-Rank: Enhancing large language models with knowledge graph for multilingual medical question answering. *arXiv preprint arXiv:2503.16131.*

Liang, J., Li, R., & Jin, Q. (2020) Semi-supervised multi-modal emotion recognition with cross-modal distribution matching. In: MM '20: The 28th ACM International Conference on Multimedia. ACM, pp 2852–2861. https://doi.org/DOI: 10.1145/3394171.3413579

Liang, C. C., Hsu, W. C., Tsai, Y. T., Weng, S. J., Liu, S. C., & Lin, C. H. (2020, July). Factors related to diabetes mellitus in the middle-aged and over in taiwan. []. MDPI.]. *Health Care, 8*(3), 242. PMID: 32751283

Liddell, K., Simon, D. A., & Lucassen, A. (2021). Patient data ownership: Who owns your health? *Journal of Law and the Biosciences, 8*(2), lsab023. Advance online publication. DOI: 10.1093/jlb/lsab023 PMID: 34611493

Lin, J. C., Jain, B., Iyer, J. M., Rola, I., Srinivasan, A. R., Kang, C., Patel, H., & Parikh, R. B. (2025). Benefit-Risk Reporting for FDA-Cleared Artificial Intelligence–Enabled Medical Devices. *JAMA Health Forum, 6*(9), e253351. DOI: 10.1001/jamahealthforum.2025.3351 PMID: 41004181

Li, Q., Qiu, C., Liu, H., Gu, J., & Luo, D. (2025b). Decoupled contrastive learning for multilingual multimodal medical pre-trained model. *Neurocomputing, 633*, 129809. DOI: 10.1016/j.neucom.2025.129809

Liu, F., Zhou, H., Gu, B., Zou, X., Huang, J., Wu, J., Li, Y., Chen, S. S., Hua, Y., Zhou, P., Liu, J., Mao, C., You, C., Wu, X., Zheng, Y., Clifton, L., Li, Z., Luo, J., & Clifton, D. A. (2025). Application of large language models in medicine. *Nature Reviews Bioengineering*, *3*(6), 1–20. DOI: 10.1038/s44222-025-00279-5

Liu, H., & Xie, Q. (2025). Applications of artificial intelligence in rehabilitation: Technological innovation and transformation of clinical practice. *SLAS Technology*, *35*, 100360. DOI: 10.1016/j.slast.2025.100360 PMID: 41161419

Liu, H., & Zhong, K. (2025). SSMIM: Semi-supervised Multimodal Interaction Model for real-time conversational emotion recognition. *The Journal of Supercomputing*, *81*(8), 897. DOI: 10.1007/s11227-025-07373-w

Liu, J., Cen, X., Yi, C., Wang, F., Ding, J., Cheng, J., Wu, Q., Gai, B., Zhou, Y., He, R., Gao, F., & Li, Y. (2025). Challenges in AI-driven biomedical multimodal data fusion and analysis. *Genomics, Proteomics & Bioinformatics*, *23*(1), qzaf011. Advance online publication. DOI: 10.1093/gpbjnl/qzaf011 PMID: 40036568

Liu, Z., Gan, C., Wang, J., Zhang, Y., Bo, Z., Sun, M., & Zhang, W. (2025, April). Ontotune: Ontology-driven self-training for aligning large language models. In *Proceedings of the ACM on Web Conference 2025* (pp. 119-133). DOI: 10.1145/3696410.3714816

Lockey, S., Gillespie, N., Holm, D., & Asadi Someh, I. (2021). A review of trust in artificial intelligence: Challenges, vulnerabilities and future directions. *Proceedings of the 54th Hawaii International Conference on System Sciences (HICSS-54)*. https://doi.org/DOI: 10.24251/HICSS.2021.664

Luo, Y., Li, W., Chen, C., Li, X., Liu, T., Niu, T., & Yuan, Y. (2025). LLM-Guided Decoupled Probabilistic Prompt for Continual Learning in Medical Image Diagnosis. *IEEE Transactions on Medical Imaging*, *44*(8), 3439–3450. DOI: 10.1109/TMI.2025.3566105 PMID: 40310742

Lv, X., Luo, J., Huang, W., Guo, H., Bai, X., Yan, P., & Li, M. (2024). Identifying diagnostic indicators for type 2 diabetes mellitus from physical examination using interpretable machine learning approach. *Frontiers in Endocrinology*, *15*, 1376220. DOI: 10.3389/fendo.2024.1376220 PMID: 38562414

Lysaght, T., Lim, H. Y., Xafis, V., & Ngiam, K. Y. (2019). AI-assisted decision-making in healthcare: The application of an ethics framework for big data in health and research. *Asian Bioethics Review*, *11*(3), 299–314. DOI: 10.1007/s41649-019-00096-0 PMID: 33717318

Ma, Y., Kolla, S., Kaliraman, D., Nolan, V., Hu, Z., Guan, Z., . . . Shickel, B. (2024). Temporal cross-attention for dynamic embedding and tokenization of multimodal electronic health records. *arXiv preprint arXiv:2403.04012.*

Macrae, C. (2025). Managing risk and resilience in autonomous and intelligent systems: Exploring safety in the development, deployment, and use of artificial intelligence in healthcare. *Risk Analysis*, *45*(4), 910–927. DOI: 10.1111/risa.14273 PMID: 38246857

Maji, P. K., Biswas, R., & Roy, A. R. (2003). Soft set theory. *Computers & Mathematics with Applications, 45*(4–5), 555–562. https://doi.org/ (03)00016-6DOI: 10.1016/S0898-1221

Maliha, G., Gerke, S., Cohen, G., & Parikh, R. B.MALIHA. (2021). Artificial Intelligence and Liability in Medicine: Balancing Safety and Innovation. *The Milbank Quarterly*, *99*(3), 629–647. DOI: 10.1111/1468-0009.12504 PMID: 33822422

Malle, F. B., & Ullman, D. (2021). A multidimensional conception and measure of human-robot trust. In *Trust in Human-Robot Interaction* (pp. 3–25). Academic Press., DOI: 10.1016/B978-0-12-819472-0.00001-0

Martinho, D., Sobreiro, P., Domingues, A., Martinho, F., & Nogueira, N. (2026, January). Ethical Responsibility in Medical AI: A Semi-Systematic Thematic Review and Multilevel Governance Model. []. MDPI.]. *Health Care*, *14*(3), 287. PMID: 41682137

Maurya, S., Asudani, D. S., Jain, J., Jaiswal, U. K., Jain, E., & Malviya, K. (2025). Evaluating the effectiveness of regression algorithms in predicting cancer progression. In *Parul University International Conference on Engineering and Technology 2025 (PiCET 2025)* (Vol. 2025, pp. 1367-1373). IET. DOI: 10.1049/icp.2025.1593

Mayer, R. C., Davis, J. H., & Schoorman, F. D. (1995). An integrative model of organizational trust. *Academy of Management Review*, *20*(3), 709–734. DOI: 10.2307/258792

McAlister, K. L., Gonzales, L., & Huberty, J. (2025). Rethinking AI Workflows: Guidelines for Scientific Evaluation in Digital Health Companies. *JMIR AI*, *4*(1), e71798. DOI: 10.2196/71798 PMID: 41343771

McInnes, L., Healy, J., & Melville, J. (2018). Umap: Uniform manifold approximation and projection for dimension reduction. *arXiv preprint arXiv:1802.03426.*

McKinney, S. M., Sieniek, M., Godbole, V., Godwin, J., Antropova, N., Ashrafian, H., Back, T., Chesus, M., Corrado, G. S., Darzi, A., Etemadi, M., Garcia-Vicente, F., Gilbert, F. J., Halling-Brown, M., Hassabis, D., Jansen, S., Karthikesalingam, A., Kelly, C. J., King, D., & Shetty, S. (2020). International evaluation of an AI system for breast cancer screening. *Nature*, *577*(7788), 89–94. DOI: 10.1038/s41586-019-1799-6 PMID: 31894144

McKnight, D., Carter, M., Thatcher, J., & Clay, P. (2011). Trust in a specific technology: An investigation of its components and measures. *ACM Transactions on Management Information Systems*, *2*(2), 1–25. DOI: 10.1145/1985347.1985353

McSherry, R., & Pearce, P. (2011). *Clinical governance: a guide to implementation for healthcare professionals*. John Wiley & Sons.

Mello, M. M., & Guha, N. (2024). *Understanding Liability Risk from Healthcare AI*.

Mennella, C., Maniscalco, U., De Pietro, G., & Esposito, M. (2023). The role of artificial intelligence in future rehabilitation services: A systematic literature review. *IEEE Access : Practical Innovations, Open Solutions*, *11*, 11024–11043. DOI: 10.1109/ACCESS.2023.3236084

Mennella, C., Maniscalco, U., De Pietro, G., & Esposito, M. (2024). Ethical and regulatory challenges of AI technologies in healthcare: A narrative review. *Heliyon*, *10*(4), e26297. DOI: 10.1016/j.heliyon.2024.e26297 PMID: 38384518

Miller, D., & Brown, E. (2018). Artificial intelligence in medical practice: The question to the answer? *The American Journal of Medicine*, *131*(2), 129–133. DOI: 10.1016/j.amjmed.2017.10.035 PMID: 29126825

Minssen, T., Gerke, S., Aboy, M., Price, N., & Cohen, G. (2020). Regulatory responses to medical machine learning. *Journal of Law and the Biosciences*, *7*(1), lsaa002. Advance online publication. DOI: 10.1093/jlb/lsaa002 PMID: 34221415

Mittal, S., & Aggarwal, Y. (2026). Evaluation of Large Language Models in the Diagnosis, Urgency Triage, and Initial Management of Ophthalmic Emergencies. *Cureus*, *18*(1). Advance online publication. DOI: 10.7759/cureus.101433 PMID: 41694895

Mittelstadt, B. (2021). Interpretability and transparency in artificial intelligence. *The Oxford handbook of digital ethics, 20*.

Mittermaier, M., Raza, M. M., & Kvedar, J. C. (2023). Bias in AI-based models for medical applications: Challenges and mitigation strategies. *NPJ Digital Medicine*, *6*(1), 113. DOI: 10.1038/s41746-023-00858-z PMID: 37311802

Moëll, B., Farestam, A., & Beskow, J. (2025). Swedish medical LLM benchmark: Development and evaluation of a framework for assessing large language models in the Swedish medical domain. *Frontiers in Artificial Intelligence*, *8*, 1538566. DOI: 10.3389/frai.2025.1557920 PMID: 40718621

Morley, J., Murphy, L., Mishra, A., Joshi, I., & Karpathakis, K. (2022). Governing data and artificial intelligence for health care: Developing an international understanding. *JMIR Formative Research*, *6*(1), e31623. DOI: 10.2196/31623 PMID: 35099403

Moss, L., Corsar, D., Shaw, M., Piper, I., & Hawthorne, C. (2022). Demystifying the black box: The importance of interpretability of predictive models in neurocritical care. *Neurocritical Care*, *37*(S2, Suppl 2), 185–191. DOI: 10.1007/s12028-022-01504-4 PMID: 35523917

Muluk, S. Y., & Olcucu, N. (2024). Comparative analysis of artificial intelligence platforms: ChatGPT-3.5 and GoogleBard in identifying red flags of low back pain. *Cureus*, *16*(7), e63580. PMID: 39087174

Mustafa, S. W., Sari, H., Asriany, A., & Hajeni, H. (2026). Transforming Workforce Development through AI-Driven Education Networks: A Pathway to Sustainable Economic Growth. In *Human-Centered Learning Design in the AI Era* (pp. 173–204). IGI Global Scientific Publishing.

Muthukrishnan, P. (2025). Artificial Intelligence and the Future of Physiotherapy: A Comprehensive Analysis of Workforce Transformation and Professional Adaptation by 2030. *Available at SSRN* 5779722. DOI: 10.2139/ssrn.5779722

Muthukrishnan, P., Shanmugalakshmi, G., & Rajadurai, S. (2025). *AI-Powered Physiotherapy: A Personalized*. Ethical, and Intelligent Rehabilitation Framework for the Posture-Disturbed Generation.

Nair, M., Svedberg, P., Larsson, I., & Nygren, J. M. (2024). A comprehensive overview of barriers and strategies for AI implementation in healthcare: Mixed-method design. *PLoS One*, *19*(8), e0305949. DOI: 10.1371/journal.pone.0305949 PMID: 39121051

Nambi, G., Alghadier, M., Mohamed, S. H. P., Aldhafian, O. R., Alshahrani, N. A., & Albarakati, A. J. A. (2024). Clinical usefulness of artificial intelligence in physiotherapy–a practice-based review. *SBV Journal of Basic. Clinical and Applied Health Science*, *7*(4), 184–188.

Natali, C., Marconi, L., Dias Duran, L. D., & Cabitza, F. (2025). AI-induced deskilling in medicine: A mixed-method review and research agenda for healthcare and beyond. *Artificial Intelligence Review*, *58*(11), 356. DOI: 10.1007/s10462-025-11352-1

Nazar, M., Unar, S., Ahmed, A., Su'ud, M. M., Alam, M. M., & Rahmat, A. (2026). Requirements Driven Explainable Artificial Intelligence Framework for Secure and Transparent Clinical Decision Support Systems. *IEEE Access : Practical Innovations, Open Solutions*, *14*, 29132–29144. DOI: 10.1109/ACCESS.2026.3664500

Nazi, Z. A., & Peng, W. (2024). Large language models in healthcare and medical domain: A review. *Informatics (MDPI)*, *11*(3), 57. DOI: 10.3390/informatics11030057

Nerella, S., Bandyopadhyay, S., Zhang, J., Contreras, M., Siegel, S., Bumin, A., Silva, B., Sena, J., Shickel, B., Bihorac, A., Khezeli, K., & Rashidi, P. (2024). Transformers and large language models in healthcare: A review. *Artificial Intelligence in Medicine*, *154*, 102900. DOI: 10.1016/j.artmed.2024.102900 PMID: 38878555

Neumann, M., & Vu, N. T. (2019) Improving speech emotion recognition with unsupervised representation learning on unlabeled speech. In: IEEE International Conference on Acoustics, Speech and Signal Processing, ICASSP. IEEE, pp 7390–7394. https://doi.org/DOI: 10.1109/ICASSP.2019.8682541

Nguyen, H. Q., Pham, H. H., Linh, L. T., Dao, M., & Khanh, L. (2022). VinDr-CXR: An open dataset of chest X-rays with radiologist's annotations. *Scientific Data*, *9*(1), 429. Advance online publication. DOI: 10.1038/s41597-022-01498-w PMID: 35858929

Nicora, G., Pe, S., Santangelo, G., Billeci, L., Aprile, I. G., Germanotta, M., Bellazzi, R., Parimbelli, E., & Quaglini, S. (2025). Systematic review of AI/ML applications in multi-domain robotic rehabilitation: Trends, gaps, and future directions. *Journal of Neuroengineering and Rehabilitation*, *22*(1), 79. DOI: 10.1186/s12984-025-01605-z PMID: 40205472

Nilsson, C. (2025). *The artificial intelligence (AI) competence paradox: how AI reshapes clinical expertise. Transforming Government: People*. Process and Policy.

Nisevic, M., Kulenovic, H., Milojevic, D., Levak, J., & Biasin, E. (2026). Regulatory challenges and liability pathways for AI-powered robots in EU medical practice. *AI & Society*, •••, 1–21. DOI: 10.1007/s00146-026-02869-2

Nivethitha, V., Daniel, R., Surya, B., & Logeswari, G. (2025). Empowering public health: Leveraging AI for early detection, treatment, and disease prevention in communities—A scoping review. *Journal of Postgraduate Medicine*, *71*(2), 74–81. DOI: 10.4103/jpgm.jpgm_634_24 PMID: 40488301

Norori, N., Hu, Q., Aellen, F. M., Faraci, F. D., & Tzovara, A. (2021). Addressing bias in big data and AI for health care: A call for open science. *Patterns (New York, N.Y.)*, *2*(10), 100347. DOI: 10.1016/j.patter.2021.100347 PMID: 34693373

Nurzynska, K., Strzelecki, M., Piórkowski, A., & Obuchowicz, R. (2025). AI in Medical Imaging and Image Processing. *Journal of Clinical Medicine, 14*(12), 4153. DOI: 10.3390/jcm14124153 PMID: 40565899

Oates, B. J., Griffiths, M., & McLean, R. (2023). *Researching information systems and computing* (2nd ed.). SAGE Publications Ltd.

Obermeyer, Z., Powers, B., Vogeli, C., & Mullainathan, S. (2019). Dissecting racial bias in an algorithm used to manage the health of populations. *Science, 366*(6464), 447–453. DOI: 10.1126/science.aax2342 PMID: 31649194

Ohu, F. C., Burrell, D. N., & Jones, L. A. (2025, October). Public Health Risk Management, Policy, and Ethical Imperatives in the Use of AI Tools for Mental Health Therapy. [). MDPI.]. *Health Care, 13*(21), 2721. PMID: 41228088

Ojewale, V., Suresh, H., & Venkatasubramanian, S. (2026). Audit Trails for Accountability in Large Language Models. *arXiv preprint arXiv:2601.20727.*

Okamura, K., & Yamada, S. (2020). Empirical evaluations of framework for adaptive trust calibration in human-AI cooperation. *IEEE Access : Practical Innovations, Open Solutions, 8*, 220335–220351. DOI: 10.1109/ACCESS.2020.3042556

Olatunji, T., Nimo, C., Owodunni, A., Abdullahi, T., Ayodele, E., Sanni, M., Aka, C., Omofoye, F., Yuehgoh, F., Faniran, T., & Dossou, B. F. (2024). AfriMed-QA: a Pan-African, multi-specialty, medical question-answering benchmark dataset. *arXiv preprint arXiv:2411.15640.*

Olawade, D. B., Plabon, S. B., Ojo, A., Ogunbona, M. A., Makanjuola, B. D., & Olasilola, R. (2026). Human in the loop artificial intelligence in healthcare: Applications, outcomes, and implementation challenges. *International Journal of Medical Informatics, 213*, 106362. DOI: 10.1016/j.ijmedinf.2026.106362 PMID: 41740273

Olawade, D. B., Weerasinghe, K., Teke, J., Msiska, M., Boussios, S., & Hatzidimitriadou, E. (2025). Evaluating AI adoption in healthcare: Insights from the information governance professionals in the United Kingdom. *International Journal of Medical Informatics, 199*, 105909. DOI: 10.1016/j.ijmedinf.2025.105909 PMID: 40198930

Olusegun, J., Oluwaseyi, J., Brightwood, S., & Temitope, O. M. (2024). *Integration of AI with electronic health records: Enhancing clinical workflows*. John Olusegun.

Pai, F. Y., & Huang, K. I. (2011). Applying the Technology Acceptance Model to the introduction of healthcare information systems. *Technological Forecasting and Social Change, 78*(4), 650–660. DOI: 10.1016/j.techfore.2010.11.007

Palama, V. (2025). A HIPAA-aware benchmark and evaluation harness for clinical LLMs to quantify hallucination, bias, and PHI leakage. *Well Testing Journal, 34*(S3), 830–849.

Palaniappan, K., Lin, E. Y. T., & Vogel, S. (2024). Global Regulatory Frameworks for the Use of Artificial Intelligence (AI) in the Healthcare Services Sector. *Health Care, 12*(5), 562. DOI: 10.3390/healthcare12050562 PMID: 38470673

Panagoulias, D. P., Palamidas, A., Virvou, M., & Tsihrintzis, G. A. (2025). A framework for evaluation and requirement extraction for fine-tuning of Large Language Models in multimodal medical diagnosis. *Knowledge-Based Systems, 326*, 113975. DOI: 10.1016/j.knosys.2025.113975

Papanastasiou, G., Dikaios, N., Huang, J., Wang, C., & Yang, G. (2024, March). Is Attention all You Need in Medical Image Analysis? A Review. *IEEE Journal of Biomedical and Health Informatics, 28*(3), 1398–1411. DOI: 10.1109/JBHI.2023.3348436 PMID: 38157463

Park, H. J. (2024a). Patient perspectives on informed consent for medical AI: A web-based experiment. *Digital Health, 10*, 20552076241247938. DOI: 10.1177/20552076241247938 PMID: 38698829

Patil, R., Heston, T. F., & Bhuse, V. (2024). Prompt engineering in healthcare. *Electronics (Basel), 13*(15), 2961. DOI: 10.3390/electronics13152961

Pedreschi, D., Giannotti, F., Guidotti, R., Monreale, A., Ruggieri, S., & Turini, F. (2019). Meaningful explanations of black box AI decision systems. *Proceedings of the AAAI Conference on Artificial Intelligence, 33*(1), 9780–9784. DOI: 10.1609/aaai.v33i01.33019780

Peixoto, H., Guimarães, T., & Santos, M. F. (2020). A new architecture for intelligent clinical decision support for intensive medicine. *Procedia Computer Science, 170*, 1035–1040. DOI: 10.1016/j.procs.2020.03.077

Perez, E., Huang, S., Song, F., Cai, T., Ring, R., Aslanides, J., . . . Irving, G. (2022). Red teaming language models with language models. arXiv preprint arXiv:2202.03286. DOI: 10.18653/v1/2022.emnlp-main.225

Pe, S., Dagliati, A., Parimbelli, E., Guerra, B. M. V., Sozzi, S., Bellazzi, R., & Nicora, G. How improper dataset split hinders model generalizability: a systematic comparison in Human Activity Recognition and exercise evaluation tasks. *Available at SSRN* 6074128. DOI: 10.1016/j.ijmedinf.2026.106464

Pesapane, F., Codari, M., & Sardanelli, F. (2018). Artificial intelligence in medical imaging: Threat or opportunity? Radiologists again at the forefront of innovation in medicine. *European Radiology Experimental*, *2*(1), 35. Advance online publication. DOI: 10.1186/s41747-018-0061-6 PMID: 30353365

Petrick, N., Chen, W., Delfino, J. G., Gallas, B. D., Kang, Y., Krainak, D., Sahiner, B., & Samala, R. K. (2023). Regulatory considerations for medical imaging AI/ML devices in the United States: Concepts and challenges. *Journal of Medical Imaging (Bellingham, Wash.)*, *10*(5), 051804. DOI: 10.1117/1.JMI.10.5.051804 PMID: 37361549

Philippe, T., Sikder, N., Jackson, A., Koblanski, M., Liow, E., Pilarinos, A., & Vasarhelyi, K. (2021). Digital health interventions for delivery of mental health care: Systematic and comprehensive meta-review. *JMIR Mental Health*, *9*(5), e35159. Advance online publication. DOI: 10.2196/35159 PMID: 35551058

Pieri, S., Mullappilly, S. S., Khan, F. S., Anwer, R. M., Khan, S., Baldwin, T., & Cholakkal, H. (2024). BiMediX: Bilingual medical mixture of experts LLM. *arXiv preprint arXiv:2402.13253*. DOI: 10.18653/v1/2024.findings-emnlp.989

Pruski, M. (2024). AI-Enhanced Healthcare: Not a new Paradigm for Informed Consent. *Journal of Bioethical Inquiry*, *21*(3), 475–489. DOI: 10.1007/s11673-023-10320-0 PMID: 38300443

Qiu, J., Lam, K., Li, G., Acharya, A., Wong, T. Y., Darzi, A., Yuan, W., & Topol, E. J. (2024). LLM-based agentic systems in medicine and healthcare. *Nature Machine Intelligence*, *6*(12), 1418–1420. DOI: 10.1038/s42256-024-00944-1

Qiu, P., Wu, C., Zhang, X., Lin, W., Wang, H., Zhang, Y., Wang, Y., & Xie, W. (2024). Towards building multilingual language model for medicine. *Nature Communications*, *15*(1), 8384. DOI: 10.1038/s41467-024-52417-z PMID: 39333468

Rahimi, B., Nadri, H., Lotfnezhad Afshar, H., & Timpka, T. (2018). A systematic review of the Technology Acceptance Model in health informatics. *Applied Clinical Informatics*, *9*(3), 604–634. DOI: 10.1055/s-0038-1668091 PMID: 30112741

Raiaan, M. A. K., Mukta, M. S. H., Fatema, K., Fahad, N. M., Sakib, S., Mim, M. M. J., Ahmad, J., Ali, M. E., & Azam, S. (2024). A review on large language models: Architectures, applications, taxonomies, open issues and challenges. *IEEE Access : Practical Innovations, Open Solutions*, *12*, 26839–26874. DOI: 10.1109/ACCESS.2024.3365742

Rajendran, G., Buchholz, S., Aragam, B., Schölkopf, B., & Ravikumar, P. (2024). Learning interpretable concepts: Unifying causal representation learning and foundation models. *arXiv preprint arXiv:2402.09236*.

Ramesh, P. (2025). AI Workflow Optimization in Clinical and Regulatory Environments. *KOS J AIML, Data Sci. Robot*, *1*(1), 1–7.

Raza, S., Radwan, A., Chaduvula, S., Alinoori, M., & Emmanouilidis, C. (2026). *Transparency in Agentic AI: A Survey of Interpretability*. Explainability, and Governance.

Richardson, J. P., Smith, C., Curtis, S., Watson, S., Zhu, X., Barry, B., & Sharp, R. R. (2021). Patient apprehensions about the use of artificial intelligence in healthcare. *NPJ Digital Medicine*, *4*(1), 140. DOI: 10.1038/s41746-021-00509-1 PMID: 34548621

Riis Hansen, E., Sagi, T., Hose, K., Lip, G., Bjerregaard Larsen, T., & Skjøth, F. (2022). Assigning diagnosis codes using medication history. *Artificial Intelligence in Medicine*, *128*, 102307. Advance online publication. DOI: 10.1016/j.artmed.2022.102307 PMID: 35534145

Rönn, T., Perfilyev, A., Oskolkov, N., & Ling, C. (2024). Predicting type 2 diabetes via machine learning integration of multiple omics from human pancreatic islets. *Scientific Reports*, *14*(1), 14637. DOI: 10.1038/s41598-024-64846-3 PMID: 38918439

Roselló Atanet, I., Tomova, M., Sieg, M., Sehy, V., Mäder, P., & März, M. (2025). Generating learning guides for medical education with LLMs and statistical analysis of test results. *BMC Medical Education*, *25*(1), 458. DOI: 10.1186/s12909-025-06978-2 PMID: 40158187

Rowe, M., Nicholls, D. A., & Shaw, J. (2022). How to replace a physiotherapist: Artificial intelligence and the redistribution of expertise. *Physiotherapy Theory and Practice*, *38*(13), 2275–2283. DOI: 10.1080/09593985.2021.1934924 PMID: 34081573

Rudin, C., Chen, C., Chen, Z., Huang, H., Semenova, L., & Zhong, C. (2022). Interpretable machine learning: Fundamental principles and 10 grand challenges. *Statistic Surveys, 16*, 1-85. 6.

Rutunda, S., Corden, G., Uwimana, A., Muhizi, J., Bayingana, C., & Otieno, G. (2025). Large language models for frontline healthcare support in low-resource settings. *npj. Digital Medicine*, *8*, 379.

Saab, K., Tu, T., Weng, W. H., Tanno, R., Stutz, D., Wulczyn, E., Carroll, A., Mahdavi, S. S., Peltz, C., & Natarajan, V. (2024). Capabilities of Gemini models in medicine. *arXiv preprint arXiv:2404.18416.*

Saeidnia, H. R. (2024). Foundations of artificial intelligence in healthcare. *Decision Making, 1*(2), 5.

Şahinbaş, K., Keskin, A., & Akçakoca, Ö. (2026). *Development of a care plan recommendation system for physical therapy patients. Pamukkale Üniversitesi Mühendislik Bilimleri Dergisi.* Advanced Online Publication.

Saldaña, J. (2013). *The coding manual for qualitative researchers* (2nd ed.). SAGE Publications.

Salim, M. S., Fu, L., Ramakrishnan, A. A., Yao, Z., & Yu, H. (2025). MedCOD: Enhancing English-to-Spanish medical translation of large language models using enriched chain-of-dictionary framework. *arXiv preprint arXiv:2509.00934.* DOI: 10.18653/v1/2025.findings-emnlp.350

Sallinen, A., Solergibert, A. J., Zhang, M., Boyé, G., Dupont-Roc, M., Theimer-Lienhard, X., Boisson, E., Bernath, B., Hadhri, H., Tran, A., & Rabbani, T. (2025). Llama-3-Meditron: An open-weight suite of medical LLMs based on Llama-3.1. In *Proceedings of the Workshop on Large Language Models and Generative AI for Health at AAAI 2025.*

Savage, C. H., Park, H., Kwak, K., Smith, A. D., Rothenberg, S. A., Parekh, V. S., Doo, F. X., & Yi, P. H. (2024). General-purpose large language models versus a domain-specific natural language processing tool for label extraction from chest radiograph reports. *AJR. American Journal of Roentgenology, 222*(4), 2330573. DOI: 10.2214/AJR.23.30573 PMID: 38230901

Sellergren, A., Kazemzadeh, S., Jaroensri, T., Kiraly, A., Traverse, M., Kohlberger, T., ... (2025). MedGemma technical report. *arXiv preprint arXiv:2507.05201.*

Sengupta, D., & Panda, S. (2026). How Clinicians Think and What AI Can Learn From It. *arXiv preprint arXiv:2601.12547.*

Shad, R., Klinton, B., & Potter, K. (2025). *The role of artificial intelligence in early disease detection: A review of current applications.* FMDB Transactions on Sustainable Health Science Letters., DOI: 10.69888/FTSHSL.2025.000361

Shafik, W., Hidayatullah, A. F., Kalinaki, K., Gul, H., Zakari, R. Y., & Tufail, A. (2026). A systematic literature review on transparency and interpretability of AI models in healthcare: Taxonomies, tools, techniques, datasets, open research challenges, and future trends. *Health and Technology*, *16*(2), 1–22. DOI: 10.1007/s12553-025-01051-w

Shah, O. I., Rizvi, D. R., & Mir, A. N. (2025). Transformer-Based Innovations in Medical Image Segmentation: A Mini Review. *SN Computer Science*, *6*(4), 375. DOI: 10.1007/s42979-025-03929-y

Shammi, S., Ghosh, P., Sutradhar, A., Shamrat, F., Moni, M., & Oliveira, T. (2025). Advances in artificial intelligence and blockchain technologies for early detection of human diseases. *IEEE Transactions on Computational Social Systems*, *12*(1), 210–237. DOI: 10.1109/TCSS.2024.3449748

Sharma, A., & Rathore, R. (2026). Secure AI in healthcare: Advanced privacy-preserving machine learning techniques for medical data. In *Artificial Intelligence and Sustainable Innovation* (pp. 244–251). CRC Press.

Sharma, D., Meshkat, S., Perivolaris, A., Kamaleddin, M. A., Teferra, B. G., Rueda, A., & Bhat, V. (2026). Reimagining psychiatric care with agentic AI: Promise, challenges, and a roadmap forward. *npj. Digital Medicine*. PMID: 41699048

Shawli, L., Alsobhi, M., Chevidikunnan, M. F., Rosewilliam, S., Basuodan, R., & Khan, F. (2024). Physical therapists' perceptions and attitudes towards artificial intelligence in healthcare and rehabilitation: A qualitative study. *Musculoskeletal Science & Practice*, *73*, 103152. DOI: 10.1016/j.msksp.2024.103152 PMID: 39067366

Shi, W., Zhuang, Y., Zhu, Y., Hazarika, D., Jin, D., & Yang, D. (2025). Retrieval-augmented generation for clinical LLMs: Reducing hallucination in high-stakes medical queries. *Journal of the American Medical Informatics Association : JAMIA*, *32*(1), 89–102. PMID: 39520711

Shool, S., Adimi, S., Amleshi, R. S., Bitaraf, E., Golpira, R., & Tara, M. (2025). A systematic review of large language model (LLM) evaluations in clinical medicine. *BMC Medical Informatics and Decision Making*, *25*(1), 25. DOI: 10.1186/s12911-025-02954-4 PMID: 40055694

Siino, M., Falco, M., Croce, D., & Rosso, P. (2025). Exploring LLMs applications in law: A literature review on current legal NLP approaches. *IEEE Access : Practical Innovations, Open Solutions*, *13*, 18253–18276. DOI: 10.1109/ACCESS.2025.3533217

Singhal, K., Azizi, S., Tu, T., Mahdavi, S., Wei, J., Chung, H., Scales, N., Tanwani, A., Cole-Lewis, H., Pfohl, S., Payne, P., Seneviratne, M., Gamble, P., Kelly, C., Scharli, N., Chowdhery, A., Mansfield, P., Arcas, B., Webster, D., & Natarajan, V. (2022). Large language models encode clinical knowledge. *Nature*, *620*(7972), 172–180. DOI: 10.1038/s41586-023-06291-2 PMID: 37438534

Singhal, K., Tu, T., Gottweis, J., Sayres, R., Wulczyn, E., Hou, L., Clark, K., Pfohl, S., Cole-Lewis, H., Neal, D., Schaekermann, M., Wang, A., Amin, M., Lachgar, S., Mansfield, P., Prakash, S., Green, B., Dominowska, E., Arcas, B. A. Y., & Natarajan, V. (2025). Toward expert-level medical question answering with large language models. *Nature Medicine*, *31*(3), 943–950. DOI: 10.1038/s41591-024-03423-7 PMID: 39779926

Singh, R. P., Hom, G. L., Abramoff, M. D., Campbell, J. P., & Chiang, M. F. (2020). Current challenges and barriers to real-world artificial intelligence adoption for the healthcare system, provider, and the patient. *Translational Vision Science & Technology*, *9*(2), 45–45. DOI: 10.1167/tvst.9.2.45 PMID: 32879755

Sisodia, D., & Sisodia, D. S. (2018). Prediction of diabetes using classification algorithms. *Procedia Computer Science*, *132*, 1578–1585. DOI: 10.1016/j.procs.2018.05.122

Smith, H., Downer, J., & Ives, J. (2024). Clinicians and AI use: Where is the professional guidance? *Journal of Medical Ethics*, *50*(7), 437–441. DOI: 10.1136/jme-2022-108831 PMID: 37607805

Soliman, A., Li, Z., & Parwani, A. V. (2024). Artificial intelligence's impact on breast cancer pathology: A literature review. *Diagnostic Pathology*, *19*(1), 38. DOI: 10.1186/s13000-024-01453-w PMID: 38388367

Song, D., Xie, W., Kong, C., Chen, J., Zhang, H., Chen, S., Gao, A., Jiang, F., Li, J., Wan, X., Li, H., & Wang, B. (2023). HuatuoGPT-II, one-stage training for medical adaption of LLMs. *arXiv preprint arXiv:2311.09774.*

Stone, P., Brooks, R., Brynjolfsson, E., Calo, R., Etzioni, O., Hager, G., Hirschberg, J., Kalyanakrishnan, S., Kamar, E., Kraus, S., Leyton-Brown, K., Parkes, D., Press, W., Saxenian, A., Shah, J., Tambe, M., & Teller, A. (2022). *Artificial intelligence and life in 2030: The one hundred year study on artificial intelligence*. Stanford University. https://doi.org//arXiv.2211.06318DOI: 10.48550

Strauss, A. T., Morgan, C., El Khuri, C., Slogeris, B., Smith, A. G., Klein, E., Toerper, M., DeAngelo, A., Debraine, A., Peterson, S., Gurses, A. P., Levin, S., & Hinson, J. (2022). A patient outcomes–driven feedback platform for emergency medicine clinicians: Human-centered design and usability evaluation of linking outcomes of patients (LOOP). *JMIR Human Factors*, *9*(1), e30130. DOI: 10.2196/30130 PMID: 35319469

Sunarti, S., Rahman, F. F., Naufal, M., Risky, M., Febriyanto, K., & Masina, R. (2021). Artificial intelligence in healthcare: Opportunities and risk for future. *Gaceta Sanitaria*, *35*(Suppl. 1), S67–S70. DOI: 10.1016/j.gaceta.2020.12.019 PMID: 33832631

Sun, C., & Harris, S. L. (2024). Reducing bias in healthcare artificial intelligence: A white paper. *Health Informatics Journal*, *30*(4), 14604582241291410. Advance online publication. DOI: 10.1177/14604582241291410 PMID: 39541598

Sunday, O. (2025). Behavioral Impacts of AI Reliance in Diagnostics: Balancing Automation with Skill Retention. *Epidemiol. Health Data Insights, 1*, ehdi014.

Sun, Z., Wong, Y., & Yeong, C. (2023). Patient-specific 3D-printed low-cost models in medical education and clinical practice. *Micromachines*, *14*(2), 464. Advance online publication. DOI: 10.3390/mi14020464 PMID: 36838164

Suresh, H., Hunt, N., Johnson, A. E., Celi, L. A., Szolovits, P., & Ghassemi, M. (2017). Clinical intervention prediction and understanding using deep networks. arXiv preprint arXiv:1705.08498.

Tack, C. (2019). Artificial intelligence and machine learningl applications in musculoskeletal physiotherapy. *Musculoskeletal Science & Practice*, *39*, 164–169. DOI: 10.1016/j.msksp.2018.11.012 PMID: 30502096

Tahavvori, A., Chelan, R. J., Aminoleslami, S., Moghadam, O. F., Haghighi, L., Abdian, Y., & Moradi, D. (2025). Large language models and ChatGPT in medical sciences: Foundations, capabilities, and challenges. *Kindle*, *5*(1), 1–222.

Taki, F. N., & Akdag, K. C. (2024). *Use of artificial intelligence in physiotherapy and rehabilitation. Current Studies in Basic Sciences, Engineering and Technology*. ISRES Publishing.

Tantowen, M., Putra, K., Isnan, M., & Pardamean, B. (2024). Principal component analysis implementation on machine learning in diabetes classification. *Commun. Math. Biol. Neurosci., 2024*, Article-ID.Cong, Y., et al. (2022).

Thakral, M., Nagpal, V., Devare, A., Devare, M. H., Ghosal, I., & Irfan, M. (2026). Education and Training for the AI-Enabled Healthcare Workforce. In *Artificial Intelligence (AI) for IT Energy Efficiency and Green AI for Environment Sustainability* (pp. 69–84). Springer Nature Switzerland. DOI: 10.1007/978-3-031-89420-6_4

Theilmann, K., Dahlem, N., Steffny, L., Podevin, D., Hartnik, J., & Greff, T. (2025, June). Towards Effective AI in Healthcare: Identifying Success Factors and the Potential of Human-in-the-Loop. In *IFIP International Conference on Artificial Intelligence Applications and Innovations* (pp. 173-188). Cham: Springer Nature Switzerland. DOI: 10.1007/978-3-031-96239-4_13

Thirunavukarasu, R., & Kotei, E. (2024). A comprehensive review on transformer network for natural and medical image analysis. *Computer Science Review*, *53*, 100648. DOI: 10.1016/j.cosrev.2024.100648

Thurzo, A., & Thurzo, V. (2025). Embedding fear in medical AI: A risk-averse framework for safety and ethics. *AI*, *6*(5), 101. DOI: 10.3390/ai6050101

Topol, E. J. (2019). High-performance medicine: The convergence of human and artificial intelligence. *Nature Medicine*, *25*(1), 44–56. DOI: 10.1038/s41591-018-0300-7 PMID: 30617339

Topuz, K., Abdulrashid, I., Davazdahemami, B., Coussement, K., & Delen, D. (2025). Developing an Interpretable Decision Support Framework for Artifact Design in Organ Transplantation. *Information Systems Frontiers*, *27*(6), 1–25. DOI: 10.1007/s10796-025-10652-9

Truong, T. D. (2025). The Evolving Synergy between AI and Human Expertise in Medical Diagnostics.

Turgunov, J. S., Rakhimova, M. O., Saidov, B. K., & Kholmatova, D. S. (2020). HUMAN-IN-THE-LOOP SYSTEMS FOR ETHICAL AI.

Uddin, J. (2025). Conversational AI in healthcare communication: Opportunities, risks, and implications for health equity. *Journal of Communication in Healthcare*, 1–4. DOI: 10.1080/17538068.2025.2594768 PMID: 41319058

Umapathi, L. K., Pal, A., & Sankarasubbu, M. (2023). Med-HALT: Medical domain hallucination test for large language models. arXiv preprint arXiv:2307.15343.

Van Der Maaten, L., Postma, E., & Van den Herik, J. (2009). Dimensionality reduction: A comparative. *Journal of Machine Learning Research*, *10*(66-71), 13.

Varkey, B. (2020). Principles of clinical ethics and their application to practice. *Medical Principles and Practice : International Journal of the Kuwait University, Health Science Centre, 30*(1), 17–28. DOI: 10.1159/000509119 PMID: 32498071

Vaswani, A., Shazeer, N., Parmar, N., Uszkoreit, J., Jones, L., Gomez, A. N., & Polosukhin, I. (2017). Attention is all you need. *Advances in Neural Information Processing Systems*, 30.

Vavekanand, R., Ali Laghari, A., & Kumar, T. (2026). Applications and limitations of large language models to integrate medical context: A comprehensive review. *Iran Journal of Computer Science, 9*(1), 12. DOI: 10.1007/s42044-025-00360-7

Vayena, E., Blasimme, A., & Cohen, I. G. (2018). Machine learning in medicine: Addressing ethical challenges. *PLoS Medicine, 15*(11), e1002689. DOI: 10.1371/journal.pmed.1002689 PMID: 30399149

Verbeek, P. P. (2011). *Moralizing technology: Understanding and designing the morality of things*. The University of Chicago Press. DOI: 10.7208/chicago/9780226852904.001.0001

Verma, A., Rao, K., Eluri, V., & Sharma, Y. (2020). Regulating AI in public health: systems challenges and perspectives. *ORF Occasional Paper, 261*, 1-46.

Verma, R. K. (2026). Federated Learning for Precision Medicine: A Blockchain-Enhanced Framework for Privacy-Preserving Predictive Analytics in Healthcare 5.0. In Shafik, W., Dutta, P. K., & Pattanaik, P. (Eds.), *The Convergence of Federated Learning and Healthcare 5.0 and Beyond: A New Era of Intelligent Health Systems. Studies in Computational Intelligence* (Vol. 1247). Springer., DOI: 10.1007/978-3-032-03985-9_28

Verma, R. K., & Kishor, K. (2024). Image Processing Applications in Agriculture With the Help of AI. In Khan, M., Khan, R., Praveen, P., Verma, A., & Panda, M. (Eds.), *Infrastructure Possibilities and Human-Centered Approaches With Industry 5.0* (pp. 162–181). IGI Global Scientific Publishing., DOI: 10.4018/979-8-3693-0782-3.ch010

Verma, R. K., Kumar, I., & Kumar, S. (2025). In Chand Kumain, S., Singh, M., Awasthi, L. K., & Singh, R. (Eds.), *"AI-driven insights: Revolutionizing satellite imagery applications," in *AI and ML Techniques in Image Processing and Object Detection* (pp. 89–104). Springer., DOI: 10.1007/978-981-96-7445-9_5

Vincent, C., & Amalberti, R. (2016). *Safer healthcare: Strategies for the real world*. Springer. DOI: 10.1007/978-3-319-25559-0

Vinnova. (2018). *Artificiell intelligens i svenskt näringsliv och samhälle - Analys av utveckling och potential* (Report No. 2018:08). Vinnova - Sveriges innovationsmyndighet.

Vrdoljak, J., Boban, Z., Vilović, M., Kumrić, M., & Božić, J. (2025, March). A review of large language models in medical education, clinical decision support, and healthcare administration. [). MDPI.]. *Health Care*, *13*(6), 603. PMID: 40150453

Wang, X., Chen, N., Chen, J., Wang, Y., Zhen, G., & Zhang, C. (2024). Apollo: A lightweight multilingual medical LLM towards democratizing medical AI to 6B people. *arXiv preprint arXiv:2403.03640*.

Wang, B., Qu, J., Li, X., Wang, C., & Bu, L. (2026). A personalized rehabilitation design method via knowledge graph-based multi-source data integration. *Advanced Engineering Informatics*, *69*, 104005. DOI: 10.1016/j.aei.2025.104005

Wang, C., Zhang, J., Lassi, N., & Zhang, X. (2022). Privacy Protection in Using Artificial Intelligence for Healthcare: Chinese Regulation in Comparative Perspective. *Health Care*, *10*(10), 1878. DOI: 10.3390/healthcare10101878 PMID: 36292325

Wang, D., & Zhang, S. (2024). Large language models in medical and healthcare fields: Applications, advances, and challenges. *Artificial Intelligence Review*, *57*(11), 299. DOI: 10.1007/s10462-024-10921-0

Wang, F., Zhang, Z., Zhang, X., Wu, Z., Mo, T., Lu, Q., Wang, W., Li, R., Xu, J., Tang, X., He, Q., Ma, Y., Huang, M., & Wang, S. (2025). A comprehensive survey of small language models in the era of large language models: Techniques, enhancements, applications, collaboration with LLMs, and trustworthiness. *ACM Transactions on Intelligent Systems and Technology*, *16*(6), 1–87. DOI: 10.1145/3768165

Wang, J., Shi, E., Yu, S., Wu, Z., Hu, H., Ma, C., & Zhang, S. (2025). Prompt engineering for healthcare: Methodologies and applications. *Meta-Radiology*, 100190.

Wang, P., Wang, A., & Wang, S. (2026). Integrating multimodal AI technologies for sports injury prediction and rehabilitation: Systematic review. *Journal of Human Sport and Exercise*, *21*(1), 22–37. DOI: 10.55860/w6j5wc21

Wang, R., Lei, T., Cui, R., Zhang, B., Meng, H., & Nandi, A. K. (2022). Medical image segmentation using deep learning: A survey. *IET Image Processing*, *16*(5), 1243–1267. DOI: 10.1049/ipr2.12419

Wang, X., Zhou, Y., & Zhou, G. (2025). The application and ethical implication of generative AI in mental health: Systematic review. *JMIR Mental Health*, *12*, e70610. DOI: 10.2196/70610 PMID: 40577783

Wang, Y., Huang, H., Rudin, C., & Shaposhnik, Y. (2021). Understanding how dimension reduction tools work: An empirical approach to deciphering t-SNE, UMAP, TriMAP, and PaCMAP for data visualization. *Journal of Machine Learning Research*, *22*(201), 1–73.

Ward, R. (2013). The application of technology acceptance and diffusion of innovation models in healthcare informatics. *Health Policy and Technology*, *2*(4), 222–228. DOI: 10.1016/j.hlpt.2013.07.002

Weiner, E. B., Dankwa-Mullan, I., Nelson, W. A., & Hassanpour, S. (2025). Ethical challenges and evolving strategies in the integration of artificial intelligence into clinical practice. *PLOS Digital Health*, *4*(4), e0000810. DOI: 10.1371/journal.pdig.0000810 PMID: 40198594

WHO. (2023). *Ethics and governance of artificial intelligence for health.* https://www.who.int/publications/i/item/9789240029200

WHO. (2025). *Ethics and governance of artificial intelligence for health: Guidance on large multi-modal models.* https://www.who.int/publications/i/item/9789240084759

Wiest, I. C., Leßmann, M. E., Wolf, F., Ferber, D., Van Treeck, M., Zhu, J., . . . Kather, J. N. (2024). Anonymizing medical documents with local, privacy preserving large language models: The LLM-Anonymizer. medRxiv, 2024-06. DOI: 10.1101/2024.06.11.24308355

World Health Organization. (2023). *Ethics and governance of artificial intelligence for health: Guidance on large multi-modal models.* World Health Organization.

Wu, C. H., Lin, J. C., & Wei, W. L. (2014). Survey on audiovisual emotion recognition: Databases, features, and data fusion strategies. *APSIPA Transactions on Signal and Information Processing*, *3*(1), e12. DOI: 10.1017/ATSIP.2014.11

Wu, C., Lin, W., Zhang, X., Zhang, Y., Xie, W., & Wang, Y. (2024). PMC-LLaMA: Toward building open-source language models for medicine. *Journal of the American Medical Informatics Association : JAMIA*, *31*(9), 1833–1843. DOI: 10.1093/jamia/ocae045 PMID: 38613821

Wu, C., Qiu, P., Liu, J., Gu, H., Li, N., Zhang, Y., Wang, Y., & Xie, W. (2025). Towards evaluating and building versatile large language models for medicine. *npj. Digital Medicine*, *8*(1), 58. PMID: 39865143

Xian, T., Mehandjiev, N., Constantinides, P., Chen, Y. W., Quboa, Q., & Kitchen, G. (2026). Clinician preferences for explainable artificial intelligence in critical care: A comparative study of interpretable models and visualizations for intubation decision support. *International Journal of Medical Informatics*, •••, 106287. DOI: 10.1016/j.ijmedinf.2026.106287 PMID: 41570512

Xiao, H., Zhou, F., Liu, X., Liu, T., Li, Z., Liu, X., & Huang, X. (2025). A comprehensive survey of large language models and multimodal large language models in medicine. *Information Fusion*, *117*, 102888. DOI: 10.1016/j.inffus.2024.102888

Xie, E., Zhao, Z., Yang, W., Li, X., Qi, L., Gao, M., Cao, Y., Fan, S., Pan, Y., & Gao, S. (2026). A plantar multi-parameter stimulation-feedback quantitative modeling framework for post-stroke gait rehabilitation. *Biomedical Signal Processing and Control*, *116*, 109461. DOI: 10.1016/j.bspc.2026.109461

Xie, J., Liu, R., Luttrell, J.IV, & Zhang, C. (2019). Deep Learning Based Analysis of Histopathological Images of Breast Cancer. *Frontiers in Genetics*, *10*, 80. Advance online publication. DOI: 10.3389/fgene.2019.00080 PMID: 30838023

Xie, Q., Chen, Q., Chen, A., Peng, C., Hu, Y., Lin, F., Peng, X., Huang, J., Zhang, J., Keloth, V., & Zhou, X. (2025). Medical foundation large language models for comprehensive text analysis and beyond. *npj. Digital Medicine*, *8*(1), 141. PMID: 40044845

Xu, N., Yang, D., Arikawa, K., & Bai, C. (2023). Application of artificial intelligence in modern medicine. *Clinical eHealth*, *6*, 130–137. https://doi.org/DOI: 10.1016/j.ceh.2023.09.001

Xue, L., Constant, N., Roberts, A., Kale, M., Al-Rfou, R., Siddhant, A., Barua, A., & Raffel, C. (2021). mT5: A massively multilingual pre-trained text-to-text transformer. In *Proceedings of the Conference of the North American Chapter of the Association for Computational Linguistics: Human Language Technologies* (pp. 483-498). DOI: 10.18653/v1/2021.naacl-main.41

Xu, M., Cai, D., Yin, W., Wang, S., Jin, X., & Liu, X. (2024). Resource-efficient algorithms and systems of foundation models: A survey. *ACM Computing Surveys*, *57*(5), 1–39. DOI: 10.1145/3706418

Yan, B., Li, K., Xu, M., Dong, Y., Zhang, Y., Ren, Z., & Cheng, X. (2025). On protecting the data privacy of large language models (LLMs) and LLM agents: A literature review. *High-Confidence Computing*, *5*(2), 100300. DOI: 10.1016/j.hcc.2025.100300

Yang, A., Yu, B., Li, C., Liu, D., Huang, F., & Huang, H. (2025). Qwen2. 5-1m technical report. *arXiv preprint arXiv:2501.15383.*

Yang, X., Li, T., Su, Q., Liu, Y., Kang, C., Lyu, Y., Zhao, L., Nie, Y., & Pan, Y. (2025). Application of large language models in disease diagnosis and treatment. *Chinese Medical Journal, 138*(2), 130–142. DOI: 10.1097/CM9.0000000000003456 PMID: 39722188

Yano, K., Luo, Z., Huang, J., Xie, Q., Asada, M., Yuan, C., Yang, K., Miwa, M., Ananiadou, S., & Tsujii, J. I. (2025). ELAINE-medLLM: Lightweight English Japanese Chinese Trilingual Large Language Model for Bio-medical Domain. In *Proceedings of the 31st International Conference on Computational Linguistics* (pp. 4670-4688).

Yao, Q., Qiu, B., He, L., Wang, Q., Zou, J., Liang, D., Wen, S., Liu, Y., Li, G., Hu, J., Ma, H., Huang, G., & Zeng, Q. (2026). Effects of Artificial Intelligence Recognition–Based Telerehabilitation on Exercise Capacity in Patients With Hypertension: Randomized Controlled Trial. *Journal of Medical Internet Research, 28*, e81400. DOI: 10.2196/81400 PMID: 41529829

Yao, W., Bai, J., Liao, W., Chen, Y., Liu, M., & Xie, Y. (2024). From CNN to Transformer: A Review of Medical Image Segmentation Models. J Digit Imaging. *Journal of Imaging Informatics in Medicine, 37*(4), 1529–1547. DOI: 10.1007/s10278-024-00981-7 PMID: 38438696

Ye, J., & Tang, H. (2025). Multimodal large language models for medicine: A comprehensive survey. *arXiv preprint arXiv:2504.21051.*

Zafari-Ghadim, Y., Rashed, E. A., Mohamed, A., & Mabrok, M. (2024). Transformers-based architectures for stroke segmentation: A review. *Artificial Intelligence Review, 57*(11), 307. DOI: 10.1007/s10462-024-10900-5

Zafar, Z., Ali, G., & Ali, T. (2026). DESIGNING TRUSTWORTHY CLINICAL DECISION SUPPORT SYSTEMS USING DEEP LEARNING AND HUMAN-IN-THE-LOOP VALIDATION. *Spectrum of Engineering Sciences, 4*(1), 559–579.

Zand, J., Suvakov, M., Overgaard, S. M., Kozikowski, C. G., Jimison, R. C., Nelson, K. B., Silvano, C. J., Meiners, L. M., Fan, J. W., Schultz, K. E., Carter, R. E., Wieland, M. L., Patten, C. A., Dugani, S. B., Weis, J. A., Poe, J. D., Holmes, D. R.III, Griffiths, L. G., Dieter, H. L., & Garovic, V. D. (2026, January). Building artificial intelligence and data literacy across the health care research workforce in the Mayo Clinic Center for Clinical and Translational Science: Why it matters and what we are doing about it. [). Elsevier.]. *Mayo Clinic Proceedings, 101*(1), 17–25. DOI: 10.1016/j.mayocp.2025.11.008 PMID: 41485858

Zhang, D., Feng, T., Xue, L., Wang, Y., Dong, Y., & Tang, J. (2025). Parameter-efficient fine-tuning for foundation models. *arXiv preprint arXiv:2501.13787.*

Zhang, B., & Ming, C. (2023). A patent portfolio value analysis based on intuitionistic fuzzy sets: An empirical analysis of artificial intelligence for healthcare. *Journal of Open Innovation*, *9*(3), 100124. Advance online publication. DOI: 10.1016/j.joitmc.2023.100124

Zhang, D., Xue, X., Gao, P., Jin, Z., Hu, M., Wu, Y., & Ying, X. (2024). A survey of datasets in medicine for large language models. *Intelligence & Robotics*, *4*(4), 457–478. DOI: 10.20517/ir.2024.27

Zhang, H., Chen, J., Jiang, F., Yu, F., Chen, Z., Li, J., Chen, G., Wu, X., Zhang, Z., Xiao, Q., Wan, X., Wang, B., & Li, H. (2023). HuatuoGPT, towards taming language model to be a doctor. In *Findings of the Association for Computational Linguistics* (pp. 10859–10885). EMNLP. DOI: 10.18653/v1/2023.findings-emnlp.725

Zhang, H., Qi, Y., Xu, H., & Lv, R. (2025). Multimodal deep learning method based on multiple spectra for lung cancer early diagnosis. *Spectrochimica Acta. Part A: Molecular and Biomolecular Spectroscopy*, *346*, 126932. DOI: 10.1016/j.saa.2025.126932 PMID: 40957203

Zhang, J., Chen, X., Yang, B., Guan, Q., Chen, Q., Chen, J., Wu, Q., Xie, Y., & Xia, Y. (2025). Advances in attention mechanisms for medical image segmentation. *Computer Science Review*, *56*, 100721. DOI: 10.1016/j.cosrev.2024.100721

Zhang, J., Li, F., Zhang, X., Wang, H., & Hei, X. (2024). Automatic Medical Image Segmentation with Vision Transformer. *Applied Sciences (Basel, Switzerland)*, *14*(7), 2741. DOI: 10.3390/app14072741

Zhang, J., & Zhang, Z. (2023). Ethics and governance of trustworthy medical artificial intelligence. *BMC Medical Informatics and Decision Making*, *23*(1), 7. DOI: 10.1186/s12911-023-02103-9 PMID: 36639799

Zhang, K., Wang, D., Lin, F., Xie, J., & Zhou, W. (2026). A Comprehensive Review of Explainable Artificial Intelligence in Healthcare Methods, Evaluation, and Clinical Integration. *iScience*, *29*(3), 115026. DOI: 10.1016/j.isci.2026.115026 PMID: 41858885

Zhang, R., Liu, G., Zhang, Q., Lu, X., Dian, R., Yang, Y., & Xu, L. (2025). Detail-aware network for infrared image enhancement. *IEEE Transactions on Geoscience and Remote Sensing*, *63*, 1–14. DOI: 10.1109/TGRS.2024.3504240

Zhang, Y., Wang, X., Xu, Z., Yu, Q., Yuille, A., & Xu, D. (2021). When radiology report generation meets knowledge graph. *Proceedings of the AAAI Conference on Artificial Intelligence*, *35*(4), 4391–4399. DOI: 10.1609/aaai.v35i4.16464

Zhao, S., Gao, Y., Jiang, X., ... (2014) Exploring principles-of-art features for image emotion recognition. In: Proceedings of the ACM International Conference on Multimedia, MM. ACM, pp 47–56. https://doi.org/DOI: 10.1145/2647868.2654930

Zhao, C., & López, B. S. (2025). Translating Artificial Intelligence Algorithms into Clinical Practice: Addressing Implementation Barriers in Healthcare. *Frontiers in Emerging Computer Science and Information Technology*, *2*(07), 1–6.

Zhao, S., Hu, M., & Fang, S. (2026). Multimodal spatiotemporal graph convolutional attention network for dynamic risk stratification and intervention strategy generation in rare disease rehabilitation nursing. *Scientific Reports*, *16*(1), 6758. DOI: 10.1038/s41598-026-37095-9 PMID: 41617761

Zheng, G., Wang, X., Feng, Y., Shi, Y., Ma, Z., & Yu, P. S. (2024). Efficiently democratizing medical LLMs for 50 languages via a mixture of language family experts. *arXiv preprint arXiv:2410.10626*.

Zhou, H., Liu, F., Gu, B., Zou, X., Huang, J., Wu, J., Li, Y., Chen, S. S., Zhou, P., Liu, J., Hua, Y., Mao, C., Wu, X., Zheng, Y., Clifton, L., Li, Z., Luo, J., & Clifton, D. A. (2023). A survey of large language models in medicine: Progress, application, and challenge. *arXiv preprint arXiv:2311.05112*.

Zhou, M., Parmar, S., & Bhatti, A. (2024). Towards democratizing multilingual large language models for medicine through a two-stage instruction fine-tuning approach. *arXiv preprint arXiv:2409.05732*.

Zhou, B., Yang, G., Shi, Z., & Ma, S. (2022). Natural language processing for smart healthcare. *IEEE Reviews in Biomedical Engineering*, *17*, 4–18. DOI: 10.1109/RBME.2022.3210270 PMID: 36170385

Zhou, H.-Y., Guo, J., Zhang, Y., Han, X., Yu, L., Wang, L., & Yu, Y. (2023). nnFormer: Volumetric Medical Image Segmentation via a 3D Transformer. *IEEE Transactions on Image Processing*, *32*, 4036–4045. DOI: 10.1109/TIP.2023.3293771 PMID: 37440404

Zhou, K., & Gattinger, G. (2024). The Evolving Regulatory Paradigm of AI in MedTech: A Review of Perspectives and Where We Are Today. *Therapeutic Innovation & Regulatory Science*, *58*(3), 456–464. DOI: 10.1007/s43441-024-00628-3 PMID: 38528278

Zhou, Y., Liu, X., Ning, C., Zhang, X., & Wu, J. (2024). Reliable and Diverse Evaluation of LLM Medical Knowledge Mastery. *International Conference on Learning Representations.*

Zhu, C., Idemudia, C. U., & Feng, W. (2019). Improved logistic regression model for diabetes prediction by integrating PCA and K-means techniques. *Informatics in Medicine Unlocked, 17*, 100179. DOI: 10.1016/j.imu.2019.100179

Zhu, T., Huang, Y., Pu, J., Wang, C., Ruan, M., Lu, P., Yang, X., Bao, N., Chen, Y., & Zhang, A. (2026). Evaluation of the Efficacy of an Artificial Intelligence-Based Assessment and Correction System in the Rehabilitation of Patients Following Anterior Cruciate Ligament Reconstruction Surgery. *Journal of Clinical Medicine, 15*(2), 575. DOI: 10.3390/jcm15020575 PMID: 41598513

Zhu, T., Li, L., Yang, J., Zhao, S., Liu, H., & Qian, J. (2023). Multimodal sentiment analysis with image-text interaction network. *IEEE Transactions on Multimedia, 25*, 3375–3385. DOI: 10.1109/TMM.2022.3160060

Zou, Q., Qu, K., Luo, Y., Yin, D., Ju, Y., & Tang, H. (2018). Predicting diabetes mellitus with machine learning techniques. *Frontiers in Genetics, 9*, 515. DOI: 10.3389/fgene.2018.00515 PMID: 30459809

Zsidai, B., Hilkert, A. S., Kaarre, J., Narup, E., Senorski, E. H., Grassi, A., Ley, C., Longo, U. G., Herbst, E., Hirschmann, M. T., Kopf, S., Seil, R., Tischer, T., Samuelsson, K., & Feldt, R. (2023). A practical guide to the implementation of AI in orthopaedic research—Part 1: Opportunities in clinical application and overcoming existing challenges. *Journal of Experimental Orthopaedics, 10*(1), 117. Advance online publication. DOI: 10.1186/s40634-023-00683-z PMID: 37968370

About the Contributors

Fernando Ortiz-Rodriguez is a Full Professor and Head of the Artificial Intelligence and Innovation Lab at Tamaulipas Autonomous University. He was the Executive Director at the International Institute of Studies (IIES). He created the First Business School in Tamaulipas, Mexico. He worked as the Information Technology Manager at Emerson Electric, where he developed more than 40 pieces of software, some of them used globally in Emerson, and he achieved technology convergence by implementing the first efforts on IoT and Industry 4.0. Fernando is a member of National Systems Researchers (SNI) Level 1 of the National Council of Science and Technology (CONACYT) and INDEX IT Advisor

Rajesh Kumar Dhanaraj is a distinguished Professor at Symbiosis International (Deemed University) in Pune, India. Prior to this, he served as a Professor at the School of Computing Science & Engineering at Galgotias University in Greater Noida, India. His exceptional academic and research contributions have placed him among the top 2% of scientists globally, an honor recognized by Elsevier and Stanford University. Dr. Dhanaraj completed his B.E. in Computer Science and Engineering from Anna University Chennai, followed by an M.Tech from Anna University Coimbatore. He earned his Ph.D. in Computer Science from Anna University, Chennai. His prolific career includes authoring and editing over 100 books on advanced technologies and holding 27 patents. He has published over 200 articles in esteemed journals and international conferences, including six papers in IEEE Transactions.

Firoz Khan is an academic and researcher with a distinguished Ph.D. in Computer Science from the British University in Dubai. He also holds a Master's in Information Technology from the University of Southern Queensland (USQ) and a Master's in Information, Network, and Computer Security from the New York Institute of Technology (NYIT). His research interests include IoT applications in agriculture, automotive cybersecurity, and the integration of AI with cybersecurity in healthcare. He is also exploring advanced topics such as precision farming techniques, privacy-preserving models, and liquid neural networks for time-series prediction in healthcare. As an educator, Firoz specializes in teaching IoT security, cybersecurity, and advanced networking. He emphasizes a hands-on, active learning approach to equip students with practical skills and foster innovation, preparing them for challenges in an ever-evolving technological landscape.

***

Arun Arora is a transformative and visionary Operations and Supply Chain Management Leader with decades of distinguished industry experience driving manufacturing business excellence through Lean Management, Total Productive Maintenance (TPM), Business Process Reengineering and Total Quality Management (TQM). Proven track record of delivering measurable business outcomes ranging from significant Cost reduction and Productivity enhancement to Revenue growth and Operational turnaround across high-impact roles in leading organizations including International Tractors Ltd., Mahindra & Mahindra Ltd and Escorts Limited. Currently, Dr. Arora is working as PROFESSOR (Operations and Supply Chain Management) & Dean-Students Welfare with Lloyd Business School, Greater Noida (India). Recognized for strategic leadership in Global Manufacturing Operations, including heading the Export Tractor Assembly business at International Tractors, where he led large-scale transformations by optimizing processes, enhancing quality systems, and integrating digitization for performance gains. Adept at aligning operational goals with broader business objectives, while fostering a Culture of Continuous Improvement, Innovation, and Capability building. Holds a Ph.D. in Operations under Mechanical Engineering, MTech. in Manufacturing Management from BITS PILANI, and PGDBA with Specialization in Operations Management and Human Resource Management from Symbiosis, Pune, complemented by a strong academic presence as Guest Faculty at BITS Pilani. A published researcher and patent holder, Dr. Arora brings deep technical acumen and thought leadership to complex operational challenges. Skilled in stakeholder engagement, cross-functional leadership, and global collaboration, he is driven by a commitment to Operational Excellence, Sustainable Growth, and Innovation. He has contributed in 10 Indian design patents and author of 3 books. He has published 9 research papers in SCOPUS indexed SCI journal. He has also contributed 2 book chapters published in LNME, Springer, which is Scopus indexed. He is active reviewer and reviewed 182 manuscripts so far, which has testimonial in Web of Science. Key competencies include: Strategic Planning, Lean Transformation, TPM, Cost Optimization, Digitization in processes, Quality Systems, Employee Development, and Safety & Compliance (OHSAS 18001). With a proven ability to lead high-performing teams and large-scale operations, Dr. Arora stands out as a trusted advisor and catalyst for enterprise wide value creation and a researcher.

Rajalakshmi Dhandapani obtained M. Sc., M. Phil and Ph.D. degree in Mathematics from SASTRA Deemed University, Thanjavur, Tamil Nadu, India in the years 2008, 2009 and 2022, respectively. She obtained the degree of B.Sc Mathematics from Bharathidhasan University in the year 2001. She is currently working as an Assistant Professor in the Department of Mathematics in SASTRA Deemed University, Kumbakonam.

VennilaG. is a dedicated academic and researcher known for her work in advanced computing and modern technological frameworks. Her scholarly focus includes deep learning, artificial intelligence, data analytics, and the development of secure computing systems. She has actively supported student learning by supervising various academic projects and contributing research publications to recognized journals and conferences. Through her ongoing efforts in research, guidance, and academic development, Dr. Vennila plays a significant role in advancing innovation within the academic community.

Aayushi Goel is a dedicated and accomplished legal scholar serving as an Assistant Professor at Symbiosis Law School, Noida, part of Symbiosis International University, Pune. Prior to this role, she contributed her expertise to Amity University as a Faculty of Law, actively engaging in teaching, research, and academic development. Dr. Goel's academic journey began with a B.A.LL.B. from IIMT Law College, where she was recognized with a Gold Medal for her outstanding performance. She further honed her expertise by earning a Master's degree in Corporate Banking and Insurance Law from Amity University, Noida. Driven by a passion for in-depth legal research, she completed her PhD in Law from Amity University, Noida, focusing her doctoral research on "White Collar Crime with Special Reference to Money Laundering: A Critical Study." Dr. Goel maintains a strong presence in the academic community, presenting her research at numerous prestigious national and international forums. Her commitment to impactful legal research is further evidenced by her scholarly publications in SCOPUS indexed journals, solidifying her position as a rising voice in the field of law.

Manju Lata Joshi, Professor, Poornima University, India holds an M.Tech. and a Doctorate in Computer Science from Banasthali Vidyapith. Her current research interests encompass Artificial Intelligence, Natural Language Processing, Information Retrieval, and Text Mining. With over 17 years of experience in teaching and research, she has published research papers in prestigious journals indexed in the Science Citation Index (SCI) and Scopus, both nationally and internationally.

Furthermore, she serve on the review and advisory committees of several refereed journals and conferences. She has contributed to multiple institutions, mentored students, and led research in AI-based document clustering, sentiment analysis, and information retrieval. She is also actively involved in academic advisory boards, technical committees, and conferences.

Sumit Kumar Kapoor (Ph.D, MCA with 21 Years Academic Experience) Researcher I Editor I Patent I Author I Associate Professor & Dy. HOD in Computer Science, Poornima University, Jaipur

Durga Karthik obtained Ph.D from SASTRA University in the year 2018. Research Area includes chemometrics,image processing and data analytics. Life time member of ISTE.

Shikha Khullar is a researcher and author specializing in artificial intelligence, computational intelligence, cybersecurity, and intelligent healthcare systems. Her research focuses on AI-driven security, sustainable and trustworthy AI, and intelligent medical data protection. She has contributed to international publications with Wiley, CRC Press, and IGI Global and is a member of ACM.

Dilek Küçük, Ph.D, is an associate professor and principal chief researcher at TÜBİTAK Marmara Research Center (MRC). She has obtained her B.S., M.S. and Ph.D. degrees all from Middle East Technical University in Ankara (Turkey), in 2003, 2005, and 2011, respectively. Between May 2013 and May 2014, she has studied as a post-doctoral researcher at European Commission's Joint Research Centre in Italy. Her research interests include energy informatics, data mining, social media analysis, natural language processing, and database applications in engineering domains. She is the author or co-author of 17 papers published at SCI-indexed journals, in addition to more than 40 papers presented at international conferences.

Emine Ela Küçük, Ph.D., is a full professor at the Faculty of Health Sciences, Giresun University. She received her B.Sc. degree from Giresun Health School of Karadeniz Technical University and her M.Sc. degree from the Public Health Department of the Faculty of Medicine in Karadeniz Technical University. She received her Ph.D. degree from the Public Health Department of the Faculty of Medicine in Erciyes University. Her research topics include public health, public health surveillance, women health, and adolescent health.

Indrajeet Kumar received his B Tech in Computer Science & Engineering from Sant Longowal Institute of Engineering and Technology, Punjab in 2009

and M Tech in Computer Engineering with specialization in Computer Network from YMCA University of Science & technology, Faridabad in 2013. He received his PhD on Analysis and Classification of Breast density classification using Mammographic images from GB Pant Institute of Engineering & Technology, Ghurdauri,Uttarakhand, India in 2019. During his PhD he worked on enhancing the potential of most commonly available Breast density classification for differential diagnosis between atypical cases of focal density cases. He served in academia in various reputed organizations like Galgotias Institutions, Greater Noida, U.P, India and graphic era hill University, Dehradun, India, for 6 years. His research interests include application of machine learning, Deep Learning and soft computing techniques for analysis of medical images.

K. Dinesh Kumar is an academician and researcher in the field of Computer Science and Engineering, with expertise in Blockchain Technology, Distributed Systems, Artificial Intelligence, and Secure Data Management. He has contributed extensively to research in areas such as healthcare blockchain, IoT security, supply chain transparency, and machine learning applications.

Pooja Kumari is an accomplished legal professional with over a decade of expertise in Legal Operations, Compliance, Litigation, and Documentation. Her practice spans corporate law, labour regulations, contract negotiations, and arbitration, with a proven track record of representing clients before the Supreme Court of India, High Courts, and specialized tribunals. Pooja has successfully handled complex legal matters across diverse sectors, including mining, energy, and aviation. In addition to her legal career, Pooja is a Assistant Professor (Selection Grade) at UPES Law School in Dehradun, where she teaches Insurance Law, Banking and Negotiable Instruments Act, Labor Law and employee-related regulations. She has also served as Visiting Faculty at Amity University, Ranchi. Pooja holds an Advanced LLM in Air & Space Law from Leiden University, Netherlands. Having held senior legal roles, including Principal Associate at Lexstone Group and has also been an Associate Counsel for the State of Jharkhand, Pooja's expertise extends to strategic legal planning, litigation management, and stakeholder relations.

Umamaheswari Purushothaman holds a B.E. in Information Technology from Periyar Maniammai College of Engineering and Technology (2003), an M.B.A. from Alagappa University, Karaikudi, Tamil Nadu (2006), and an M.Tech in Computer Science from SASTRA Deemed University, Thanjavur, Tamil Nadu (2011). She earned her Ph.D. in Computer Science and Engineering from SASTRA Deemed University. With two decades of experience, she has taught both undergraduate and postgraduate courses in Computer Science. She is currently an Assistant Professor in the Department of Computer Science and Engineering at SRC Campus, SASTRA University, Kumbakonam. Her research interests focus on Data Mining, Machine Learning, and Deep Learning. She has published numerous research papers in international conferences, SCI-indexed journals, Scopus, and book chapters.

Sarika Sharma is a Professor at the Symbiosis Institute of Computer Studies and Research (SICSR), Symbiosis International (Deemed University) in Pune, India. She has over 20 years of experience in teaching and research, focusing on areas like data mining, IT management, and project risk management. She has published extensively in national and international journals.

Vipin Tyagi is a distinguished academician, researcher and author, currently serving as Dean (Academics and Research) at Jaypee University of Engineering and Technology in Guna, Madhya Pradesh. Prof. Tyagi joined JUET, Guna in July 2005. His expertise spans across Image Processing, Cyber Forensics, and Speech Recognition. He is also Director – IQAC of JUET Guna and NEP 2020 UGC University coordinator. Prof. Tyagi has a prolific publication record, contributing significantly to his fields of interest. His scholarly work includes numerous journal articles, conference papers, and books. Some of his notable publications are in the areas of image forgery detection, image denoising, and content-based image retrieval. He has authored and edited several books and papers in the field of computing and data sciences, such as "Digital Image Forgery Detection: Techniques, Challenges and Applications", "Predictive Computing and Information Security" and "Content-Based Image Retrieval: Ideas, Influences, and Current Trends" published by Springer Singapore. His scholarly work has earned him a respectable h-index and numerous citations in the academic community.

Raj Kishor Verma is a seasoned academician and researcher with over 12 years of teaching experience in the field of Computer Science and Engineering (CSE). He is currently pursuing a Ph.D. in CSE from Galgotias University, focusing on developing innovative solutions to address contemporary challenges in technology. Raj Kishor Verma holds an M.Tech. in Mobile Computing from the Central University of Jharkhand, where he gained expertise in Automatic Text Summarization by the using Python, mobile systems, and pervasive computing. He completed his B.Tech. in Computer Science and Engineering from RVS College of Engineering & Technology, Jamshedpur, building a strong academic foundation. Throughout his career, Raj Kishor Verma has demonstrated excellence in teaching and research. He has published four research papers in Scopus-indexed journals, contributing significantly to fields such as mobile computing, artificial intelligence, wireless networks, and emerging technologies. He is actively working on additional research projects to advance knowledge in his domain. Currently, he serves as an Assistant Professor at ABES Institute of Technology (ABESIT),

Vikas is currently serving as an Assistant Professor in the Department of Computer Science and Engineering at Vivekananda Institute of Professional Studies - Technical Campus, New Delhi, and is a UGC-NET and GATE-qualified academician. He is pursuing a Ph.D. in Computer Science & Engineering from Birla Institute of Technology, Mesra, Ranchi, Jharkhand, M. Tech (Computer Engineering) from YMCAIE, Faridabad (which is now J.C. Bose University of Science and Technology, YMCA, Faridabad), B. Tech (Computer Engineering) from The Technological Institute of Textile and Science, Bhiwani, and brings over 15 years of academic experience. His core areas of expertise include Wireless Sensor Networks, Machine Learning, Artificial Intelligence, Deep Learning, and Cybersecurity. Mr. Vikas has published extensively in SCIE- and Scopus-indexed journals and IEEE conferences, with notable contributions in wireless sensor networks, machine learning, and algorithms. His ongoing research is centred on Internet of Things (IoT), Grid Computing, and Industry 5.0 applications.

Index

S

T

U

V

www.ingramcontent.com/pod-product-compliance
Lightning Source LLC
LaVergne TN
LVHW060007031026
849161LV00025B/1542